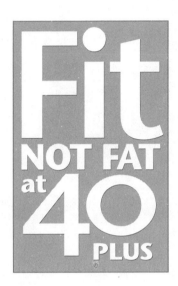

Fit
NOT FAT
at 40
PLUS

The Shape-Up Plan That
Balances Your Hormones,
Boosts Your Metabolism,
and Fights Female Fat in
Your Forties—*and Beyond*

by the Editors of
PREVENTION Health Books
for Women

RODALE

Printed in the United States of America

Rodale Inc. makes every effort to use acid-free ∞ , recycled paper ♲ .

The Fitness Level Chart on page 68 is reprinted with permission from www.shapeup.org—the Web site of Shape Up America! in Washington, D.C.

The YMCA sit-and-reach test on page 70 is reprinted with permission from ACSM's Guidelines for Exercise Testing and Prescription, © Lippincott, Williams & Wilkins, 2000.

Cover design by Carol Angstadt
Interior design by Rita Baker
Illustrations by Julie Johnson

Library of Congress Cataloging-in-Publication Data

    Fit not fat at 40-plus : the shape-up plan that balances your hormones, boosts your metabolism, and fights female fat in your forties—and beyond / by the editors of Prevention Health Books for Women.
        p.   cm.
    Includes index.
    ISBN 1–57954–559–9   hardcover
    ISBN 1–57954–598–X   paperback
    1. Physical fitness for women.   2. Middle aged women—Health and hygiene.   3. Weight loss.   I. Title: Fit not fat at forty-plus.
    II. Prevention Health Books for Women.
    RA778 .F493   2002
    613'.04244—dc21   2002006953

Distributed to the book trade by St. Martin's Press

2   4   6   8   10   9   7   5   3   1   hardcover
2   4   6   8   10   9   7   5   3   1   paperback

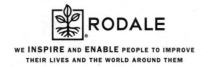

RODALE

WE **INSPIRE** AND **ENABLE** PEOPLE TO IMPROVE
THEIR LIVES AND THE WORLD AROUND THEM

FOR PRODUCTS & INFORMATION
WWW.RODALESTORE.COM
WWW.PREVENTION.COM
(800) 848-4735

About *Prevention* Health Books

The editors of *Prevention* Health Books are dedicated to providing you with authoritative, trustworthy, and innovative advice for a healthy, active lifestyle. In all of our books, our goal is to keep you thoroughly informed about the latest breakthroughs in natural healing, medical research, alternative health, herbs, nutrition, fitness, and weight loss. We cut through the confusion of today's conflicting health reports to deliver clear, concise, and definitive health information that you can trust. And we explain in practical terms what each new breakthrough means to you so you can take immediate, practical steps to improve your health and well-being.

Every recommendation in *Prevention* Health Books is based upon reliable sources, including interviews with qualified health authorities. In addition, we retain top-level health practitioners who serve on the Rodale Books Board of Advisors to ensure that all of the health information is safe, practical, and up-to-date. *Prevention* Health Books are thoroughly fact-checked for accuracy, and we make every effort to verify recommendations, dosages, and cautions.

The advice in this book will help keep you well-informed about your personal choices in health care—to help you lead a happier, healthier, and longer life.

Notice

CONTENTS

ACKNOWLEDGMENTS

Heartfelt thanks to the many fitness professionals who recognize the unique fitness needs of women over 40 and contributed their advice and expertise to the program offered in this book. The editor and publisher especially want to thank the following individuals for the hours of time and high levels of attention they devoted to making sure this book offers a safe, effective, and motivating plan for women who want to get fit—and stay fit—at age 40 and beyond.

Michele Olson, Ph.D., professor of health and human performance at Auburn University in Montgomery, Alabama

Amy Campbell, R.D., a certified diabetes educator and program coordinator of the Fit and Healthy weight-loss program of the Joslin Diabetes Center at Harvard University

Arthur Weltman, Ph.D., director of the exercise physiology program at the University of Virginia in Charlottesville

Selene Yeager, certified personal trainer, fitness instructor, *Prevention* magazine contributing editor, and author of *Selene Yeager's Perfectly Fit*

PHOTO CREDITS

Courtesy of Rosanna Pittella: page 308 (before)

Courtesy of Stephen Lacko: page 308 (after)

Courtesy of Accusplit: page 312

Courtesy of Grace Penny: page 330

Courtesy of Benoit Built Inc.: page 349

Mitch Mandel/Rodale Images: pages 176–184, 186–196, 198–208, 210–223, 227, 229–237, 239–241, 245, 247–249, 251–256, 258–266, 276, 279, 297

Resistance band courtesy of Bodylastics International

Weights courtesy of Lei Weights

Exercise capri tights courtesy of Athletica

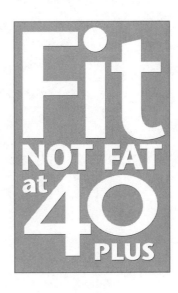

IT'S NEVER TOO LATE TO SHAPE UP

Those "Over the Hill" birthday cards aren't fooling you—in many ways, once you hit 40, you are in the prime of your life. The kids are getting more independent, freeing you up for your own pursuits. You've settled into a comfortable space with your job and your relationship. You have more time for friends, hobbies, romance, and, most important, yourself.

You're more confident than ever—and part of that confidence is knowing that you want to look and feel your best. Regardless of some physical changes—the beginnings of hormonal surges, slightly creaky bones, maybe a little more "squish" around the middle—you still have more than half of your vibrant, active life ahead of you. In the grand scheme of things, you're a young woman—so how can you stay that way? What can you do to take full advantage of these vigorous, exciting, prime-time years?

With the right food, exercise, and stress management plan, your forties can find you healthier and more attractive than ever. Data from the Women's Health Lifestyle Project suggests that women who exercise moderately and eat low-fat diets can prevent weight gain in the years leading up to and during menopause. Good eating habits and exercise can also ward off the high blood pressure, high blood sugar, and elevated blood lipids that can accompany those extra 10 pounds that seem to cling on to the belly for dear life.

The good news is, even if you've smoked, drunk, eaten chips with abandon, and shirked exercise for the past 3 decades, you can still whip yourself into nearly as good shape as the woman who has practiced a healthy lifestyle for her entire life.

"It's never too late to start," says George Vaillant, M.D., professor of psychiatry at Harvard University and Brigham and Women's Hospital in Boston and author of *Aging Well*. Researchers believe that beginning an endurance exercise program as late as 65 or 70 can help lower your health risks—so you can look at this plan as a big head start!

This book will be your guide to navigating hormonal changes, metabolism shifts, and life's intervening hassles. With this plan, nothing will keep you from losing weight and getting fit.

A Fitter You, Inside and Out

It's not your imagination. Maintaining your weight after 40 *is* tougher than it was when you were 20. Beginning at age 40, most women lose about ½ pound of muscle and gain 1½ pounds of fat each year. This may not seem like much on paper, but after 10 years and 15 pounds, it can add up.

Don't blame yourself—blame basic biology. Several pesky factors, like lessening estrogen, a slowing metabolism, and, yes, that constant bedeviler stress—all seem to be conspiring against you. By your 4th decade, you may also have accumulated some pains or ailments that can limit your activities, and therefore your ability to follow weight-loss plans geared for women in their twenties and thirties.

That's where this book comes in: It doesn't matter if you have back problems, knee pain, arthritis, asthma, diabetes, or even just a chronic lack of willpower. You name it, and the Fit Not Fat Program has a customized, personalized plan that will work for you.

And while you're whittling away your waist, you can take great pleasure in the fact that losing pounds now also makes you more likely to prevent breast cancer, lower your risk of diabetes, and even live longer. Not bad side effects of dropping a few dress sizes.

Your Personal Fit Not Fat Strategy

Sometimes it helps just to hear you're not alone. In part 1, Shape Shifting at 40-Plus, you'll learn the latest scientific findings about the biological ins and outs that all women face as they round the corner of 40 years. You'll get the full details of the changes your body is going through, changes you may be sensing without knowing their cause. Just when you thought you'd never get the same weight-loss results you once did, this cutting-edge research into the causes of post-40 weight gain offers brand-new, more effective solutions.

Speaking of solutions, if you're ready to dive right into your program, you can head straight to part 2, Your Personal Fit Not Fat Strategy. First read chapter 5, How Fit Are You Now? to take a snapshot of your current fitness level. These markers will give you benchmarks that can help you set your goals and shape your strategy.

You'll take those goals with you into chapter 6, Building Your Master Plan. The Master Plan is your week-by-week, individual strategy to get the most powerful results out of the Fit Not Fat Program. You'll set motivating goals in three areas—eating, exercise, and relaxation—each one a key to efficient, long-lasting weight loss. A handy Master Plan chart (page 76) helps pull together all of these segments into one fully integrated program for fast, permanent, total-body change.

Incorporating all of these steps progressively is the best way to achieve results, but feel free to modify to suit your own needs and schedule. Just use the chart in the book, or a modified weekly plan of your own, to create a plan that works for you and in-cludes the components that you feel most strongly about.

The first component of your program, part 3's 40-Plus Eating Plan, was designed by Amy Campbell, R.D., a certified diabetes educator and program coordinator of the Fit and Healthy weight-loss program of the Joslin Diabetes Center at Harvard University. The seven steps in her delicious, flexible eating plan work together, yielding more energy, fewer cravings, and fast, safe, permanent weight loss. Based around the days of the week, this quick-start, easy-to-learn plan also helps you prevent diabetes, cancer, and heart disease and will set you on the path to a thinner, fitter you—for life. To make cooking and shopping a snap, check out the 14-day menu planner of mouthwatering, interchangeable meals and snacks (page 391)—each day's menu works in perfect sync with the Fit Not Fat Food Plan.

You know that exercise is the fountain of youth—the problem is fitting it in when you have the energy and motivation to do it. The second segment of the Fit Not Fat Program, part 4's 40-Plus Exercise Plan, starts with chapter 8, What's the Best Exercise for You? The quizzes in this chapter determine your fitness personality, the style that will allow you choose the best exercise for you from the wide menu of convenient options in the Fit Not Fat Basics: Blast Calories and Burn Fat, Sculpt and Strengthen Muscles, and Increase Flexibility and Balance. Discover new fitness options along with every exercise you've ever loved—such as aerobic classes and weight training, Pilates, tai chi, and yoga—with special sections that get right to the heart of your problem areas: belly, butt, thighs, and more. If you have special considerations, like a bum knee or a bad back, not to worry—four chapters of customized fitness prescriptions are tailored just for you. Use your Master Plan strategy to map out your week's workouts, and you'll automatically have a well-balanced, trainer-approved program to burn calories, tone your muscles, and add grace and flexibility that adjusts to *your* life and *your* goals.

When you hear about the third component of the Fit Not Fat Plan, part 5's 40-Plus Relax and Recharge Plan, you may be tempted to think it's an indulgence. But many leading researchers now agree that stress management and ongoing motivation are two of the key factors that determine a woman's success in long-term weight loss. That's right—bubble baths will help peel off pounds. Browse through dozens of favorite escapes and antistress strategies, and sign up for your mandatory daily "me" time sessions on the bottom row of your Master Plan chart.

To round out your complete Fit Not Fat Program, you'll need a good set of tools to help you on your way. In addition to the 14-day menu planner, part 6 also includes a Calorie, Fat, and Fiber Counter and Shopping Guide—a trove of information that boasts more than 500 common and name-brand foods, with their calorie, fat, and fiber content, conveniently tabulated and charted for easy reference. The Shopping Guide, organized from "fit" to "fat" choices, helps you make the best choices between similar items, so every bite adds up to pounds lost.

Now, are you ready to give Mother Nature a run for her money? Defy time, hormones, and gravity with the Fit Not Fat Program, and you'll see what a difference a week can make!

PART 1

SHAPE SHIFTING AT 40-PLUS

"WHAT'S HAPPENING TO MY BODY?"

At first glance, the statistics can look a bit grim: In the 3 decades leading up to menopause, the average woman can expect to gain 29 pounds. That means someone who weighed a svelte 120 pounds at age 17 will edge toward 149 by the time she turns 47.

Even if you've had the best of intentions, you may feel as though those pounds showed up overnight—between ages 34 and 47 alone, we generally add 10.5 pounds to our frames. Consequently, many 40-plus women find themselves out of shape, but in different ways—and gaining extra pounds is sometimes just the beginning of the changes. Learning the background of your special situation can give you the information you need to make your plan the most effective it can be.

Take Shelly, Suzanne, Janet, Marie, and Colleen, five hypothetical but typical women in their middle years. At 40, Shelly is the youngest of the women, and she doesn't consider herself overweight. Yet Shelly knows her waist is thicker than average and not well-defined, giving her figure a boxy look that makes it difficult for her to find clothes that fit. To make matters worse, she's convinced her once taut backside is droopy. Lately, she feels like she's morphed into a rectangle.

In her mid-forties, Suzanne was once what doctors call a classic "pear shape." She's always carried her weight in her hips, thighs, and backside, and her waist remained small. In recent years, the 45-year-old has weathered two major crises—her husband's unexpected death and a daughter's emotional breakdown. In the ensuing stress, not only has Suzanne gained weight, but she's also become "apple-shaped." Her weight having migrated to her middle, Suzanne feels some days like she can't even find her waist anymore.

Once tall, broad-shouldered, lean, and athletic, Janet faces her own battle of the bulge. At 51, she weighs about as much as she used to, but somehow she feels fat and flabby. Her stomach isn't nearly as flat as it was. She also notices that she gets winded easily and can't run as fast as she once could. She just doesn't seem to have the strength or agility to ski, play tennis, or heft sacks of compost around her yard the way she used to.

Back in her twenties and thirties, Marie, now 55, turned heads with her classic hourglass shape. She gained a few pounds after having children—but not many. Then, in her late forties, Marie had a hysterectomy. Overnight, it seemed, her curves turned to rolls. Now she finds herself lamenting that her shape will never be the same again.

Colleen's fight against flab started when she was a girl, before she graduated from junior high school. While her lean friends downed fries, burgers, and shakes without gaining an ounce, the same foods made Colleen pack on the pounds. As a young woman, Colleen lost weight easily when she dieted, shedding pounds the way another woman might slip off a sweater. Yet now, at 58, no amount of dieting budges the stubborn flab. Colleen also has osteoporosis, and her slight stoop accentuates her rounded belly.

These women may face different challenges, but they have much in common. Like millions of other women at midlife, all five feel heavier and less shapely as the birthdays add up. Worse, all seem to be accumulating fat where they mind it the most—in their midsections. They're also not alone there.

"In my experience, the number one complaint of aging women is fat in the abdomen," remarks Ann Grandjean, Ed.D., executive director of the International Center for Sports Nutrition in Omaha, Nebraska.

When we're not armed with the proper information, extra weight and fat—plus age-related changes in metabolism, hormone levels, muscle tone, strength, bone density, joint flexibility, endurance, and balance—can help bring on a midlife fitness crisis at age 40 and beyond. Let's review these changes one at a time, and then learn how to tackle them by working *with*—instead of against—our bodies' natural processes.

Shifting Body Fat Ratios

Consider Janet, the 51-year-old who says she looks and feels flabby. She weighs the same as she did on her wedding day 25 years ago, yet she feels lumpy and out of shape.

Janet's core issue is her body's changing ratio of fat to muscle. By nature, our muscle mass peaks around age 30. Starting at around age 40, each year inactive women lose nearly ½ pound of muscle and gain about 1½ pounds of fat. That means a woman who's 80 has only about a third of the muscle mass she boasted when she was 40.

Between ages 20 and 60, the average person gains 20 to 30 pounds of fat, but the proportion of fat becomes more dramatic, says Glenn Gaesser, Ph.D., professor of exercise physiology at the University of Virginia in Charlottesville. "It's not unusual for a person to lose 10 pounds of muscle and gain 40 pounds of fat, with the scale showing a gain of 30 pounds," he says.

A decline in growth hormone that comes with aging may also play a role in the loss of muscle mass. Scientists don't yet fully un-derstand all the factors, but they do know that growth hormone increases muscle and decreases fat.

A second factor is inactivity. Like a lot of women, Janet simply doesn't work out as much as she did in her twenties, thirties, and forties. Because we lose muscle if we don't use it, Janet's lean muscle mass is shrinking as her fat stores increase. Lean muscle is denser than fat and takes up less room, so Janet feels bigger even though the number on her bathroom scale doesn't budge.

Protecting Muscle Tone

Beginning when we're around age 25, muscles left to their own devices will gradually become smaller and weaker. Each muscle consists of fibers, individual strands of tissue. Without regular exercise, these fibers shrink, or atrophy. According to researchers at the American College of Sports Medicine, unless we exercise regularly, we lose about 10 percent of our muscle by age 50, and the rate of muscle loss only accelerates from there.

Women are especially prone to losing upper-body strength—that is, our arms can be weaker than our legs. That's because women have fewer and smaller muscle fibers than men do. But resistance training can recruit the muscle fibers that are directly responsible for maintaining muscular strength.

In that way, losing muscle strength and tone isn't a given. When Miriam Nelson, Ph.D., director of the Center for Physical Fitness, School of Nutrition Science Policy, at Tufts University in Boston, studied 39 post-menopausal women, she found that those who performed strength training twice a week—including women in their eighties and nineties—were measurably stronger. After a year, the women, on average, nearly doubled the weight they were able to lift, from 7.7 pounds to a little over 14 pounds. In essence, they had totally reversed this effect of aging on their bodies.

One concern many women voice about weight training is a fear of "bulking up," but don't fret—you will not look like a steroid-charged bodybuilder if you start to work out. Strength training will simply tone your muscles and maintain the muscle you have, Dr. Grandjean says. As a bonus, you'll prevent embarrassing "bat wing" arm flab.

Belly Be Gone!

Some women gain all their weight in their bellies, giving them an apple shape. Even women who manage to maintain their weight at 40-plus may notice a thickening middle. They wear the same size skirts and jeans, but their waistbands and belts are tighter. Or they have to go up one size just to accommodate an expanding middle.

Abdominal obesity is more than a fashion headache. It can increase a woman's risk of diabetes, high blood pressure, heart disease, and certain cancers. When researchers from the University of Minnesota followed more than 30,000 women between ages 55 and 69 over a dozen years, they made a startling discovery: The overweight women who carried extra pounds around their waists were more likely to die during that time period than overweight women who carried their extra weight all over their bodies.

Scientists believe one of the reasons abdominal fat is so dangerous is because the type of fat that settles around your waist is metabolized, or burned, differently than the fat that causes heavy thighs. Abdominal fat

FITNESS MYSTERIES

Why are my waist, hip, and other measurements up to an inch larger when I use a metal measuring tape than when I use a cloth or vinyl tape?

A metal tape measure is simply not made to work in a circular way around the curves of a woman's body, says Pauma Deaton, consumer information specialist for the Prym-Dritz Corporation in Spartanburg, South Carolina, a leading manufacturer of sewing notions. "Metal tapes are meant to measure a flat surface. So if you use a cloth tape and a metal tape, you're going to come up with different numbers," she says.

Deaton advises women to measure themselves with vinyl or cloth tapes only. Vinyl tends to be more accurate because it's less likely to stretch than old-fashioned cloth tapes.

contributes to higher levels of cholesterol and fatty acids in the blood and higher blood pressure, thereby increasing a woman's risk of heart disease.

But how do women like Suzanne, who start out life as pears, morph into apples? The answer, some scientists say, may rest in stress. The stress hormone cortisol, released during trying times, is associated with abdominal fat—which in turn is strongly linked to heart disease, stroke, high blood pressure, and diabetes. (For a more detailed description of how and why this occurs, see chapter 4.)

Winning the Metabolic War

Metabolism is the very essence of what keeps you alive. Your body produces heat when you perform even the simplest tasks, like walking the dog or sleeping peacefully. Metabolism, also known as the basal metabolic rate (BMR), is the total heat (expressed in units of calories) our bodies produce through physical activity and normal body functions such as breathing, circulation, and tissue repair.

The rate at which your body consumes and expends energy also affects your weight and shape. Put simply, metabolism is a matter of "calories in, calories out." Your body extracts energy, measured in calories, from the fat, protein, and carbohydrates that make up food and beverages—which in turn take part in a complex series of biochemical reactions.

Many factors—your height and weight, age, stress levels, even hormones—influence your basal metabolic rate. In general, the younger you are, the higher your BMR. During childbearing years, your monthly cycle also consumes a good deal of energy, says Madelyn Fernstrom, Ph.D., director of the Weight Management Center at the University of Pittsburgh Medical Center Health System. But when you skip periods—say, during perimenopause—your body loses out on the calorie expenditure of ovulation and your metabolism slows.

The potential shift from less muscle to more fat that we discussed earlier also affects metabolism. Compared with fat, muscle is an energy-gobbling powerhouse. Fatty tissue, found in greater amounts in women then in men, simply doesn't have muscle's metabolic get-up-and-go.

"If you don't have as much lean muscle tissue as you used to, your metabolic rate will go down," says John Acquaviva, Ph.D., an exercise physiologist who is an assistant professor of physical education at Roanoke College in Salem, Virginia. "Lean muscle tissue requires calories every minute, even when we're sleeping. But fat doesn't require any energy. In fact, it's simply energy that's waiting to be used."

"Every decade, your metabolic rate—that is, your calorie requirement—drops up to 5 percent," Dr. Fernstrom says. That means if you continue with the same activity level and lifestyle in your forties that you had in your twenties, and you don't alter your food intake, you will gain weight. That's why you need a *new* plan—one that works with your post-40 metabolism. (For more information on the effect of metabolism on weight gain, see chapter 2.)

Mastering The Hormone–Weight Connection

As women get older, the endocrine system—including glands that produce the hormones that regulate our metabolic rate—naturally becomes less efficient.

Two of the key players are estrogen, a female hormone that's produced mainly in the ovaries, and progesterone, which is also vital to a woman's healthy reproductive system.

Both estrogen and progesterone levels drop during perimenopause, the years leading up to what our mothers called "the change."

Contrary to popular belief, menopause does not automatically increase weight, and neither does taking hormone replacement therapy. Declining estrogen levels may instead whet a woman's appetite, which can lead to weight gain, says Eleftheria Maratos-Flier, M.D., associate professor of medicine at Harvard Medical School and head of the section on obesity at the Joslin Diabetes Center, both in Boston. "Although more studies are needed, it appears that as you decrease estrogen stimulation, you increase your appetite because estrogen suppresses appetite," says Dr. Maratos-Flier.

FIT FLASH

Lack of Exercise, Not Menopause, Is to Blame for Weight Gain

Many factors contribute to weight gain at midlife, but contrary to popular belief, menopause isn't to blame.

When investigators at the New England Research Institutes followed more than 400 premenopausal women in their fifties for 3 years, they discovered that menopause in itself doesn't trigger weight gain. Hormone replacement therapy didn't pack on the pounds either, the study found. The results of this research confirm the findings of earlier studies on weight gain in menopause.

While menopause doesn't pack on the pounds, some lifestyle choices do. The factor most consistently connected to weight gain in midlife women is a dearth of exercise. Studies have shown that postmenopausal women are less active than women who haven't stopped menstruating. Inactivity, combined with a metabolism growing more sluggish with each passing year, can result in extra pounds.

Kicking the cigarette habit is also a major factor in weight gain among older women, although doctors stress it's far better to carry a few extra pounds than keep a tobacco habit.

Another, more directly contributing factor to midlife weight gain may be the fat-regulating hormone leptin, which appears to decline as we age. Leptin—derived from the Greek word *leptos*, or "thin"—lives up to its name by reducing food intake and increasing the energy we "spend."

The results of one study in Italy concluded that leptin indeed declines during aging. "A woman over 50 may have a lower leptin level than a younger woman even if they share the same body mass index (BMI)," says Dr. Maratos-Flier. Although this effect is also seen in men, it is more pronounced in women. (You're thinking, So what else is new?)

A fourth hormone is probably the more common cause of our weight gain after 40. The American Association of Clinical Endocrinologists reports that 17 percent of women ages 60 and older have low levels of thyroid hormone, a condition known as hypothyroidism. (For more information on the impact hormones can have on 40-plus weight gain, see chapter 3.)

The Battle for Bone Density

Declining levels of estrogen may have indirect effects on weight gain, but their effects on bone density, posture, and appearance are well-established. In adolescence, estrogen works in concert with other growth-promoting hormones to trigger a growth spurt, prompting girls to grow taller practically overnight. In adulthood, it promotes the de-posit of new bone, which in turns maintains the skeleton's normal density. Think of estrogen as a bone "coach." It spurs our bodies to make strong, new bone—and it limits the work of osteoclasts, large cells that break down, or weaken, bone by releasing calcium from bone into the bloodstream.

Yet declining estrogen isn't the only cause of declining bone density or osteoporosis, the brittle-bone disease of aging. Inactivity is another big factor. When we work out, the impact "stresses" bones, and in this case, stress is a good thing—it strengthens the skeleton.

When we don't exercise or when we eat too little calcium-rich food and too little protein, we increase our risk for osteoporosis, which is characterized by porous, lightweight bone that looks something like a sponge. The more porous bone is, the more susceptible it is to breaking. Women are especially at risk—one out of every two women will break a bone because of osteoporosis sometime after the age of 50. As we get older, the complications arising from hip fractures become more serious, leading to the death of about 35,000 Americans a year; only about a third of men and women who break a hip fully recover.

Weak bones can also impact a woman's appearance. Women with osteoporosis, like Colleen, often develop kyphosis, a hunched back triggered by early osteoporosis. As the spine curves in and shoulders droop, the stomach can protrude, creating a potbelly—

probably not the effect you're going for. Luckily, the Fit Not Fat Food and Exercise Plans ensure that you'll have your calcium and exercise bases covered.

Keeping Joints Flexible

How many of us can remember bending over to touch our toes without even thinking twice? If you can still do all the poses on our yoga video, you can thank your joints, the sites where two or more bones, tendons, or ligaments meet. Joints not only hold our skeletons together; they also render them flexible, allowing the full range of motion we need for everyday activities.

Yet joints, too, are vulnerable to the effects of aging. Unless you make a deliberate effort to stay nimble, the tendons (connecting muscle to bone) and ligaments (connecting bone to bone) gradually grow more rigid, and then weaken and shorten. As a result, your flexibility declines.

The more you stretch throughout the day, the more likely you'll tune in to your body's natural desire to move your muscles and joints, and the more flexible you'll be. Stretching helps muscles regain some of their suppleness.

Plus, the longer you stretch, the better. When scientists at Brigham Young University in Provo, Utah, studied the stretching habits of a group of healthy older men and women (the average age was 85), they found that those who stretched for 60 seconds increased

FIT | FLASH

Challenging Your Bones Cuts Fracture Risk

You may enjoy walking in the neighborhood, dancing around your house, or even long stretches of strenuous gardening, and each of these activities does indeed burn calories. But to build stronger bones, you may need to *shock* them.

Research from the University of Cambridge Institute of Public Health and Primary Care in England found that these moderate activities did not reduce the estimated fracture risk in 5,210 people studied. However, researchers found that 2 hours a week of high-impact activities, such as step aerobics, jogging, and tennis, did reduce estimated hip fracture risk by 33 percent in men and 12 percent in women.

To build bone, try to constantly push it to work harder, says Christine Snow, Ph.D., professor of exercise and sports science and director of the bone research lab at Oregon State University in Corvallis. "While walking can help maintain bone mass, it doesn't build bone," she explains.

Walking is still great exercise, but to maximize your bone-building benefits, make sure to add weight training and/or moderate- to high-impact activities to your routine.

HOW THEY DID IT

She Whittled Her Waist with All-Weather Exercise

For years, Carole DeMartino of Bloomfield, New Jersey, thought she was addicted to food, destined to be heavy forever. When she cast off her bad habits and fad diets for a truly healthy style of living, she lost 120 pounds, slimming down once and for all.

It was like leading a double life, foodwise. At work, I'd delicately nibble a salad for lunch and pass on snacks, but at home I'd eat with wild abandon: a bag of chips with sour cream, a stack of crackers with peanut butter and marshmallow, a big dinner followed by butter almond ice cream, popcorn, and more. I put a lock on the fridge and then would break in at 2:00 A.M. I felt addicted to food.

I tried lots of fad diets: Hollywood, rotation, cabbage, protein, even a 9-month fast on coffee, corn, and rice. I lost 120 pounds but developed ulcers, then regained all the weight. I lost and gained hundreds of pounds over the years. I thought I'd be heavy forever.

My wake-up call came at 51, after I put my 5-foot-4-inch body on a scale and the needle teetered at 265 pounds! A horrible feeling settled over me. I was a borderline diabetic with high cholesterol and hypertension. Now I was also severely obese.

I knew undoing the damage would be tough at menopause, thanks to hormone fluctuations. Still, I had new resolve. For 2 weeks I ate only fruits, vegetables, and fish, eating to my heart's content so that I wouldn't feel hungry. Next, I added whole grains, low-fat dairy, beans, and nuts.

My plan was simple: no calorie counting, no food weighing. No more following someone else's strict diet. I was making healthy choices in moderation, and creating my own healthy lifestyle, something I could stick with forever.

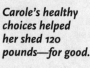

Carole's healthy choices helped her shed 120 pounds—for good.

Then I did something that I'd never done as an adult: exercise. The first day, it was a mere walk around the block, which winded me. Still, I walked every day, slowly increasing my time and distance. Soon there were no excuses. When it rained, I walked at the mall. When it got too hot, I jogged laps in our backyard pool. When it got too cold, I danced like a maniac to rock music in the basement. I added daily strength training with free weights and a resistance band and never looked back—or needed a gym!

I still vividly recall the day that I first saw definition in my arms, 6 months into my own weight-loss program. In 2 years, I happily lost a whopping 120 pounds, whittled 15 inches off my waist, and traded in my 44DD industrial-strength bras for sexier 36Cs.

Today, at 59, I feel my best ever. I walk a mile in 13 minutes, wear a two-piece swimsuit, and can dance until the last song is played.

their flexibility and range of motion nearly twice as much as groups who stretched for 15 seconds or 30 seconds or who didn't stretch at all. (See chapter 11 for fun, easy stretching workouts to incorporate into your day.)

Boosting Energy and Endurance

When women turn 40 and older, it's not unusual to feel they don't have the energy to do activities they've done all their life, says Betsy Keller, Ph.D., associate professor and chair of the department of exercise and sports sciences at Ithaca College in New York. The prospect of adding an hour-long aerobics class to your daily schedule may seem daunting, but even women who work out may feel less able to keep up with others or work out as intensely as they're used to.

Luckily, this lag in energy is completely reversible. The culprits behind low energy are those tendencies to lose muscle, gain body fat, and become less physically active as we get older. Any increase in muscular strength and endurance is likely to pay off in major energy dividends—not to mention how much easier it is to lug around fewer pounds! (For tips on boosting energy with nutrition, breathing exercises, and small changes in exercise training, see chapter 15.)

Maintaining a Sense of Balance

If you fell off your bike as a kid, you probably just picked yourself up, ran to Mom for some Mercurochrome, and went back to play with your friends. As you get older, you may fall more easily—perhaps for no reason. Losing your sense of balance can have serious consequences. Falls are the leading cause of injury for older adults. For women especially, poor balance combined with brittle bones, weak muscles, and inflexible joints can result in a life-altering injury, making it difficult to participate in everyday activities such as getting out of a chair or walking.

But why is staying upright a problem? As you age, your inner ear loses sensitivity, decreasing its ability to detect changes in balance, says Steven Wolf, P.T., Ph.D., a professor of rehabilitation medicine at Emory University School of Medicine in Atlanta, who studies changes in balance among older men and women. In addition, your eyesight may weaken, nerve cells become less sensitive, and the reaction time and flexibility of your muscles may decrease.

"The earlier individuals can be made aware of keeping their senses 'sharp,' the better they can become at delaying the adverse impact that dealing with conflicting or multiple stimuli might have on balance control," says Dr. Wolf. (For details on maintaining balance as part of your overall fitness program, see chapter 11.)

You Can Be Fit, Not Fat, at 40-Plus

While it is true that middle age is a prime time to gain weight, extra pounds are not a given.

"For a long time, it was thought that weight gain was a normal, essential part of aging," says Dr. Grandjean. "That fatalistic, this-is-going-to-happen-no-matter-what attitude comes from the picture we have in our brains of a frumpy 40-year-old sitting around and getting fat—it simply doesn't have to be that way."

Data from a well-known study called the Women's Healthy Lifestyle Project provides strong evidence that women who eat low-fat diets and exercise moderately can prevent weight gain during what doctors call the "menopausal transition." What's more, women can change their lifestyles to prevent thicker middles and avoid high blood pressure, high blood glucose, and elevated blood lipid levels.

Starting with part 2 of this book, Your Personal Fit Not Fat Strategy, we'll help you design a program that will enable you to tackle, and even reverse, many of the previously dreaded changes associated with midlife. Every eating recommendation and exercise plan has been formulated with *your* body, your needs, your life, in mind. Turn to page 60 to get started now, or read the rest of part 1 for more information about how your body is negotiating these changes.

CHAPTER 2

STOKE YOUR METABOLISM

What do overloaded trains and women over 40 have in common?

A freight-and-physics challenge.

Consider this: There was a time, maybe a half-century ago, when railroads finagled a way around overloaded trains or engines facing mountainous terrain. If the company plied a train with too much weight, workers hitched it to an engine up front and then hitched another engine behind the train to give it added momentum up steep hills.

Your metabolism works something like a train engine. In midlife, metabolism slows like an overloaded train facing a heck of a hill. Although the metabolic train slows, it doesn't have to grind to a halt. All it needs is a little extra push.

IS THIS YOUR PROBLEM?

Seven Signs of a Flagging Metabolism

Not sure whether a slow metabolism is responsible for weight gain? To help identify if any metabolic factors are at work, ask yourself these questions.

1. Is it difficult for you to keep track of how many calories you're eating?

Most women have no idea how many calories they're eating—or how many they really need. To calculate how many calories your body burns each day, take your weight in pounds and divide by 2.2 to get kilograms. Then multiply that result by .9 to get the number of calories you burn each hour. Multiply that figure by 24—and voilà! That's the number of calories you burn each day.

One way to lose weight is to cut your calories by 250 each day, then "spend" another 250 calories in exercise. A 150-pound woman walking at a rate of 4.5 miles an hour, for example, burns approximately 7.2 calories per minute. If she walks 35 minutes a day, she'll exercise off approximately 250 calories.

2. Do you customarily rely on very low calorie diets or other crash diets to lose weight?

Crash diets that promise the world may slow your metabolism and are a formula for failure.

"The more you diet, the greater your metabolism decreases," says Miriam Nelson, Ph.D., director of the Center for Physical Fitness, School of Nutrition Science Policy, at Tufts University in Boston. Eating too few calories—say, 800 to 1,200 a day—can compromise your metabolism.

Don't jump directly from an 800-calorie-a-day diet to 1,500 or more calories, though. "Instead, gradually increase the caloric intake over 1 or 2 weeks," says John Acquaviva, Ph.D., an exercise physiologist and assistant professor of physical education at Roanoke College in Salem, Virginia. If you're eating a 750-calorie diet now, inch up to 900 calories for a few days, Dr. Acquaviva advises. Then eat about 1,000 calories for another few days, and so on, until you've reached 1,500 calories, the number *Prevention* magazine recommends for safe, permanent weight loss.

3. Have you given up on exercise completely since you have no time for formal workouts?

You needn't don your sweats and spend an hour or two working out. It's perfectly acceptable to burn your calories in short spurts of movement. "Some lean women simply stop taking elevators and walk more," says Michael Jensen, M.D., an endocrinologist and professor of medicine at the Mayo Clinic. "They'll do those extra little things to expend the extra energy." Incorporating these bite-size miniworkouts into your day helps you accumulate burned calories, no matter what you're wearing.

4. Do you have a sedentary job (as an office worker, for example) and hobbies (such as reading and needlework), with little opportunity for either aerobic exercise or weight-bearing effort?

A century ago, nearly one-third of the effort expended in factory and farm work was fueled by human muscle. Today life is quite different. Machines now do the work that was once routine for our great-grandmothers. Nutritionists say that modern technology has replaced physical activity and is probably the single biggest factor in obesity.

Women with desk jobs must make a conscious effort to get their hearts pumping and their muscles working. Think of maintaining your body's muscle mass as having a large nest egg in the bank that will serve you well in years to come.

Remember, muscle burns more calories than fat, and muscles grow stronger and bigger when they are exercised frequently. On the other hand, muscles shrink and lose strength if they aren't challenged. When you exercise, your muscle investment grows, and their calorie-burning power is more than money in the bank; it's actually compounding interest that gets you to your weight-loss goal faster. Conversely, if your muscles are idle, they will shrink, and, just as if you were drawing from your savings every week, leave you in a tough spot down the road.

5. Do you favor running, walking, or other forms of aerobics but avoid doing any kind of weight training?

When you stick solely with aerobics, you're spending more time trying to achieve less impressive results than you could get with a combination of aerobics and weight training. "When the numbers on the scale begin to creep up, you have to change the way you eat and exercise," says Madelyn Fernstrom, Ph.D., director of the Weight Management Center at the University of Pittsburgh Medical Center Health System. "When you exercise, don't merely increase your calorie output by working out harder," she says. "Maintain your muscle mass by lifting weights. Your muscle mass atrophies unless you work at it."

(continued)

IS THIS **YOUR PROBLEM?** *(cont.)*

Before beginning a weight-lifting program, check with your doctor first, then start slowly. If you have a preexisting health condition, an exercise physiologist or certified trainer can help you design a program that works for you.

6. Have you successfully exercised away excess pounds but found yourself slacking off as you get closer to your goal weight?

This temptation is a common mistake. As you drop pounds and move within reach of your goal weight, you should actually exercise *more* because your trimmer body burns fewer calories. Think of those 20 pounds you've ditched as a 20-pound backpack. "If you carried a 20-pound backpack around with you every day, you'd burn an extra 200 calories a day at least," says Dr. Jensen. "If I took that backpack away and you didn't do anything different, you'd be burning 200 fewer calories a day. The only way you could make up for not carrying that extra weight around is to do more than you'd previously done."

7. Are you taking antidepressants or other mood-regulating medicines, or anti-histamines, or steroids?

These medicines can either slow your metabolism or stimulate your appetite, or both, says Dr. Fernstrom. Older classes of antidepressants—such as Elavil or Zyprexa, an antipsychotic drug—can be particularly challenging. Other potential troublemakers include insulin and oral diabetic drugs. Both make your body more efficient at using calories—insulin, for example, is the hormone that helps you store fat for the times you need it. So, if you take insulin or diabetic drugs, your body becomes more efficient at holding on to fat, and you waste fewer calories.

Doctors often take weight into consideration when prescribing medication dosage, and even a modest gain or loss can lead to a change in your present treatment, so it's important to keep your doctor informed. In the meantime, you can offset your metabolic efficiency by boosting your energy output with increased exercise. For starters, add a 10- or 15-minute walk to your day after work or during your lunch hour.

A Crash Course on Metabolism

Don't curse your metabolism. You need it for every breath you take.

All forms of life—from simple algae in a backyard swimming pool to your dog or cat to the human body—depend on hundreds of carefully regulated, and simultaneous, chemical reactions to stay alive.

When your body digests food, it breaks down the carbohydrates, fats, and proteins you eat into smaller compounds that are absorbed by the blood.

▶ Carbohydrates (found primarily in fruits, vegetables, grains, potatoes, and candy, for example) break down into glucose.

▶ Fats (from either vegetable oils like olive oil or animal fats like butter) break down into fatty acids and glycerol.

▶ Proteins (from fish, meat, poultry, eggs, dairy food, and beans, for example) break down into amino acids.

Carbohydrates, protein, and fat contain calories. Fiber is a form of carbohydrate that produces no calories and aids in weight control by providing bulk, which makes food more filling.

Your basal metabolic rate (BMR) is the number of calories you expend to sustain life—the energy spent to keep the heart beating, the lungs expanding, or the body humming along at a healthy 98.6°F. But you also expend energy when you move—walk, run, cycle, garden, dance, chase a bus, or work out at the gym.

Both the conversion of food to energy and your body's use of that energy—your metabolism—play a key role in weight control. If you take in more energy than your body needs, you gain weight. It doesn't matter if all those extra calories came in the form of a double cheeseburger, two extra slices of garlic bread with spaghetti, a second pat of butter slapped on your mashed potatoes, or a glass or two of wine with dinner every night. Extra calories in all forms—protein, fat, carbohydrates, and alcohol—add up to weight gain.

If your body has an excess of calories from any source, it rearranges them into stores of fat and carbohydrates, to be drawn upon between meals and overnight in between fuel deliveries. If you take in more energy than you burn, you gain weight as body fat.

A Natural Slowdown in Metabolism

Almost imperceptibly at first, a woman's metabolic train slows as the birthdays add up.

Somewhere in her thirties, a woman's metabolism approaches a big hill and starts to slow about 5 percent every decade. That means that if a moderately active 35-year-old woman ate a set number of calories a day to maintain a weight of 140 pounds, she might gain weight eating the same number of calories at age 45.

COOL TOOL

BodyGem

By 2003, you'll be able to wake up, check your metabolism, and calculate how many calories you can eat without gaining an ounce with a small, store-bought device called BodyGem. Until then, simply seek out one of the 150 facilities that now offer metabolic testing with this breakthrough invention.

The BodyGem is a light, portable device that measures the rate at which you burn oxygen and calculates your resting metabolic rate (RMR)—how many calories your body burns just staying alive. Your resting metabolism accounts for about 60 to 70 percent of the calories you use every day. It's the number that lets some skinny people indulge worry-free while others must watch every crumb.

WHAT THE EXPERT SAYS: "Trying to lose weight without knowing your RMR is like balancing your checkbook without knowing how much money you're spending," says former Olympic trainer and exercise physiologist Jay T. Kearney, Ph.D., vice president of clinical affairs at HealtheTech, the maker of the BodyGem in Golden, Colorado. "Your RMR also changes over time, especially as you lose weight. That's why people hit frustrating plateaus when they diet. By checking your RMR every few weeks, you can continually adjust your diet and exercise routine to lose weight steadily and consistently."

PURCHASING TIPS: The BodyGem test is currently available in select gyms and spas. The testing typically costs around $65.

For many women at midlife, the weight gain is so gradual they don't notice it until they try to slip into their "skinny" jeans and can't close the zipper. Or they find they need to notch their belt at the next larger hole.

"If you gain 1 pound a year, after a year it won't seem like much, but after 10 years, it adds up," says Geoffrey Redmond, M.D., endocrinologist and director of the Hormone Center of New York and president of the Center for Health Research, both in New York City, and the author of *The Good News about Women's Hormones.*

The only way to burn calories over and above your basal metabolic rate is to expend more effort. Regular, intentional, calorie-burning exercise goes a long way to counteracting the falloff in metabolism that occurs at midlife. (Chapter 9 shows you how.)

Scientists don't yet know why, but African-American women have lower basal metabolic rates than Caucasian women, according to a study from the National Institutes of Health. "It may turn out that African-American woman may need to exercise longer, more frequently, and with greater intensity than others to keep the weight off," says Jana Klauer, M.D., a research fellow at the New York Obesity Research Center at St. Luke's–Roosevelt Hospital and Columbia University.

When it comes to metabolism, the sexes aren't equal either. One study at Jean Meyer USDA Human Nutrition Research Center on Aging at Tufts University in Boston found that women's "resting energy expenditure"—the number of calories expended on day-to-day activities—declined significantly as they aged, but the decline wasn't nearly so noticeable in aging men.

Hormones, too, influence metabolism in various ways. Cortisone and hydrocortisone are crucial to regulating the metabolism of proteins, carbohydrates, and fats. Insulin from the beta cells of the pancreas triggers cells to take in glucose and amino acids. And a hormone called thyroxine responds to another hormone, called thyroid-stimulating hormone (TSH), to prompt many cells to increase their metabolic rate, their growth, even their heat production.

FIT | FLASH

Aging Doesn't Have to Mean Muscle Loss

The muscle loss that we attribute to aging may come down to our habits declining, not our years passing. Researchers from the University of Texas Medical Branch at Galveston tackled the long-held scientific belief that we lose muscle as we age because muscle proteins inherently start breaking down faster than we can create them. When they injected 48 men at rest (half average age 70, half average age 28) with amino acids (building blocks for muscle), muscle breakdown was similar in both groups.

"The actual problem may be that older people's eating and exercise habits deteriorate and/or they have more trouble using protein from food," says lead researcher Elena Volpi, M.D., Ph.D., assistant professor of medicine at the University of Southern California in Los Angeles.

While this research was done on men, it may have implications for women, too. Researchers are investigating a number of possible therapies, but for now an exercise program and a wise diet may be the answer. Dr. Volpi recommends that older adults get plenty of protein in the form of meat, fish, and, if necessary, supplements (ask a registered dietitian), as well as exercise (lift weights or walk) 2 or 3 days a week. That alone can help stem the typical muscle loss of 5 pounds a decade.

Muscle Matters

As if they don't have it easy enough sometimes, men hold a metabolic edge over women because they have more muscle, and muscles are the "workhorses" of the body, says Ann Grandjean, Ed.D., executive director of the International Center for Sports Nutrition in Omaha, Nebraska. Consider the case of Janet, the former college athlete introduced in chapter 1 who felt "fat" even though she hadn't gained weight. Like many women, she had gained fat and lost muscle over the years.

Janet weighed 140 pounds at age 35. At that time, 23 percent of her body consisted of fat. (Experts consider 23 to 33 percent body fat healthy for women ages 40 to 59). Back then, 32 of Janet's 140 pounds were fat. The rest—108 pounds—consisted of bone, muscle, water, and internal organs. By the time Janet reached age 51, her body fat had increased from 23 percent to 30 percent, yet her weight had remained the same. Her body now contains 42 pounds of fat, 10 more pounds of fat than at age 35. At the same time, Janet had lost approximately 5 pounds of muscle.

When women gain fat and lose muscle, two things happen.

▶ Fat isn't as dense as muscle, so any fat gained takes up more space than muscle. Even if you haven't gained weight on the scale, your body can appear larger, and your clothing size may even increase.

▶ Because muscle burns more calories than fat, your metabolism slows and you burn fewer calories, which can contribute to weight gain if you don't make adjustments in your calorie consumption.

Janet worries that if she isn't extraordinarily careful about what she eats, she will gain weight—and with good reason. The amount of lean body mass you have is an important factor in determining the rate at which you burn calories. If lean body mass drops, metabolism drops. Every pound of muscle a woman loses slashes the number of calories she burns by as many as 30 calories a day. If she loses 10 pounds of muscle over 3

BESTBET

Grab Some Weights

For the metabolism booster that keeps going and going, you can't beat weight training.

In one study, Miriam Nelson Ph.D., director of the Center for Physical Fitness, School of Nutrition Science Policy, at Tufts University, had men and women strength train three times a week. On average, they increased their metabolisms by 15 percent—that's 200 to 300 extra calories their bodies were burning *every* day.

A bonus: "Even though they were strength training 3 days a week, they would have to eat those extra calories 7 days a week to maintain the same weight," Dr. Nelson says. Now, that's a gift that keeps on giving!

decades, she could burn 300 fewer calories each day, or a whopping 2,100 fewer calories each week. By the time she celebrates her 55th birthday, she could have lost as many as 15 pounds of muscle, and now burn 450 fewer calories each and every day.

What this means for Janet—and other women in their forties and fifties—is that maintaining muscle mass is critical as the birthdays add up. Lean muscle matters because there's so much of it. Calorie-burning muscle accounts for approximately 40 percent of the body mass of a normal-weight woman—that's 56 pounds for a 140-pound woman like Janet—so it's a major factor in energy.

Here's some good news: Because muscle mass is linked directly to metabolic rate, women can give their metabolic engines a boost with weight training and other forms of exercise that builds muscle.

Are You Eating Too Little?

As a young woman, Colleen (the 58-year-old introduced in chapter 1) lost weight easily when she crash dieted, shedding pounds so quickly, she began to feel invincible. Sometimes it's easier for busy women to skip exercise, opting for yet another 800-calorie-a-day crash diet instead. Yet the older you get, the less productive crash dieting is. Dieting alone results in a loss of some lean weight—that is, muscle—in addition to fat. But if the weight is regained by returning to a normal diet, it will be in the form of fat. This is known as

the "yo-yo effect." Therefore, like so many other women who have crash dieted, Colleen may find it difficult to lose weight now that she is older since she has increased her body's proportion of fat to muscle. Losing lean tissue has simply made it more difficult to burn an optimal number of calories.

Crash diets send an SOS to the metabolism, practically screaming, "You're in starvation mode!" Sensing that food is scarce, the body conserves its reserves, slowing the metabolism to hold on to what it has until the next big meal comes along.

"Humans first evolved in conditions of feast or famine," Dr. Redmond says. "If they killed an animal in ancient times, people could eat a lot, then often they went a long while before they saw food again."

Men and women who gained or retained weight were more likely to survive than thin folks who weighed 98 pounds dripping wet and never gained an ounce. Even now, millions of years later, when food is plentiful for our population, that "calorie-conserving" mechanism still exists, triggering our bodies to slow their metabolic rates when we eat little or nothing.

Crash diets and very low calorie diets also deplete the body of calorie-burning muscle. Confronted with a dramatic decrease in calories, the body draws upon glycogen in the liver and fatty acids from fat stores to power the cells' work. After several hours, though, the liver's glycogen stores are depleted.

Conquer "Gym Phobia"

If you haven't gone to a gym for years—or you've never set foot in one—your first time can be intimidating, especially if you're not comfortable with your body, the equipment, or the people who work out there.

Don't assume everyone else at the gym will be a hardbody, says Karen Coleman, Ph.D., a health psychology expert at the University of Texas in El Paso. A lot of Americans now weigh more than they should, so chances are, you'll be joining people of all shapes and sizes. To get over your anxiety and enjoy your workouts, experts offer women over 40 this special advice.

START OUT BY WORKING OUT AT HOME. "If women aren't very confident in their ability to go to a gym, they might want to purchase weights and start at home," says Heather Hausenblas, Ph.D., assistant professor at the University of Florida in Gainesville, who works in health and exercise psychology. "When they feel comfortable at home, maybe they'll have confidence to do it in the gym."

SHOP AROUND. You'll be giving a gym your business, so it should meet your needs as a customer, Dr. Coleman says. Start by visiting workout centers in your area listed in the yellow pages or on the Internet. Look for one that's convenient to your home or office, and think about when you'd most like to work out—what's the traffic like at that time? What are the best routes to get there quickly?

TAKE A LOOK AROUND FIRST. Does the equipment look modern and comfortable? Do you see other women who are your age and fitness level? Can staffers help you get

---

While many of the body's cells depend on fatty acids to fuel their work, the red blood cells and cells of the nervous system need glucose. In fact, the brain and nerve cells consume about two-thirds of the total glucose the body uses each day, 400 to 600 calories in all.

To supply the red blood cells, brain, and nerves with glucose after the glycogen is gone, the body opts for biology's version of plan B: It breaks down muscle and liver tissue to make the glucose it needs.

The metabolic catch-22? As the lean, protein-rich liver breaks down and shrinks, it works less in order to "spend" less energy. The same is true of muscles: As they waste away, they also work less and demand less fuel. Metabolism, in effect, grinds to a crawl.

As metabolism slows, fat loss also slows, so much that dieters on crash diets or very low calorie plans lose less fat than they would on a sensible reduced-calorie program. In most cases, this means that crash dieters who see big losses on the scale may actually lose less fat than dieters who opt to eat—and enjoy—more food.

the most of your time in the gym? Prepare a list of questions that are most important to you, and know that no issue is too small: Are there fresh towels for everyone's use? Are the showers clean? What's the music like? These will all impact your enjoyment, and consequently your commitment to working out.

CONSIDER A FEMALE-ONLY GYM. You may feel more at ease in a facility that's open only to female clients and instructors, if available, Dr. Coleman says. Some coed gyms also offer separate men's and women's sections.

GET EXPERT HELP. Ask a qualified instructor at the gym to show you, as soon as possible, how to safely and effectively use all the equipment. Body alignment is critical and can save you time and effort down the road. Ideally, the instructor should be certified by the American College of Sports Medicine or the National Strength and Conditioning Association. Most gyms offer an orientation session as part of your joining package.

If you're turned off by perky young instructors who wouldn't know a stretch mark from a stretch limo, look for a staffer who's closer to your age and build. You may be able to identify with her more easily, says Dr. Coleman.

GO AT OFF-PEAK HOURS. If you've been avoiding the gym because you like your privacy, off-peak hours are ideal. You may have the place more to yourself, and you can pick and choose your equipment based on your preference, not just on which pieces have the shortest lines. Usually the busiest times at the gym are lunchtime and after-work hours, but stop by and peek in four or five different times to gauge which crowd level is best for you.

Low-carbohydrate diets also trigger the body to draw upon its glycogen stores to provide glucose to the cells. Once those glycogen reserves are gone, the body turns to protein, its only remaining source of glucose. Although low-carbohydrate diets are high in protein—focusing on lots of fish, meats, and cheese—the body still breaks down lean tissue, like muscle, to meet its energy needs. Luckily, consuming a satisfying 1,500 calories a day will help most women avoid the slowdown in metabolism that occurs with low calorie intake.

Morning, Noon, or Night: Just Do It

Aside from burning calories, exercise also boosts your metabolism—and depending on when you do it, it could have even more potent calorie-burning power. In one study, done at the University of Chicago, scientists discovered that male athletes who exercised at 6 o'clock in the evening or late at night, around 1 o'clock, showed significant increases in levels of cortisol and thyrotropin—two hormones that are critical in energy metabolism. Those who exercised in the

Why do I gain weight every time I quit smoking, and what can I do about it?

While there's no question that some men or women who quit cigarettes can gain weight in the short term, we're not exactly sure why, says Douglas E. Jorenby, Ph.D., associate professor of medicine and director of clinical services at the Center for Tobacco Research and Intervention at the University of Wisconsin Medical School in Madison. Unfortunately, there's a chance a woman who quits will gain 5 to 10 pounds.

Exactly how nicotine affects the metabolism is still murky, but doctors do know smokers tend to weigh less than nonsmokers of the same height. "It's as if when a person smokes, her body wants to defend a lower weight," Dr. Jorenby says.

On the other hand, once they've experienced the initial weight gain, many people find that they more easily adopt healthy habits when they quit, like increasing exercise, cutting out extra sodas or coffee, or making different food choices. All of these new replacement habits will mean longer-lasting, *healthier* weight loss in the future.

To counteract the initial weight gain, start or step up your exercise efforts as soon as you quit. Exercisers report less frequent and less severe nicotine cravings than sedentary men and women. Nicotine gum is another good option, says Dr. Jorenby. Talk to your doctor about various smoking cessation products.

Any way you look at it, you're still better off quitting than smoking. You'd have to be severely obese to stress your heart the same way smoking one pack of cigarettes a day stresses it.

morning or afternoon had much smaller increases in the same hormones and smaller drops in blood glucose. (Comparable studies still need to be done on women.)

"Although the effects of exercising late at night were the most extreme, we also saw significant increases of cortisol and thyrotropin in evening exercisers," said Orfeu Buxton, Ph.D., a postdoctoral fellow in endocrinology at the University of Chicago and lead author of the study. "Right now, we're not sure what that means. But we do know the differences in the hormone levels are very large depending on whether you exercise at night or evening, or early in the day."

While Dr. Buxton said it's premature to recommend exercising at one time of day over another, he will say his study broke ground by looking at the hormonal effects of exercising at night. "Right now, what's important is getting exercise in at some part of the day," says Dr. Buxton. "It will be years before we know if evening is definitely better." Until we know more, most experts agree that the best time to exercise is when *you* have the time and the energy and are most likely to actually do it.

That "Magic Pill" Is All Hype

An old marketing axiom dictates, "Find a need and fill it." Enter supplements touted for their alleged ability to boost metabolism and burn calories, aiding in weight loss—such as ephedra (also known as ma huang), tiratricol, and others.

These miracle cures aren't so miraculous—or safe—after all.

"Most of the studies show they have virtually no effect, or the effects are insignificant," says John Acquaviva, Ph.D., an exercise physiologist and assistant professor of physical education at Roanoke College in Salem, Virginia. For example, you may only burn an extra 25 or 30 calories a day. When you burn a total of 2,000 calories a day, that's nothing. "If you're burning 30 more calories a day through taking these products, it's not worth the risk," says Dr. Acquaviva.

One study—conducted by the Department of Medicine at the University of California, San Francisco, and the California Poison Control System in San Francisco—found that dietary supplements containing ephedra alkaloids (ma huang) cause high blood pressure, heart palpitations, and central nervous system abnormalities in some people. Some deaths have also been linked to this controversial supplement. Almost half of the 140 cases the scientists examined for the study were considered "definitely or probably related or possibly related" to the use of the dietary supplements. The most common problem was high blood pressure, but researchers also documented strokes and seizures.

"For women who have underlying medical conditions they didn't know about, this stuff can be very dangerous," says Miriam Nelson, Ph.D., director of the Center for Physical Fitness, School of Nutrition Science Policy, at Tufts University in Boston.

The Food and Drug Administration (FDA) warns that "metabolism-boosting" products containing tiratricol, also known as triiodothyroacetic acid (TRIAC), marketed through health food stores, gymnasiums, and fitness centers, is a potent thyroid hormone that can trigger heart attacks and strokes. Other side effects include insomnia, sweating, nervousness, and diarrhea.

Just because a product claims to be "herbal" or "natural" doesn't mean it's safe or effective. At best, products so labeled could be a waste of money. At worst, serious damage to one or more vital organs could occur, especially when used with other drugs. Since over-the-counter supplements and herbal remedies are not regulated by the Food and Drug Administration, they can put "miraculous" language on their labels to entice you.

The best news is, the most effective means to boost your metabolism—building muscle—is *free* and widely available today. As you design your Master Plan in chapter 6, be sure to look through chapter 10 to learn how to build, strengthen, and tone your muscles—and blast extra calories, even while you sleep!

CHAPTER 3

ESCAPE HORMONE HAVOC

No program for staying fit not fat at 40-plus would be complete without mentioning our dear friends hormones. Implicated in everything from night sweats to teary jags to bursts of sexual friskiness, these powerful and influential wizards also play a large role in influencing our weight and body composition, either directly or indirectly.

Produced by glands, organs, tissues, and even some individual cells, dozens of hormones and hormonelike chemicals are coursing through your body at any given time. At least 20 of them are secreted by nine major glands of your endocrine system, the body's main hormone factories. Although hormones are produced only in tiny amounts, their impact on the human body is enormous. These vital messengers get their name from a Greek word that means "to set in motion," and they work in concert with the nervous system to choreograph the work of the body's cells.

The ovaries, for example, secrete the estrogen that controls our menstrual cycles but also produce testosterone, which influences muscle and bone growth. Your pancreas secretes insulin, a metabolic hormone, and the pituitary gland secretes a growth hormone that made us grow steadily taller as children and helps us maintain our muscle bulk as adults. In a highly evolved and very complex way, these hormones and others influence your height, weight, shape, and size; your energy levels; and your metabolism.

Let's look at how each one can shift as a woman approaches and travels through midlife.

Thyroid: The Energy and Weight-Loss Hormone

A small gland that generally weighs less than an ounce, your thyroid sits just below your Adam's apple, or larynx. The small, butterfly-shaped gland controls your metabolism's every move, from the rate at which your heart beats to how fast you burn calories.

The thyroid hormones thyroxine, also known as T_4, and triiodothyronine, T_3, regulate metabolism, while the thyroid hormone calcitonin works with parathormone, a hormone secreted by the parathyroid glands, to regulate the body's calcium level. The body works hard to maintain steady and consistent levels of both T_3 and T_4 within very narrow limits. Too low a level results in *hy-*

pothyroidism; too much results in *hyper-*thyroidism.

A common disorder that affects far more women than men, hypothyroidism can begin when the body develops antibodies—protein warriors that usually protect us from disease—against its own gland. Most people with thyroid disease have no symptoms, or the symptoms are subtle enough to go unnoticed or be attributed to another condition. Symptoms include loss of energy, parched skin, muscle weakness, cramps, a slow heart rate, and hair loss.

"With hypothyroidism, the body sees the thyroid as foreign tissue and attacks it," says Geoffrey Redmond, M.D., endocrinologist and director of the Hormone Center of New York and president of the Center for Health Research, both in New York City, and the author of *The Good News about Women's Hormones.* Because thyroid hormones stimulate energy production, a deficiency leaves you tired and lethargic. Metabolism slows, and you burn the foods you eat at a lower rate. Think of a once raging campfire that burns logs more slowly as the flames wane. With your body burning carbs, fats, and proteins at a slower rate, weight can accumulate even if you exercise and follow a low-fat diet.

Like most autoimmune diseases, thyroid disease strikes more women than men. In fact, hypothyroidism affects women 5 to 10 times more often than men. The chance that

(continued on page 37)

IS THIS YOUR PROBLEM?

Maybe Hormones Really Are to Blame

If you can't seem to lose weight no matter how hard you try—or if you're just plain too tired or weak to even think about working out—you may have an undiagnosed hormone imbalance. Ask yourself these questions to help determine if your body chemistry is working against you. With help from your doctor, you can get on track.

1. Are you lethargic, depressed, and unable to lose weight? Do you find yourself frequently cold or constipated, have irregular or heavy periods, or find yourself forgetful or unable to concentrate? Do you find you're losing some of your hair, feel like your voice is different, or notice your skin has a yellow tone?

You may have hypothyroidism, an easily missed yet treatable disease. A woman's symptoms depend on how long she's lacked sufficient levels of thyroid hormones and how severe her shortage is. Symptoms, such as fatigue and changeable moods, can be particularly vague in the disease's early stages. As the thyroid gland gradually declines in function, you may complain that you can't stand the cold, or experience memory problems. Finally, when your thyroid function is severe, you might realize that your voice has changed or you're losing more hair than usual.

Other signs to look for: muscle cramps, dry skin, and hoarseness. If your thyroid gland enlarges, you may have difficulty swallowing or sometimes feel like you're choking.

A number of tests can detect low thyroid output, but the most important are those that measure TSH and free T_4. If a sluggish thyroid is in fact responsible for your problems, simple and safe medication can help.

2. Are you age 40 or older, overweight, and inactive or have a family member who has diabetes? Are you African-American, Native American, or Hispanic? Are you thirstier and urinating more than you used to? Are you unusually hungry?

You're at higher risk for type 2 diabetes if you fit those demographics or already have symptoms. The signs of type 2 diabetes are likely to develop gradually over months or years, and fully half of type 2 diabetics aren't even aware they have it.

If you are at risk for diabetes or have any of these symptoms, ask your doctor to test you for diabetes. A normal fasting plasma glucose level is less than 110 milligrams per deciliter, measured on two occasions. The American Diabetes Association recommends that all women be tested at age 45, then retested every 3 years if the results are normal.

To prevent type 2 diabetes, exercise regularly, lose weight if you carry extra pounds, and eat at least 25 to 35 grams of dietary fiber each day. Exercise increases the efficiency of insulin's action on cells. It can also help you lose weight. Avoid skipping meals or sitting down to huge feasts because both can trigger dramatic fluctuations in glucose.

3. Is the skin on your neck or under your breasts and armpits velvety, slightly raised, and darkened?

You may have acanthosis nigricans, or AN, a skin condition associated with insulin resistance, obesity, and the propensity to develop type 2 diabetes. Only women with very high insulin levels or a condition called polycystic ovary syndrome develop AN.

Women with AN notice thickened or darkened skin in the collar region of their necks or other areas of the skin exposed to mild friction. The skin doesn't itch; it merely looks as if it's dirty and you haven't washed in a while.

If you lose weight, the appearance of your skin may improve in as little as 2 weeks. There are currently no drugs to treat acanthosis nigricans, but there is a drug on the market that may help nondiabetic women with insulin resistance shed extra pounds in midlife. In one study at the New York Medical College in Valhalla, overweight nondiabetic women who took the diabetic drug metformin (Glucophage) while on a carbohydrate-modified diet of no more than 1,200 to 1,600 calories a day lost an average of 19.2 pounds after a year. Obese women fared even better, losing an average of 33.2 pounds. If you're overweight or have acanthosis nigricans, ask your doctor whether you are a good candidate for this drug.

4. Have you suddenly gained weight around your waist and developed elevated blood pressure at the age of 40 after having been slender all your life or despite the fact that you work out regularly?

You may have syndrome W, a cluster of symptoms that includes weight gain in your abdomen, intermittent high blood pressure, HDL cholesterol abnormalities, intense hunger, and high insulin levels. Women with syndrome W have normal blood glucose levels, but elevated insulin levels.

If you have the symptoms of syndrome W, talk to your doctor about testing for insulin abnormalities. This can include a fasting insulin (a result greater than 12 is abnormal) or a glucose tolerance test with insulin levels.

(continued)

IS THIS **YOUR PROBLEM?** *(cont.)*

Harriette Mogul, M.D., an endocrinologist at the New York Medical College in Valhalla who treats many premenopausal and menopausal women with these symptoms, advises that you request an IGFBP-1, a simple single blood test that she first reported as a marker of insulin resistance. If tests show that your insulin levels are elevated, discuss with your doctor possible treatment with the diabetes drug metformin (Glucophage). Dr. Mogul also recommends that women with syndrome W limit themselves to four or five servings of carbohydrates each day, shun all sources of sugar, and eat a high-fiber diet filled with vegetables and low-sugar fruits. Fruits to avoid: bananas, mangoes, orange juice, and dried fruits.

5. Have you noticed excess facial and body hair? Do you have trouble losing weight even on a low-fat diet?

Among other signs, facial or abdominal hair in women who find it hard to lose weight may be a sign of polycystic ovary syndrome (PCOS). A genetic tendency may be at work, but weight gain and insulin resistance play key roles in perpetuating PCOS, a cause of infertility. Occurring most often in women of reproductive age, it usually begins in the teen years. The condition is identified in women after age 40 only if doctors have missed diagnosing it earlier. But if PCOS turns out to be your problem, this is one instance where the Fit Not Fat Food and Exercise Plans may help.

6. Are you taking cortisone for asthma or arthritis?

In addition to the effects of certain hormones produced by your body, taking synthetic hormones—such as Prednisone for asthma, rheumatoid arthritis, or osteoarthritis—for extended periods can cause significant weight gain. Prednisone is a corticosteroid, a family of drugs related to a naturally occurring hormone called cortisol, produced by our adrenal glands. Cortisol reduces inflammation, and so do corticosteroid drugs. When corticosteroids are inhaled into asthmatic lungs, injected into a painful tendon or joint for arthritis, or applied to inflamed skin as creams, they generally cause few side effects. The same is true for corticosteroid pills taken for a short period. However, if they are taken as pills for extended periods or are given intravenously, they can trigger weight gain because they stimulate appetite and cause the body to retain fluids.

Corticosteroids also cause protein to break down and be converted into sugar. The sugar, in turn, is converted into fat that collects in the face and abdomen. Used long term, high doses of corticosteroid drugs may cause osteoporosis, high blood pressure, and diabetes. However, in some serious medical conditions, corticosteroids might be lifesaving, despite these risks. *Never* cease any prescription medicine before consulting with your doctor first.

a woman will develop hypothyroidism increases with age. One statewide study in Colorado found that while about 4 percent of the women participating who were 18 to 24 years old had below-normal thyroid function, the incidence was more than double—in fact, about 10 percent—among women ages 45 to 54. The authors also found that most of the women who had hypothyroidism were unaware they had the disease.

Hyperthyroidism, a less common thyroid disorder, is also seen more often in women than men, particularly women in their thirties and forties. Graves' disease, which affected former First Lady Barbara Bush, is the most common form of hyperthyroidism. Symptoms of an overactive thyroid include weight loss, irritability and nervousness, muscle weakness, sleep distur-

bances, feeling warm or hot much of the time, protruding eyes or vision problems, irregular menstrual periods, and an enlarged thyroid, known as goiter. Curiously, if a midlife woman's fatigue is caused by a thyroid problem, it's more likely due to an overactive thyroid than an underactive one. High levels of thyroid hormones, Dr. Redmond says, shift the body's metabolism into high gear, stimulating chemical energy production so much that the body cannot use the extra energy efficiently. The result? Sometimes crushing fatigue.

Insulin Resistance: Warning Sign of Diabetes

When a lack of exercise or a sound eating plan contributes to weight gain, those excess pounds can lead to resistance to insulin. Se-

---

BESTBET

Consider a Thyroid Test

If you are bone tired after an easygoing day or can't seem to lose weight no matter how much you cut back on food and step up exercise, ask your doctor to test you for a thyroid hormone deficiency.

"I recommend that women start getting tested at the age of 35, then go in for testing every 5 years, since hypothyroidism is more common in women and increases with age," says Geoffrey Redmond, M.D., endocrinologist and director of the Hormone Center of New York and president of the Center for Health Research, both in New York City, and the author of *The Good News about Women's Hormones*. It's especially important to be tested prior to planning for pregnancy since normal thyroid levels are vital for the health and development of the fetus.

"Symptoms are not always a good way to tell because some people who are fatigued or sluggish or get cold easily have normal thyroid levels, and some people have no symptoms but have abnormal levels," says Dr. Redmond. "If you have symptoms, definitely get tested. But even if you don't have symptoms, get tested. It's in your best interest."

creted by cells in a portion of the pancreas known as the islets of Langerhans, insulin regulates levels of glucose in the blood.

The body breaks down carbohydrates—found primarily in fruits, vegetables, breads and grains, potatoes, and sweet treats such as doughnuts—into glucose, our main source of fuel. Lipids, or fats, are broken down into fatty acids and glycerol, and proteins—such as chicken, fish, and cheese—are broken down into amino acids. Insulin is the key that unlocks, or binds with, receptors on the body's cells. Once insulin has unlocked the door, the glucose passes freely from the blood into the cell, where it is either stored for use in the future or used for energy.

Insulin resistance develops gradually over time. The pancreas churns out its usual amount of insulin, but the insulin can't unlock the doors to the cells. To keep the blood's glucose level normal, the pancreas churns out even more insulin.

Insulin resistance typically develops gradually in overweight, inactive women. Most overweight women, in fact, have high insulin levels, although most people with insulin resistance produce enough insulin to maintain near-normal blood glucose levels. No one knows what causes insulin resistance, but some scientists believe a defect in specific genes may trigger both it and type 2 diabetes. Scientists do know obesity and a sedentary lifestyle aggravate insulin resistance.

Insulin resistance is unhealthy because it can lead to elevated levels of triglycerides, blood fats that can lead to heart disease. Also, women with insulin resistance tend to have too little HDL cholesterol, the healthy form of cholesterol that protects us from unhealthy fat deposits on the arteries' walls.

Usually the body naturally makes all the cholesterol it needs and maintains it at a normal level. But many factors—including your genes, diet, and age—can influence the level. When a woman eats red meat or other foods that contain cholesterol or saturated fat, the extra cholesterol can form deposits on the walls of the arteries, which can eventually lead to chest pain called angina, heart attack, or stroke. This can also happen if her body makes too much cholesterol or can't maintain the levels in a normal range. Having high levels of another kind of cholesterol—low-density lipoprotein, or LDL cholesterol—makes the deposits worse, but having high levels of the good, high-density lipoprotein, or HDL, protects women against arteriosclerosis, or deposits, because it removes cholesterol from the lining of the arteries.

Diabetes: Getting Fit Can Help

While it's difficult to know for sure, estimates suggest that one out of four Americans with insulin resistance will develop type 2 diabetes. And virtually all diagnosed type 2 diabetics have insulin resistance. With insulin resistance, glucose can't get into the body's cells, so it builds up in the blood.

Resistin: The Hormone behind Insulin Resistance?

Scientists have long known of the connection between obesity and diabetes but haven't understood how the extra weight influenced the body's metabolism of sugar. Now they may have a key clue.

Researchers at the University of Pennsylvania School of Medicine discovered that fat cells produce a hormone—resistin—that interferes with insulin's important work.

The scientists happened upon resistin as they studied a new class of anti-diabetic drugs called thiazolidinediones, or TZDs. The scientists knew that TZDs trigger a receptor in fat cells, but they weren't sure how. Looking for an explanation of how TZDs worked, they screened fat cells to look for a gene that was essentially paralyzed by the drugs—that's when they happened upon resistin.

Upon further investigation, the scientists found that levels of resistin were higher in obese mice. They decided to try making antibodies against the hormone, and when they gave the antibodies to obese mice, the animals' blood sugar levels and insulin action improved.

Inspired, the scientists treated normal-weight mice with resistin and found that the hormone impaired the healthy animals' insulin action. Stay tuned for more developments on this newly discovered hormone.

The symptoms of type 2 diabetes develop gradually over months or even years, and some women have no symptoms. If symptoms are present, they may include fatigue, frequent infections, blurry vision, and slow healing of wounds and sores. If a woman has had the disease for several years, she may notice that she's become very thirsty because the extra glucose draws water out of the body's tissues and into the blood. Sensing the additional water in the blood, her kidneys transform it into more urine than usual, and this leads to dehydration. A chronic disease, uncontrolled diabetes can lead to complications such as nerve damage, foot problems, and arteriosclerosis.

Obesity is one of the major risk factors associated with type 2 diabetes: more than 80 percent of women with type 2 diabetes are overweight or were once overweight. Though type 2 diabetes was once considered a disease of midlife, women are being diagnosed with it at younger and younger ages— a powerful link to the corresponding increase in obesity among women in their twenties and thirties.

Exercise is an essential part of diabetes control. "Blood glucose levels can drop 20 to 30 percent after a single exercise session," says Cathy Mullooly, director of exercise physiology at Joslin Diabetes Center in Boston.

Mullooly recommends that you aim to walk at least three or four times a week at a slow or moderate pace for 20 to 30 minutes. (To help control blood sugar, follow the Fit Not Fat Exercise Plan in part 4.)

As you lose weight, your body will likely become more sensitive to the insulin your pancreas makes, Dr. Redmond says. If you're overweight and have insulin sensitivity, losing even 10 to 15 percent of your current body weight—20 to 30 pounds if you weigh 200 pounds—can increase your cells' sensitivity to insulin. If you're currently on insulin or medication for diabetes, your dosages may need to be adjusted as you lose weight.

Syndrome X: Metabolism Gone Awry

Researchers at Stanford University coined the term *syndrome X* to explain a quartet of disorders—diabetes, obesity, high blood pressure, and abnormal blood fats. This concept, also called the metabolic syndrome, has been expanded to include many symptoms, such as central and abdominal obesity and elevated heart rate, among others. But the underlying metabolic defect that links, and most probably precedes, all of these disorders is insulin resistance. Syndrome X is associated with a condition known as polycystic ovary syndrome, or PCOS, a cause of irregular menstrual periods and infertility in women of childbearing age. Women with PCOS have insulin resistance but lack other

features of syndrome X—high blood pressure and blood fat abnormalities—and they typically have fat deposits all over, rather than just in the abdomen. But the underlying defect, insulin resistance, puts them at risk to later develop syndrome X and diabetes.

High-fat or high-carbohydrate diets may be responsible for syndrome X, but exercise and weight loss can be powerful medicine. Losing weight generally triggers a drop in triglyceride levels and often raises levels of HDL, the "good" cholesterol that removes fat deposits from arteries. Studies show that weight loss, through a reduction of calories and increased exercise, can also make the body more sensitive to insulin, decrease fat around the abdomen, and lower blood pressure.

Syndrome W: A Female-Only Fat Problem

Some women who watch their weight and exercise religiously report a dramatic change in their bodies soon after they celebrate their 40th birthdays. They complain of fatigue and weight gain, particularly extra flab around the waist. They cut back on calories and notch their exercise routines into high gear, yet still can't lose weight. Their doctors notice a rise in their once normal blood pressure readings. Their appetite and cravings for carbohydrates shoot up dramatically.

"The vast majority of women with midlife weight gain tell me that they notice a

FIT
| **FLASH**

Burn Calories to Lower Your Risk of Breast Cancer

Whether you vacuum, wait tables, or jog, you're beating your breast cancer odds, according to Canadian researchers from the University of Alberta in Edmonton and the University of Calgary in Alberta. When scientists surveyed 2,470 women, half with breast cancer and half without, they found that postmenopausal women who had done the *most* moderate activity, such as cleaning or assembly work, throughout their lives had a 30 percent lower risk of breast cancer than those who had done the *least*. Though recreational exercise didn't show a benefit, it's because these women didn't do much exercise or organized sports, says study author and Alberta Cancer Board epidemiologist Christine Friedenreich, Ph.D. Other research has shown significant risk reduction with vigorous recreational activities such as jogging and sports.

"What matters is total energy expenditure," says Dr. Friedenreich. "The more calories you burn over time, the better." Researchers speculate that activity protects by lowering high-risk hormones as well as by preventing weight gain, which itself is a risk factor for breast cancer.

dramatic change in their ability to maintain their weight with diet and exercise after turning 40," says Harriette Mogul, M.D., an endocrinologist at the New York Medical College in Valhalla, who treats many pre-menopausal and menopausal women with these symptoms. "Women don't say, 'It starts at age 38.' They don't say, 'It starts at age 45.' They say '40.'"

Mogul dubbed the disorder that causes this constellation of symptoms "syndrome W" and says it's a precursor to the better-known syndrome X, or metabolic syndrome. The W represents the four key characteristics of the condition: women, weight gain, an increased waist size—dubbed "waist gain"—and "white coat hypertension," the modest

rise in blood pressure seen in some women visiting doctors' offices.

Keep an eye out for some of these clues that you may have syndrome W.

▶ You've gained 20 pounds or more since your twenties, and the weight is concentrated around your abdomen or hips.

▶ You're an avid exerciser but still can't lose weight.

▶ Your waist measurement increased 2 inches or more since your twenties, or your skirt/pant size increased two sizes or more.

▶ You are prone to bingeing once you start to eat, especially after eating sweets and starches.

▶ Your blood pressure is significantly higher than it used to be (140/85 mg/dl may be high for you), and it seems to be particularly high when you go to the doctor.

"In my practice, at least 95 percent of the women with syndrome W exercise more than three times a week, and they've always been very healthy," says Dr. Mogul. "Yet they have high blood pressure for the first time in their lives, or higher elevations than ever."

In her study of women with syndrome W, Dr. Mogul made another discovery. Tests showed that the women had high insulin levels—pointing to insulin resistance—despite perfectly normal blood glucose levels. Dr. Mogul is convinced insulin is at the heart of the women's increased waist size and other symptoms. The powerful hormone can constrict blood vessels, laying the groundwork for cardiovascular damage. But Dr. Mogul explains that doctors generally measure only blood sugar and not insulin, so the association between weight gain and insulin resistance is missed, especially in women with mild weight gain and subtle changes in blood pressure. The disorder isn't detected early on, and women are advised simply to eat less and exercise more.

"The blood sugar levels can be normal—normal for years," she says. "But if caught early, syndrome W is treatable with dietary changes and, if necessary, medication that can lower weight, improve the metabolic pro-

FIT | FLASH

Exercise Keeps Women Fit and Hot Flash–Free

Exercise, how it loves us—let us count the ways: it can improve blood sugar levels in diabetics; it's one of the best weapons to maintain bone mass in the war against osteoporosis, the bone-thinning disease of older women; and, of course, it's great for controlling weight. Now it turns out that exercise helps with hot flashes, moods, and concentration, too!

Two Australian studies that looked at relieving symptoms of menopause without drugs found that women who exercised regularly were less likely to complain of related symptoms, such as hot flashes and night sweats.

A similar study found that women who *deliberately* worked up a sweat were more likely to have brighter moods than their sedentary sisters. Women who worked out also reported fewer memory and concentration problems.

The researchers concluded that while hormone replacement therapy can ease severe symptoms of menopause and protect a woman's health down the line, exercise may significantly reduce distress, too.

file, and delay or possibly prevent diabetes and heart disease."

Dr. Mogul treats women with syndrome W with a carbohydrate-modified high-fiber diet that eliminates sugars and limits patients to four or five servings each day of carbohydrates. Women with syndrome W should also avoid high-sugar fruits, such as bananas, mangoes, dried fruits, orange juice, and pineapple, and instead choose low-sugar citrus fruits, like grapefruit, and berries.

Most women with syndrome W also require the diabetes drug metformin (Glucophage), which improves insulin resistance. In one study, Dr. Mogul found that 80 percent of women treated with metformin improved. In addition to making the body more receptive to the actions of insulin, metformin reduces appetite and food intake and cuts down on the free fatty acids in a woman's bloodstream—a cause of insulin resistance.

As women lose weight, their appetite diminishes and their blood pressure drops. Their fatigue disappears, too. "All of the women feel better," Dr. Mogul says. If you feel you may be at risk for syndrome X or W, talk to your doctor and schedule a complete physical, including blood tests that measure insulin activity.

Estrogen: Another Key to Internal Fitness

Nearly every cell, organ, and tissue in a woman's body—including the brain—contains estrogen receptors, the little locks that open to let the hormone in. Estrogen, in fact, affects about 300 tissues in a woman's body. It not only spurs a woman's sexual development and prepares the uterus for the implantation of a fertilized egg; it also protects her bones and probably her heart.

The most potent form of estrogen is called estradiol. Other, less powerful estrogens are estriol and estrone. Although most estrogens are produced in the ovaries, body fat, skin, and muscle can make them, too.

Estrogen defends our bones. While best known for its effect on the reproductive system, estrogen is a bone protector, and bone strength is a key marker of fitness. Estrogen inhibits the work of osteoclasts, or cells that weaken bone, and prompts a woman's body to make healthy, new bone. Lacking estrogen, a woman's bones break down more quickly than they once did, and lose calcium. This can trigger osteopenia, a loss of bone, and eventually to osteoporosis, a more severe brittle bone disease.

The weaker or more porous a bone is, the more likely it is to break. Thanks to osteoporosis, one out of every two women will break a bone sometime after the age of 50. Some women, even at an advanced stage of osteoporosis, don't even know they have the disease until they break a wrist or hip in a seemingly innocent fall. Some women have been known to suffer a compression fracture of the spine simply by lifting a bag of groceries! A number of these fractures can trigger kyphosis, the hunched back of osteoporosis.

It's particularly important that midlife women maintain—or build—the bone they have. Following the Fit Not Fat Exercise Plan—especially weight-bearing aerobic exercise and strength training—is an excellent way to build bone mass. Working out strengthens bone, and strong bone is a critical key to longevity and long-term freedom of movement.

Estrogen may protect the heart. Estrogen also contributes to internal fitness by acting directly on blood vessels to prevent deposits of fat from gathering inside arteries, possibly reducing a woman's risk of developing heart disease. Experts say estrogen also protects the heart indirectly by lowering the levels of bad cholesterol and fats that circulate in the blood and lurk like sinister thugs waiting to do damage. What's more, estrogen cleverly raises the levels of HDL, or good cholesterol, which protects the heart against disease by removing deposits from artery walls.

Estrogen gives us curves. The loss of estrogen during menopause doesn't just lead to hot flashes. It can also change a woman's shape. Before menopause, fat tends to concentrate in the thighs and hips. That tendency is related to lipoprotein lipase, or LPL, an enzyme produced by fat cells that prompts the body to store calories as fat. In women, fat cells in the thighs, hips, and breasts secrete LPL. Men tend to secrete LPL in the fat cells in the stomach area.

FIT | FLASH

Exercise Preserves Ovarian Health

Next time you're ready to drop out of your aerobics class or jump off the treadmill early, stick it out for the sake of your ovaries. Regular exercise may help protect you from ovarian cancer.

In a study at the University of Pittsburgh, researchers looked at the exercise histories of 2,100 women and found that those who hiked, biked, or did a similar form of physical activity at least 4 hours a week were 27 percent less likely to develop ovarian cancer than women who exercised less than 1 hour a week. And moderately active women—who exercised between 1 and 4 hours weekly—still had a 15 percent reduction in ovarian cancer risk.

Why? Exercise keeps weight down, for one, which lowers your overall risk of cancer. More specifically, exercise lowers levels of the reproductive hormones linked to ovarian cancer.

If you think it's too late in life for you to get moving, think again. High levels of physical activity will help protect your ovaries at *any* age.

After menopause, when estrogen levels fall dramatically, women tend to put on pounds (due to lifestyle changes, not menopause per se). Some of this extra weight may be deposited as fat over the abdomen. The redistribution of fat is perhaps partly due to the loss of estrogen, along with a decrease in exercise and reduced muscle tone and other factors. (Another cause may be that as estrogen decreases, larger amounts of insulin circulate in the bloodstream, allowing too much glucose to enter the cells and be stored as fat.) This shifting of fat can be dangerous since central fat is associated with increased risks for heart disease and diabetes. "Estrogen tends to keep fat on the hips, breasts, and bottom, and these areas lose fat when estrogen drops," Dr. Redmond says. "The net effect is less of an hourglass shape."

One option that can serve many purposes is replacing that missing estrogen. Hormone replacement therapy, or HRT, comes in many natural and synthetic forms. Some women take HRT in the form of a patch, a gel, or vaginal tablets or devices like a vaginal ring or an IUD because those forms of estrogen are less likely than oral estrogen to trigger gallstones or blood clots. Estrogen patches are designed to release the hormone slowly over time, and many women get good results with them. In studies of female twins in England and Australia, HRT was associated with less abdominal fat. (Hormone replacement may not be advisable for all women, so be sure to discuss all the potential benefits and risks with your doctor.)

Note that if you work out regularly and use an estrogen patch, your doctor may need to adjust your dosage because exercise can alter the amount of hormone your skin absorbs. "Absorption of the drug is dependent on all of the patch sticking to the skin," Dr. Redmond explains. Tiny wrinkles will not make much difference, but separation from the skin will. If you see the patch has separated from your skin or has sweat under it, you should change it. Or time patch changes for after exercise. "Women should be able to judge a problem by an increase in hot flashes," he adds. If you notice a difference, talk to your doctor.

Testosterone: A Muscle and Bone Builder

Starting at about age 40 or so, as a woman approaches and passes through perimenopause, her estrogen levels wane and levels of progesterone, a companion hormone, decline. But she also loses some testosterone. Testosterone isn't just a male hormone that puts that come-hither look into your husband's eyes. Females, too, produce the chemical, but in significantly lower amounts. In adolescent girls, for example, testosterone that's released by the ovaries and the two adrenal glands is responsible for the development of pubic hair and contributes to growth of muscles and bones.

Research says having a hysterectomy doesn't cause weight gain. So how come I've gained 15 pounds since having mine?

The change in production of hormones such as estrogen and testosterone that occurs when the ovaries are removed was thought to contribute to weight gain, especially the accumulation of abdominal weight after removal of the ovaries. In fact inactivity following surgery, combined with a natural slowdown in metabolism, is at fault.

Hysterectomy is surgical removal of the uterus. During a simple hysterectomy, doctors remove only the uterus. During a radical hysterectomy, fallopian tubes, ovaries, and lymph glands are removed, too. Radical hysterectomy is usually performed for endometrial cancer and advanced cervical cancer.

"Weight fluctuations are common after any kind of surgery," says Geoffrey Redmond, M.D., endocrinologist and director of the Hormone Center of New York and president of the Center for Health Research, both in New York City, and the author of *The Good News about Women's Hormones*. "After surgery, there is weight loss. Then the body needs to repair itself and needs to store food to rebuild itself. Perhaps sometimes it overshoots and gains too much weight."

Lack of exercise, coupled with the natural slowdown in metabolism that tends to occur at midlife, also plays a role. Every woman who goes through abdominal surgery needs time to recover, so it may take time to get back to your previous level of fitness, says Dr. Redmond.

To beat post-hysterectomy weight gain, get back into your exercise program as soon as your doctor gives you the go-ahead, and don't give up on your long-range fitness goals.

Though the ovaries stop producing estrogen during menopause, they continue to produce small amounts of testosterone, which can be converted in body fat to estradiol (a principal form of estrogen). Nevertheless, declines in testosterone are also linked to atrophy of both muscle and bone and a decrease in sexual drive.

While there's no evidence yet that women need supplemental testosterone after menopause, some experts feel that a combination of estrogen and a small amount of testosterone may help to increase bone mass as well as improve mental alertness, energy level, and sometimes sexual drive. There's even preliminary evidence that some women who take testosterone as part of their hormone replacement therapy could experience a decrease in body fat. Ask your doctor if he or she thinks testosterone replacement might be right for you.

Growth Hormone: The Muscle Booster

As we accumulate years, we also lose some of our growth hormone, a product of the pitu-

HOW THEY DID IT

First Step toward Diabetes Control: Toss Out All the Sausage

An environmental health specialist a few months shy of her 39th birthday, Jacqueline Bellinger was carrying about 310 pounds on her 5-foot-9-inch frame when doctors diagnosed her with type 2 diabetes. She eagerly embarked on an eating and exercise program that has brought her weight down to 158 pounds and changed her life for the better.

I was diagnosed with diabetes in July 1995. It didn't come as that big a surprise because there's an awful lot of diabetes in my family—both type 1 and type 2. When I was diagnosed, my fasting blood sugar was 263. You're considered to have diabetes if it is 126 milligrams per deciliter or more. No wonder I was feeling lousy.

I met with a diabetes educator and nutritionist. The first thing we did at home was empty the larder. A few of my friends and relations made out handsomely with things like Polish sausage and 12-ounce steaks. After about 6 months, I lost my taste for things like rich meats. I would rather eat just a little lean meat and fill up on vegetables.

I immediately started with just a 30-minute walk every day, too. That started peeling the weight off pretty quickly. But walking is not practical in eastern Washington in the winter, so I now use a cross-country ski machine and an exercise bike for 45 minutes in the morning and 30 minutes before I go to bed at night. I walk a lot when I'm on vacation. To me a vacation is no fun without it!

Today my blood sugar measurements are in the near-normal range. Technically, I'm a type 2 diabetic, but my pancreas doesn't make much insulin. That means I must be especially careful to exercise regularly and eat wisely to keep my blood sugar levels stable.

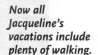

Now all Jacqueline's vacations include plenty of walking.

I work hard to exercise and eat healthful foods because I'd like to protect my eyesight and my kidneys—and both feet. I've seen the complications of diabetes firsthand in members of my father's family. Two of my uncles ended up blind, and I haven't gotten off scot-free. I have some kidney damage. But if I keep my blood sugar at near-normal levels, I can reduce my chances of developing further complications. So far, I don't need pills.

And my hard work is paying off. I feel so much better now. When you feel better physically, you feel better emotionally. It's also great fun going to shop. They didn't use to make large-size clothes for teenagers in the 1970s. Now I'm wearing all the fun stuff I didn't wear years ago: tie-dyes and flared jeans.

itary gland that increases the body's ratio of muscle to fat. Growth hormone plays a critical role in a little boy's or girl's growth and development, but its importance doesn't disappear with childhood. It appears to play a role not only in muscle and bone strength but also in body composition. Growth hormone stimulates production of a substance called insulin-like growth factor, or IGF-1. Made by the liver, IGF-1 flows through the bloodstream, searching for IGF-1 receptors on the surface of the body's cells, including muscle cells. It signals the muscle cells to grow in number and size.

Scientists believe that a decline in growth hormone plays a role in the aging process of some men and women—but don't run out just yet and sign up for costly injections of human growth hormone. The synthetic preparations of GH are prescribed only for children and adults who have a deficiency of the hormone due to damage to the pituitary gland.

For anyone else, the medical risks far outweigh any gains, says Craig D. Rubin, M.D., a geriatrics specialist who is professor of internal medicine at the University of Texas Southwestern Medical Center in Dallas. In healthy people, growth hormone injections can cause swelling from water retention, an increase in blood glucose, high blood pressure, and carpal tunnel syndrome, among other side effects. Although there is no evidence to suggest that excess growth hormone increases the risk of cancer, the connection remains controversial.

"There's never been a study of true value, as far as I know, that shows growth hormone made a significant functional change" in a person's life, Dr. Rubin says. "There's not been a situation where a person was weak and couldn't do the activities of daily living and suddenly took growth hormone and was robust."

While research shows that growth hormone can increase the amount of muscle in some individuals, the increase isn't any more, and may be less, than the increase in muscle seen with exercise, Dr. Rubin says. And, he adds, an overwhelming amount of evidence shows that exercise wards off several chronic diseases associated with sedentary living.

Yes, ladies, the jury is in—exercise (along with a healthy diet) is the closest thing we have to a cure-all. Get started today. (Turn to chapter 6 to begin formulating your Master Plan.)

CHAPTER 4

DE-STRESS YOUR FAT CELLS

Life in the 21st century poses new kinds of stresses—terrorist alerts, bioterrorism threats, and economic downturns, to say nothing of the usual traffic jams, deadlines, and, for many, impossible demands.

Researchers are discovering that women are exposed to more stress than men and are more sensitive to its effects. For example, a telephone survey sponsored by the National Sleep Foundation found that nearly half of all adults surveyed reported symptoms of insomnia in the few nights immediately after the September 11, 2001, attacks on the World Trade Center and the Pentagon. And women, it found, reported more difficulty sleeping than men did.

Stress can not only wreak havoc on your skin, your nerves, and your relationships—chances are good it's also helping pack on, and keep on, the pounds.

IS THIS YOUR PROBLEM?

Is Stress Making You Fat?

Not sure why your midsection is expanding by the day? Ask yourself these questions for clues into causes that could be eluding you.

1. Do you often feel anxious, cynical, or depressed?

Your outlook may be contributing to a thicker waistline. In a study from the North American Association for the Study of Obesity that looked at middle-aged and elderly men and women, researchers found a link between cynicism and anxiety and higher waist-to-hip ratios. Among women, depression and spare tires were linked; among men, anger was linked to higher abdominal fat.

"These emotions may increase levels of cortisol, a hormone that seems to steer fat to the abdomen," says study author Tracy L. Nelson, Ph.D., M.P.H., assistant professor in the department of health and exercise science at Colorado State University in Fort Collins.

Another study, at Duke University in Durham, North Carolina, found that high hostility levels are linked to larger waists and higher body mass index. Still other research has shown that people with high levels of hostility have a higher output of both cortisol and adrenaline in response to anger, and that they down more calories than those with lower hostility levels.

2. Are you struggling to make ends meet—or do you think you are?

Researchers in Sweden found that men who were lower on the socioeconomic scale were more likely to have potbellies and higher cortisol levels in response to perceived stress.

Whether chronic and low-grade or sudden and acute, stress can change your weight, your shape, or both. Perhaps you've experienced the stress-induced feeding frenzies that drive you to binge on chocolate or chips at the end of (or during) a hellish day? Those cookies may feel like medicine, but they're *literally* headed straight for your belly, posing special risks above and beyond overall weight gain.

A Tale of Crises, Cookies, and Cortisol

Remember Suzanne, the 45-year-old we met in chapter 1? Formerly pear-shaped, Suzanne not only gained weight at midlife; she's also changed shape. She's grown a spare tire around her middle.

At the same time that's happening, her life has also been changing dramatically. Last year

3. Are you a caregiver or a working mom with kids? Do you have health problems of your own?

Both single and married working mothers face higher stress levels, not so much in their factories or offices but in the home.

Studies show that caregivers of mentally or physically challenged relatives are also at risk for chronic stress. If you take care of a highly dependent patient, have a tense relationship with the patient, are low-income, or are African-American, you are at higher risk for severe stress or stress-related illnesses. One reason African-Americans are more vulnerable is that they tend to be in poorer health than Whites and, as a result, face greater stress as caregivers.

4. Do you feel powerless to change things?

When it comes to stress, the sort that makes us feel powerless may be the most dangerous. "Psychological stress of the kind that we can't do anything about seems to lead to the greatest production of cortisol. And an increase in cortisol stimulates the uptake of fat into abdominal fat," says Cynthia K. Buffington, Ph.D., associate professor in the department of medicine at the University of Tennessee (UT) Health Science Center and director of research at the Obesity Wellness Center of the UT Medical Group, both in Memphis. Women, she adds, seem to be most vulnerable to the kind of stress that makes us want to throw our hands up in despair.

A sense of belonging could just be an antidote to abdominal fat. One study of adolescents and young adults in Finland suggests social support may protect against

(continued)

Suzanne's husband died driving on a snow-covered road when another motorist lost control of his car. Three months ago, Suzanne's college-age daughter collapsed from an emotional breakdown that stemmed from her anguish. And today Suzanne just learned that her elderly father, who lives with her, has prostate cancer that has spread to his bones.

It's the Chernobyl of bad days, the kind of over-the-top crisis that can broadside a woman with the force of a runaway truck. Numb, speechless with grief, and angry to boot, Suzanne falls into a common trap: She hauls out the hot fudge and Häagen-Dazs. She eats and eats and eats, as if all the chomping could grind her problems into a powder that would just blow away.

As her world implodes, Suzanne's

IS THIS YOUR PROBLEM? *(cont.)*

abdominal fat and its health risks. Other research shows that older people who are actively connected with their adult children are protected against the health tolls of major stressors such as lower social class or low income.

5. Do you always seem to be hungry?

Studies in rats suggest that cortisol is directly involved in the ability of a "satiety" hormone, leptin, to regulate the sense of satiety, or fullness. Induced by stress, excess levels of cortisol coursing through your system may be quelling the appetite-suppressing effects of leptin. Stress-related secretion of cortisol may make leptin less effective, leading to what one expert calls "leptin resistance." When leptin loses its punch, men and women feel hungrier and, in turn, eat more.

6. Are you reaching for high-carbohydrate foods like cookies and cakes more than you used to?

Your cravings may be stress-induced, says Mary Dallman, Ph.D., professor of physiology at the University of California, San Francisco, who studies the effects of repeated stress on animals. She discovered that rats that were stressed and had higher-than-normal

---

middle expands, a ring of abdominal fat that puts her at increased risk for both type 1 and type 2 diabetes, heart disease, even cancer—and changes her pear-shaped body to a rounded, less defined apple.

The experiences of women like Suzanne are part of the growing evidence of what scientists are discovering in laboratories and medical offices around the world: Chronic stress can lead to the sustained release of the stress hormone cortisol, which helps to pack pounds around some women's waists.

Cortisol can actually help "remodel" women's bodies. "So many women go from pears to apples and accumulate fat in their abdomens rather than their buttocks," says Mary Dallman, Ph.D., professor of physiology at the University of California, San Francisco, who studies the effects of repeated stress on animals. If a woman eats for comfort when she's stressed, she's actually setting herself up for a double whammy: She already has high cortisol levels, and then she eats carbohydrates, which releases more insulin, the fat storage hormone. This combination steers fat directly to her tummy.

Let's look at the complex interaction of several factors that make that happen.

levels of cortisol ate more than rats that were stressed and had normal levels of cortisol. Dr. Dallman also found that stressed rats with high cortisol levels chose foods with high levels of sucrose, one form of sugar.

7. Do you smoke or drink heavily?

Abdominal obesity is linked to heavy drinking and tobacco smoking. In contrast, the fat that dimples your thighs or arms—doctors call this "peripheral obesity"—isn't connected to smoking or heavy alcohol consumption.

Many smokers say they light up to manage stress and relieve tension. Some smoke to halt depressing thoughts and moods. Research indicates that alcoholics are also much likelier to smoke than others.

As with smokers and tobacco, heavy drinkers report turning to alcohol to reduce their stress. Some women pour themselves too many glasses of wine or sip too many martinis, thinking it will help them cope with—and disengage from—their troubles. Ironically, the drinking may snowball into a source of stress itself because it increases both appetite and cortisol levels, adding more abdominal weight in the process.

The Science behind Stress-Induced Fat

Stress is inevitable—and natural. When Suzanne learned of her father's fatal prognosis, her body responded to stress the same way her body would if she were hiking in the wild and encountered a protective mother bear with her cubs. Facing the bear, Suzanne would instinctively retreat, slowly walking backward toward safety, as her adrenal glands released epinephrine, cortisol, and other stress hormones.

Next, she would sprint to a run, her heart rate shooting up, her pupils dilating, and her blood racing to her muscles. All those changes efficiently enable her body to fight—or flee—in a time of severe stress.

Suzanne probably doesn't encounter protective mother bears very often, but as she faces the devastating losses in her personal life, she endures an onslaught of cortisol just the same. With her body reacting the same way to bad news that it would to physical danger, the released cortisol mobilizes her stored fat to prepare her body to bolt from danger. Once it's on the move, that fat can do some serious damage to the body's critical systems.

How Stress Inflates a Spare Tire

Unfortunately, in the absence of an imminent physical threat, this stress-induced outpouring of cortisol goes to waste—and to waist.

"If we don't engage in the fight-or-flight response, all of this extra fat that was mobilized but not burned up migrates to the stomach," explains stress expert Redford Williams, M.D., professor of psychiatry at Duke University Medical Center and director of the Behavioral Medical Research Center in Durham, North Carolina.

BESTBET
_____

Breathe with Purpose

Fitness expert Meg Jordan, R.N., Ph.D., a medical anthropologist at the Health Medicine Institute in Walnut Creek, California, who founded *American Fitness* magazine, calls the breaths we take our "life force." Taking a moment to breathe with purpose, she says, bathes your brain in oxygen, clears away the cobwebs—and takes you to the calming "still point" inside yourself.

To reach your still point, pay close attention to your breath as it moves through your nose or mouth, down your throat, into your lungs, and out of your body. Take note of how your breath sounds and feels. If your mind wanders away from your breath, don't fret about it. Return your focus to your breathing. In a few minutes, your breath will slow to a nice, even rhythm, calming you in the process.

Here's why. Abdominal fat has more cortisol "receptors" than other kinds of fat, says leading stress researcher Elissa E. Epel, Ph.D., a postdoctoral scholar in psychiatry at the University of California, San Francisco. That means that abdominal fat is extra-sensitive to hormones and responds to stress hormones by accumulating fat. "During times of stress, if you secrete a lot of cortisol, fat's going to be stored in your abdomen rather than on your hips," she explains.

Some of the strongest evidence of the cortisol–abdominal fat connection comes from doctors' understanding of both a hormonal disorder called Cushing's syndrome and the eating disorder anorexia nervosa. Triggered by prolonged exposure of the body's tissues to cortisol, Cushing's syndrome causes severe fatigue, weak muscles, high blood pressure, high blood sugar levels, plus upper-body obesity and skinny arms and legs. And although anorexics are painfully thin, they traditionally have "sky-high" levels of cortisol, leading to an increased proportion of abdominal fat, Dr. Dallman says.

In a study of 59 healthy premenopausal women, Dr. Epel and her colleagues found that those with rounder bellies secreted more cortisol and performed poorly on laboratory stress tests, compared with women without spare tires. In fact, women with high waist-to-hip ratios—that is, whose waist and hip measurements were similar—perceived the

The Stress–Insulin Connection

Faced with an onslaught of stress, many women reach for high-fat, high-carbohydrate treats such as hot caramel and Ben & Jerry's. Yet fatty sweets like those can lead to a classic double whammy. High-fat diets trigger the body to produce even more of the stress hormone cortisol. And high-carbohydrate treats such as cake, candy, and ice cream trigger the body to produce a lot of insulin, a vital hormone that regulates the levels of glucose in the blood—and promotes fat storage.

Produced in the pancreas, insulin nudges muscle cells to absorb glucose, which are then converted into energy. Think of insulin as the body's glucose police force. It prevents too much glucose from loitering around our bodies—and it ensures that the tissues that need glucose get it.

The presence of both cortisol and insulin activates an enzyme called lipoproteinlipase, or LPL, which promotes the storage of fat, says stress researcher Elissa E. Epel, Ph.D., a postdoctoral scholar in psychiatry at the University of California, San Francisco.

Exposed to free fatty acids from broken-down abdominal fat, the liver increases its production and output of glucose and finds itself less able to clear insulin from the blood.

Over time, all the extra insulin circulating in the blood causes the muscles and other insulin-sensitive tissues to resist insulin's actions. Insulin resistance, in turn, triggers a rise in blood sugar levels, setting a woman up for type 2 diabetes.

challenges as "more threatening" and reported more chronic stress.

The bottom line is, dealing with saddlebags or heavy thighs might just be healthier than having a potbelly and skinny legs. Dr. Epel's study also found that overweight women with extra weight that was spread throughout their bodies adapted to the stress, and their cortisol levels dropped. In contrast, slender women with round tummies didn't adapt—they continued to secrete significantly more cortisol in response to familiar challenges in the lab, compared with slender counterparts who carried weight at their hips.

The Dangers of Ab Fat

Scientists believe deep abdominal fat may also behave differently than the subcutaneous fat resting just under the skin or fat dimpling our thighs.

"Abdominal fat is quicker to break down and spew the by-products of fat metabolism—including fatty acids—into the blood," says Wendy Kohrt, Ph.D., professor of medicine in the division of geriatric medicine at the University of Colorado in Denver, who has studied the link between abdominal fat and stress.

What makes abdominal fat so dangerous is its proximity to the portal vein, the vein that feeds into the liver. "If blood flowing through fat goes directly to the liver, any substances released by the fat reach the liver in much higher concentrations" and the liver works harder to detoxify the blood, explains Geoffrey Redmond, M.D., endocrinologist and director of the Hormone Center of New York and president of the Center for Health Research, both in New York City, and the author of *The Good News about Women's Hormones*.

What's more, when your liver is exposed to high amounts of free fatty acids, it increases the likelihood that you will develop diabetes, heart disease, high blood pressure, even stroke, says Cynthia K. Buffington, Ph.D., associate professor in the department of medicine at the University of Tennessee (UT) Health Science Center and director of research at the Obesity Wellness Center of the UT Medical Group, both in Memphis.

One study of more than 44,000 women between ages 40 and 65 done at Brigham and Women's Hospital and Harvard Medical School in Boston found those with waists measuring larger than 28 inches had a two- to three-times-higher risk for coronary heart disease than women who had smaller waists. Numerous other studies have shown that abdominal fat is linked to high blood pressure and glucose intolerance. (When a person has impaired glucose tolerance, her blood glucose levels are higher than normal, but not high enough for a diagnosis of diabetes.) Another study, published in the *American*

Do You Have Stress Fat?

Women who are otherwise lean but develop a paunch of abdominal fat are more likely to have cortisol-related fat, says Nancy Adler, Ph.D., professor of medical psychology, director of the Health Psychology Program, and director of the Center for Health and Community at the University of California, San Francisco, and a leading expert on socioeconomic status and its impact on health.

Most women who have excess abdominal fat know it. Their skirts no longer fit, they have trouble snapping their jeans, and they can't tuck in their blouses, even if their weight stays the same. If you're still not sure whether your abdominal fat poses a problem, hit the sewing box for your tape measure.

"The most useful way to gauge your risk is a simple waist measure," says Glenn Gaesser, Ph.D., professor of exercise physiology at the University of Virginia in Charlottesville. "For women, a waist measurement of 35 inches or larger is where you begin to see increased risk for elevated blood glucose levels, higher blood pressure, and elevated blood lipid levels." (It's 40 inches for men.)

FIT | **FLASH**

In the Long Run, Weight Control Is More Fun

Research suggests that the longer men and women maintain a significant weight loss, the easier and more fun it becomes. A study at the University of Pittsburgh School of Medicine of more than 900 adults who lost an average of 62 pounds found that people who had kept their trim figures for an average of 7 years reported that they expended less effort dieting and maintaining their weight.

In fact, the longer the individuals had maintained their weight loss, the more pleasurable they found staying slim. And those that had gained back some of the weight had regained less.

The researchers speculate that the longer we keep off our excess weight, the more satisfaction we'll have and the less effort we'll feel is needed. In other words, the longer you maintain a weight loss, the easier—and more fun—it becomes.

Journal of Epidemiology, suggests apple-shaped women have a higher risk of developing breast cancer, particularly if they've gone through menopause.

Conquering Your Stress Appetite

OK, so we know stress eating is bad for us—so why is it so hard to stop? One possible explanation: Cortisol itself may also stimulate appetite.

Scientists know that when the body perceives danger, the hypothalamus, a gland in the brain, secretes corticotrophin-releasing factor, or CRF, a hormone that suppresses appetite. One theory holds that if cortisol lingers in the body but the hypothalamus halts the release of CRF, which opposes the actions of cortisol, that person will be hungry as her body recovers from stress.

There was a time when this hunger served a real survival purpose. "It makes sense evolutionarily because if you've just burned off a tremendous amount of energy running away from a predator, you need to start replenishing those depleted energy stores," Dr. Epel says.

Dr. Epel found that women who released high levels of cortisol when they were stressed ate more when they were under the gun, although she is careful to say the effect of cortisol is not very strong. Although the presence of high levels of cortisol itself would not lead directly to weight gain, the extra calories the women in the study ate could have easily led to added pounds.

For example, after Suzanne's husband died and her father got sick, Suzanne turned to high-carbohydrate treats, especially at night. She was no longer satisfied with healthy shakes of skim milk, fruit, and flaxseed. She was seduced by a high-calorie quartet: cakes, cookies, ice cream, and candy.

Until we can learn to handle stress effectively, these cravings will remain a part of a vicious circle. "Psychological distress alters neurochemicals in your brain, and that in turn leads to an increase in appetite and an increase in carbohydrate cravings," says Dr. Buffington, an expert on psychological distress and its link to obesity and disease. Chowing down on carbs sends insulin levels skyrocketing, which in turn coaxes the body to hang on to fat—and around and around it goes.

Where it will stop, we still don't know. Another theory about the stress–fat connection contends that stress increases the release in the brain of a naturally occurring opiate that reduces our perception of pain and anxiety associated with stress—and increases food intake. Some researchers speculate that the stress-related release of cortisol may also be linked to the body's resistance to leptin, a hormone that keeps our appetites at bay.

As with other developments in this up-and-coming field, many questions remain. But what we do know is that learning to handle stress can be an effective weight-loss tool all by itself. That's why stress relief forms one-third of the Fit Not Fat Master Plan. While you're formulating your Master Plan (in chapter 6), be sure to take a spin through part 5, The 40-Plus Relax and Recharge Plan, to learn strategies that can help you tackle and defeat that stress fat once and for all.

PART 2

YOUR PERSONAL FIT NOT FAT STRATEGY

CHAPTER 5

HOW FIT ARE YOU NOW?

If you're considering investing in a mutual fund, stock, bond, or other investment, you certainly will consider its current purchase price. But you'll also size up other important numbers: the high and low prices for the year, past performance, dividends, yield, price-to-earnings ratios, potential earnings, and so on. No single number gives you the true picture of the health of that potential investment.

Just as numbers help you to size up a potential investment, certain numbers enable you to track your nutritional, physical, and mental fitness. Before you begin the Fit Not Fat Plan, it's essential to get a sense of where you stand now. Not only will these measurements will help you set your eating, exercise, and stress management goals; they'll also help you determine you how quickly you'll reach your goals. They'll even give you proof of your progress as you go along.

"Measuring your 'before and after' fitness levels is very motivating," says J. Andrew Doyle, Ph.D., associate professor and exercise physiologist at Georgia State University in Atlanta, and an American College of Sports Medicine–certified exercise test physiologist. If you ever reach a plateau—a bear market, so to speak—taking a look at your long-term performance may help keep you from getting discouraged.

Ideally, everyone would have access to all of these tools and could delight in watching their changing numbers reflect their increasing fitness. But everyone does not have access, nor does everyone need to do *every* calculation. In order to set weight-loss goals in the Fit Not Fat Plan, you'll need to evaluate your current eating, exercise, and stress management levels. Those levels boil down to the results of five basic tests: Daily Calorie Intake; Aerobic Fitness; Muscular Endurance; Flexibility; and Stress Resistance. (Each of these tests is designated below with a star.)

★ Daily Calorie Intake

Losing weight is all about accounting—it basically comes down to calories in and calories out. But every woman has slightly different calorie and nutrient budgets, and quantifying these differences is the key to success in any weight-loss program.

The following chart is a tool to help you get a handle on how many calories you should eat, depending on your activity level,

in order to reach your weight-loss goal. First, write a list of everything you eat for 3 days, keeping track of calories. (The Fit Not Fat Calorie, Fat, and Fiber Counter and Shopping Guide, page 352, is a handy reference.) Tally up the total calories for each day, and take the average of the three. This is your current caloric intake.

Now find your current weight on the chart. The most permanent weight loss happens at a rate of 1 to 2 pounds per week, maximum. If you go any faster, you work against your own metabolism and ultimately set yourself up to rebound. The best strategy is to set minigoals of 10 pounds of weight loss at a time. (For example, if you want to go from 160 to 140, you first shoot for 150, and then 140.) This will give your body enough time to adjust to the decreased calories without going into starvation mode, which would make it start to hoard calories—definitely not something you want. Trace your finger across the chart from your current weight to the best description of your activity level—that's the number of calories you need to eat in order to lose your first 10 pounds.

WHAT TO AIM FOR: Experts suggest limiting yourself to deficit of 250 to 500 calories each day to lose weight at a safe rate, so if your current calorie intake is much higher than the chart's, cut down slowly. Start by trimming 250 calories a day for a week; move down another 250 each week until you reach

Your Daily Calorie Goal Chart

CURRENT WEIGHT	MINIGOAL WEIGHT	ACTIVE	MODERATELY HIGH	MODERATE	LOW
110	100	1,800	1,500	1,300*	1,100*
120	110	1,980	1,650	1,430*	1,210*
130	120	2,160	1,800	1,560	1,320*
140	130	2,340	1,950	1,690	1,430*
150	140	2,520	2,100	1,820	1,540
160	150	2,700	2,250	1,950	1,650
170	160	2,880	2,400	2,080	1,760
180	170	3,060	2,550	2,210	1,870
190	180	3,140	2,700	2,340	1,980
200	190	3,320	2,850	2,470	2,090
210	200	3,500	3,000	2,600	2,200

1. **High activity level:** You have a physically demanding job, engage in regular sports, or work out more than 5 hours a week.
2. **Moderately high:** You get 3 to 5 hours of activity a week.
3. **Moderate:** You're active less than 3 hours a week.
4. **Low:** You don't engage in regular physical activity.

Prevention magazine recommends that you do not go below 1,500 calories per day.

the level listed on the chart. Bear in mind that you can always speed up your weight loss by increasing your activity level—which, as a bonus, bumps up the calories you're allotted!

Once you have your current caloric goal nailed down, you can enter it in "This week's daily calorie goal" on your Master Plan (page 76). Reevaluate your calorie goals after every 10-pound weight loss.

Body Mass Index

Your scale weight alone is like a stock price. Without other information, it's of limited use as a fitness marker. Your body mass index— a ratio of your weight to height—is more useful as a marker of weight-related health risks in populations as a whole, says Bonita Marks, Ph.D., assistant professor of exercise and sport science at the University of North Carolina in Chapel Hill.

WHAT TO AIM FOR: According to the National Institutes of Health, a normal BMI falls between 18.5 and 24.9. A BMI higher than 25 is a sign that you're overweight, and a BMI higher than 30 indicates obesity.

To determine your BMI, consult the accompanying chart. Recheck your BMI every 2 to 3 months.

Body Fat Percentage

Your BMI is a good start, but it doesn't tell you how much of your body is fat and how much is bone, muscle, internal organs, and water. In fact, BMI could even exaggerate your health risk if you're very muscular. So a high BMI may be just a "warning flag," suggests Dr. Marks. You'll also need to seek out

Body Mass Index (BMI) Table

HEIGHT	WEIGHT (IN POUNDS)													
4'10"	91	96	100	105	110	115	119	124	129	134	138	143	148	153
4'11"	94	99	104	109	114	119	124	128	133	138	143	148	153	158
5'0"	97	102	107	112	118	123	128	133	138	143	148	153	158	163
5'1"	100	106	111	116	122	127	132	137	143	148	153	158	164	169
5'2"	104	109	115	120	126	131	136	142	147	153	158	164	169	174
5'3"	107	113	118	124	130	135	141	146	152	158	163	169	175	180
5'4"	110	116	122	128	134	140	145	151	157	163	169	174	180	186
5'5"	114	120	126	132	138	144	150	156	162	168	174	180	186	192
5'6"	118	124	130	136	142	148	155	161	167	173	179	186	192	198
5'7"	121	127	134	140	146	153	159	166	172	178	185	191	197	204
5'8"	125	131	138	144	151	158	164	171	177	184	190	197	203	210
5'9"	128	135	142	149	155	162	169	176	182	189	196	203	209	216
5'10"	132	139	146	153	160	167	174	181	188	195	202	207	215	222
5'11"	136	143	150	157	165	172	179	186	193	200	208	215	222	229
6'0"	140	147	154	162	169	177	184	191	199	206	213	221	228	235
BMI	19	20	21	22	23	24	25	26	27	28	29	30	31	32

Source: National Heart, Lung, and Blood Institute

your body fat percentage, keeping in mind that the human body needs a certain amount of fat to function properly. "Knowing your body fat percentage allows you to determine if you have a healthy ratio of muscle to fat," Dr. Doyle notes.

However, finding your body fat percentage is not as simple as stepping on a scale, Dr. Doyle says. The available methods simply *estimate* the amount of fat, and the numbers these methods provide may be

BESTBET

Get Your Body Fat Measured

Carry your bathroom scale to your closet and hide it in the back—and do it without a bit of guilt.

"We tend to focus on the scale weight too much instead of other things," says J. Andrew Doyle, Ph.D., director of the applied physiology lab at Georgia State in Atlanta. When you step on a scale, it has no idea *what* it's measuring. Two women could have the exact same height and weight, but the first is carrying around too much fat, while the second is very muscular.

Instead of focusing on how much you weigh, have your body fat measured by a trained professional at a local gym or the exercise physiology lab at a nearby university, Dr. Doyle says.

If you still feel compelled to pull the scale out of the closet, limit yourself to one weigh-in per month. Anything more isn't especially useful.

right on the money or slightly off, depending on a number of factors.

Probably the most accurate method is "hydrostatic weighing"—where you're weighed while under water. Most likely, you'll need to visit a university's exercise department for this test, says Dr. Doyle. If that's too much of a hassle, you can likely find these two simpler options at a local gym.

Skin-fold testing. A tester pinches folds of skin at various body sites and measures their thickness with calipers. "For men, the most common sites used are chest, abdomen, and thigh. For women, the back of the arm (triceps), hip, and thigh are most often measured," says Dr. Doyle. Taken as an equation, the composite of these measurements indicates your body fat percentage.

Skin-fold testing isn't as easy to perform as it looks. It requires a lot of training and practice to do accurately, he says. Ask the gym manager to see proof that your tester is certified through the American College of Sports Medicine (ACSM), or has a college degree from an exercise science program, and has done plenty of these tests.

Making note of your skin-fold thicknesses is a useful way to track your progress on the Fit Not Fat Plan. They should grow smaller over time as you become fitter.

Bioelectrical impedance analysis. A simple device that may look like a bathroom scale passes a tiny current through your body.

COOL TOOL

Body Fat Monitors

Tempting as it may be, a home body fat monitor isn't the best way to estimate your percentage of body fat, say experts.

"Bioelectrical impedance is based on the body's resistance to a small amount of electrical current," says H. N. Williford, Ed.D., department head of physical education and director of the Human Performance Laboratory at Auburn University in Montgomery, Alabama, who works with body fat monitor testing. The current flows freely through tissues with a large amount of water, like muscle, and slower through tissues with low water content, like fat. Thus, the faster the current flows, the lower your body fat percentage. This method is accurate only if you're optimally hydrated, you haven't eaten within 4 hours of testing, you're well-rested and have not exercised within 12 hours before the test, and you've gone to the bathroom within 30 minutes of testing—all very specific criteria.

Body fat monitors sold for home aren't as accurate as professional models and may mislead you into thinking you're either fatter or slimmer than you are. They don't take into account the variations that go into determining what's ideal for you, such as body frame type (small to medium), height, weight, body mass index (BMI), athletic ability, health, and age.

If you want to know your true body fat percentage, see a professional. Good places to check include a nearby university or a health club with trainers who are skilled at assessing body fat with research-quality skin-fold calipers. You can also see an exercise physiologist or licensed dietitian.

Even then, don't obsess over the percentages, or you'll get easily discouraged. "A woman may lose 2 to 3 pounds of body fat, but it can take 3 months for even a high-quality body fat tool to register the change," says Michele Olson, Ph.D., professor of health and human performance at Auburn University.

Many trainers and physicians use these regularly in their practices.

Because fat conducts electricity poorly, compared with fat-free tissue, the device can estimate how much of your body consists of fat by analyzing the speed at which the current travels through your body. However, to get an accurate reading, before the test you must avoid eating and drinking for 4 hours; avoid alcohol and caffeine; abstain from exercise for 12 hours; and use the restroom. If used properly, it's about as accurate as the skin-fold test, Dr. Doyle says.

Don't bother rechecking your body fat more frequently than every 3 months, Dr. Doyle suggests. The margin of error is greater than the change you're likely to have made in a shorter period of time.

WHAT TO AIM FOR: According to Shape Up America!, a national fitness organization, 23 to 33 percent is the healthy body fat percentage for women ages 40 to 59. For women ages 60 to 79, the healthy range is 24 to 35 percent.

Waist Measurement

A measuring tape will provide you with another useful figure regarding your figure.

According to the National Institutes of Health (NIH), your waist circumference is a sign of how much abdominal fat you're carrying around; having a large amount of abdominal fat can raise your risk for conditions such as diabetes, high blood pressure, and heart disease.

To measure your waist circumference, feel down your side under your arm until you find where the top of your hipbone meets soft tissue. This will probably be even with your belly button. Loop a tape measure around your belly just above that bone. Make sure it's parallel with the floor all the way around your body.

Breathe normally, and be sure not to cinch it tight to get a smaller number.

WHAT TO AIM FOR: A waist circumference of 35 inches or less. If your waist measurement is greater than 35 inches

FITNESS MYSTERIES

Why do so many girls and young women in their teens and twenties who never work out have board-flat stomachs and wear midriff-baring crop tops, while I do 100 situps a day and still have a bulging belly now that I've hit 40? It's not fair!

Those washboard abs you see in music videos and exercise equipment commercials reflect two physical attributes: strong, toned muscles and an absence of overlying fat to conceal them, says Kathy Sward, Ph.D., clinical assistant professor in exercise physiology and programming director for the health enhancement program of the University of Pittsburgh Medical Center.

Toning the muscles requires plenty of exercise like situps or crunches, which any woman can do regardless of her age. But even a normal amount of body fat—say, 23 percent—might be enough padding to cover those abs, Dr. Sward says. And if you've been pregnant, your abdomen may have undergone changes not seen in younger women who haven't yet borne children, sparing them a belly bulge even if they don't work out. So comparing yourself with women 20 or 30 years your junior isn't realistic. If you must, judge your body on how you compare with other women your age.

That said, faithfully following the Fit Not Fat Exercise and Food Plans in this book can go a long way toward giving you a pleasing torso, even if you can't pass yourself off as 20 years old at the beach.

FIT | FLASH

Exercise Turns Back the Clock

Think you'll never feel as good as you did in your twenties? Think again.

One landmark study suggests that if you work out for 6 months, you can feel as fit as a 20-year-old. In 1966, researchers took five men in their twenties, recorded their fitness levels, and submitted them to 3 weeks of bed rest to test its effects. The researchers then put them on an 8-week exercise program and recorded their resulting fitness levels. In 1996, the men returned for retesting. Now in their fifties and more sedentary, their average weight had climbed 25 percent, body fat had doubled, and aerobic capacity had dropped 11 percent. They followed the same exercise program: 1 hour of walking, jogging, or cycling, four or five times a week. After 24 weeks, all five regained the baseline cardiovascular fitness levels they had achieved in their twenties.

While this study was done on men, the results could be promising for everyone. "It's never too late to exercise and combat the effects of aging," says study coauthor Benjamin Levine, M.D., medical director of the Institute for Exercise and Environmental Medicine at Presbyterian Hospital in Dallas.

Motivating note: The bed rest proved more damaging to the men's aerobic fitness than the 30 years of aging!

and your BMI is between 25 and 29.9, you have a high risk of developing problems. A BMI between 30 and 39.9 puts you at a very high risk.

★ Aerobic Fitness

One of the standard tests of the fitness of your heart and lungs requires you to simply run or walk 1.5 miles as fast as you comfortably can. How much time and effort it takes for you to cover that ground indicates how well your heart and lungs can do their jobs—and how ready you are to jump into your Fit Not Fat Exercise Plan.

The following test is offered by Shape Up America! and devised by the Cooper Institute in Dallas. Find a 1.5-mile course, such as a running track or other safe, flat surface. Or drive along a lightly traveled stretch of flat pavement and measure out 1.5 miles, using your car's odometer. Then run or walk the course at a comfortable pace and time yourself. Don't push yourself too hard. You should be tired at the end, but not weak and sick to your stomach.

WHAT TO AIM FOR: Use the following chart to determine your aerobic fitness level based on your age. If you need to improve,

Aerobic Fitness Test (Run/Walk 1.5 Miles)

FITNESS LEVEL	TIME		
AGE	40–49	50–59	60 PLUS
SUPERIOR	Less than 14:32	Less than 15:58	Less than 16:21
MODERATE	14:33–16:12	15:59–17:14	16:22–18:00
MINIMAL	16:13–17:29	17:15–18:31	18:01–19:02
UNFIT	More than 17:30	More than 18:32	More than 19:03

Source: The Shape Up America! organization

following the guidelines for aerobic exercise in chapter 9 will increase aerobic fitness.

★ Muscular Endurance

Women tend to have less upper-body strength than men do. A good way to check the endurance of muscles in your upper arms, shoulders, and chest is by doing pushups, says Kathy Sward, Ph.D., clinical assistant professor in exercise physiology and programming director for the Health En-hancement Program of the University of Pittsburgh Medical Center.

She recommends the following test and scores, from the American Council on Exercise, but adds that if you can't perform at these levels, don't fret—this is the starting point. Simply jot down the results of this test, and use them to set your Fit Not Fat Exercise goals and to compare with your progress. The more you use your muscles, the greater your muscular endurance will be.

Muscular Endurance Test (Maximum Number of Pushups)

	SCORE		
AGE	40–49	50–59	60–69
EXCELLENT	More than 24	More than 21	More than 17
ABOVE AVERAGE	15–23	11–20	12–16
AVERAGE	11–14	7–10	5–11
BELOW AVERAGE	5–10	2–6	1–4
POOR	Less than 4	Less than 1	Less than 1

Source: The Personal Trainer Manual of the American Council on Exercise

FIT | FLASH

Staying in Shape at Menopause Is Simply a Matter of Choice

In yet another study confirming that menopause does not sentence women to weight gain, the University of Pittsburgh Women's Healthy Lifestyle Project began following more than 500 premenopausal women, average age 47, as they edged into "the change." About half of them continued whatever they were doing. The others were instructed to eat less saturated fat and cholesterol, reduce their calorie and fat intake, and increase their physical activity.

Four-and-a-half years later, the group that lived healthier had lost weight, while the other women had gained more than 5 pounds on average. What's more, LDL, or "bad" cholesterol, had increased by a smaller amount among the first group, and waist circumference had shrunk more.

The researchers concluded that making these lifestyle choices can keep women healthy and fit, even as they go through menopause.

Though you can do the pushups with your knees, instead of your toes, on the ground, the test won't give as good a result since your knees are bearing some of the load. Your hands should be shoulder-width apart, your back and entire body should be straight from shoulders to toes, like a plank, and you should lower yourself until your chest is a fist's width from the floor. Exhale as you pushing yourself up.

WHAT TO AIM FOR: Use the Muscular Endurance Test to determine if your muscles are up to snuff, based on your age. (These guidelines are specifically for women.)

Bone Density

Women can lose up to one-fifth of their bone mass in the 7 years after menopause, according to the National Osteoporosis Foundation. Since bone loss—osteoporosis—doesn't cause symptoms until you've lost substantial amounts of bone, you may not even know if your bones are growing ever thinner until a minor fall leaves you with a hip, wrist, or spinal fracture.

That's why having a bone scan, starting before you officially reach menopause, to check bone density is an essential marker of fitness. These painless, safe tests can measure the bone density of your wrist, spine, hip, finger, heel, or shin.

There are several ways to measure bone density, but the current gold standard is the dual energy x-ray absorptiometry (DEXA), which compares your bone density with that of young women at peak bone mass and expresses it as a T-score.

You should get a bone mineral density (BMD) test if you're in menopause or past it and haven't been tested, or if you're in your thirties or forties with at least one of the following risk factors: You've broken a bone from minor trauma; you have a condition associated with bone loss, like hyperthyroidism; or you've been taking medications that can cause bone loss, like corticosteroids or antiseizure medication.

WHAT TO AIM FOR: Bone mineral density (BMD) within 1 standard deviation (SD), or a T-score above -1, of a young "normal" adult is normal. A BMD with a T-score between -1 and -2.5 is a sign of low bone mass (osteopenia). A BMD with a T-score at or below -2.5 establishes that you have osteoporosis.

Calcium and weight-bearing exercise can prevent bone loss, but they don't rebuild lost bone. Current osteo medications can prevent fractures and even build back some bone. If you discover you have low bone density or osteoporosis, make sure your doctor discusses the pros and cons of prescription therapies with you, including hormone replacement therapy, alendronate (Fosamax), calcitonin (Miacalcin), and raloxifene (Evista).

★ Flexibility

There is no single best way to test your overall flexibility (although getting out of a subcompact car after a long road trip comes close). However, the sit-and-reach test will give you some sense of the flexibility of your lower back, hips, and hamstrings. Here's how to do it.

Find a partner to assist you. Lay a yardstick on the floor and place a foot-long piece of tape straight across it at the 15-inch mark. Sit down with the yardstick between your legs, with your heels touching the edge of the tape and spread about 10 inches apart.

Slowly reach forward and slide your fingertips down the yardstick as far as possible. Keep your hands even with each other, and

Flexibility Test (Sit-and-Reach)

	SCORE			
AGE	36–45	46–55	56–65	GREATER THAN 65
WELL ABOVE AVERAGE	22	21	20	20
ABOVE AVERAGE	19	18	17	17
AVERAGE	17	16	15	15
BELOW AVERAGE	15	14	13	13
WELL BELOW AVERAGE	12	10	9	9

Source: Guidelines for Exercise Testing and Prescription, of the American College of Sports Medicine

keep them in contact with the yardstick. Be sure not to hold your breath or press your knees down or allow them to bend upward during the test. Have your partner read your score, which is the most distant point your fingertips can reach on the yardstick.

WHAT TO AIM FOR: Use the guidelines in the chart opposite to determine how flexible you are. To develop and improve, follow the advice in chapter 11. Repeat the test every 3 months and record your score, to track your improvement.

Balance

How well you can keep your body in control while you're moving or standing still is yet another marker of fitness after 40.

You don't have to perch on a unicycle or dance across a balance beam to test your balance. Simply stand for as long as possible on one foot without support. You may want to stand near a solid object that you can grab in case you lose your balance. Write down your time, then try the test on the other foot.

WHAT TO AIM FOR: There's no specific time on which to gauge yourself. Simply take a base measurement. Practice the balance improvement exercises starting on page 239, then recheck yourself every month.

★ Stress Resistance

As discussed in chapter 4, if you can't tame a belly bulge, stress in your life may be to blame. Released under stress, the hormone cortisol can prompt you to eat more, and it promotes fat storage in your abdomen.

Measuring your level of stress can be a subjective thing, but the quiz on the following page can help you quantify that stress and determine how well you are currently coping with it. It can also help you set your Fit Not Fat Relax and Recharge goals as well. The quiz was devised by Leah J. Dickstein, M.D., professor of psychiatry and associate dean for faculty and student advocacy at the University of Louisville School of Medicine, who has studied and taught women's and men's stress issues for more than 20 years.

WHAT TO AIM FOR: Ideally you'll be able to answer true to at least 10 out of these 15 questions, Dr. Dickstein says. Each highlights an important factor—including sleep, respect, companionship, safety, and personal opportunities—that we need in our lives to make us resilient to stress.

But no matter how many of these factors you're missing, from one to 15, think about how you can make them a part of your life, she urges.

You now have a clear picture of where you stand in comparison to your goals. Your next step is to take the information you've gleaned and the goals you've set and plug them into your Fit Not Fat Master Plan. You're almost ready to begin!

Stress Resistance Test

1. I regularly have meaningful contact with friends and family.   True ☐   False ☐

2. I sleep at least 7 hours each night.   True ☐   False ☐

3. If I can't or don't want to do a task someone asks me to do, I can say "Sorry, but no."   True ☐   False ☐

4. Sexual harassment is not a problem for me in my workplace.   True ☐   False ☐

5. Physical or mental domestic violence is not a problem for me at home.   True ☐   False ☐

6. My time management skills allow me to get my duties done efficiently.   True ☐   False ☐

7. I know how to delegate tasks and chores to other people so I don't have to do them all.   True ☐   False ☐

8. I feel that people really listen to me and understand what I'm telling them.   True ☐   False ☐

9. There is no artificial barrier keeping me from advancing at my workplace.   True ☐   False ☐

10. I'm surrounded by "men and women of good conscience," people with power who enable me to access the fair opportunities I deserve.   True ☐   False ☐

11. I don't have another woman in my life who is a "queen bee"— pushy and demanding and needing to be the most important and only woman in control.   True ☐   False ☐

12. I have a positive attitude that I'm worth being treated respectfully.   True ☐   False ☐

13. I stay aware of my health, fitness, nutritional, spiritual, and creative needs, and I make sure any health problems are appropriately handled.   True ☐   False ☐

14. I have an outlet that allows me to practice my faith, whether it be informal quiet prayer or a worship service I attend.   True ☐   False ☐

15. I have an outlet for my creativity, whether it's an activity like playing the piano, decorating lampshades, or writing poetry.   True ☐   False ☐

CHAPTER 6

BUILDING YOUR MASTER PLAN

If you look closely, you'll find it behind the greatest dinner parties, vacations, and business ventures. The key to most successes, big or small, is a well-constructed plan.

Your weight-loss efforts are no exception. To achieve results, you'll need some direction, and the Fit Not Fat Master Plan is your customized road map to a slimmer, fitter, healthier you.

With the Fit Not Fat Plan, flexibility is paramount. For optimal results, follow the Master Plan strategy, including each of the program's three components, to effectively build on your achievements week by week. Or feel free to design your own plan, picking the elements that work best for you—just use the Master Plan chart (on page 76), or create your own version, to keep track of your progress so you'll know exactly when to celebrate your triumph.

Starting Your Journey: Setting the Goals

To know where you're headed, you have to know where you're starting from. The best place to begin is with the measurements you took in chapter 5. In your journal or on a sheet of paper, write each of your five key benchmarks—daily calorie intake (based on weight), aerobic fitness, muscular endurance, flexibility, and stress resistance. (While you may not use every one of these in setting your main goal, each can come into play when you begin to do your weekly Master Plan strategy sessions.)

Underneath these, write down any fitness or weight-loss goals you may have. Maybe you want to look skinny for your 25th-year high school reunion. Maybe the doctor told you losing 20 pounds would help your blood pressure. Maybe you just want to get back into your favorite jeans or keep your thighs from rubbing together or run up the stairs without feeling like you're going to collapse. Whatever your goals are, write them all down, keeping them as specific as possible.

Before you go any further, be kind to yourself and do a little reality check. Try to separate "achievable goals" from "frustrating fantasies." In other words, if one of your goals is to get a body like Britney Spears, try shifting it toward someone in the ballpark but still motivational—like, say, Susan Sarandon. Go down your list with a positive but realistic eye, and locate the achievable goals.

Now, looking at the list that's left, if you had to pick just *one* of these goals, which would it be? If you have trouble narrowing it down, close your eyes and envision each goal coming true—which one would make the biggest difference in your life? Which goal would make you happiest?

Got one? Okay. Circle it—this is now your Main Fit Not Fat Plan Goal.

Quantifying and Timing Your Goals

Any good goal, at its root, can be broken down into numbers. Losing a certain number of pounds is a no-brainer—the math is built right in. Even if you want to drop a pants size, you'll probably need to shed a certain number of inches in your waist, hips, and thighs. (Look for the measurement information on a catalogue order form—that should give you a gauge for comparison.)

When your goal is something nonspecific, like "I want to show my ex-husband how hot I look at my niece's wedding," you can still break that down numerically. What does "hot" look like? Is it a size 10 dress? A few inches off the waist? A 5-K walkathon completed the day before?

Once you have your number, you can set a timeline for your program. Let's say you want to lose 10 pounds in all. If you check back with your daily calorie intake reading, you'll notice that you have to cut 250 to 500 calories a day to lose 10 pounds. Experts say that losing weight at a rate of 1 to 2 pounds a week will result in the safest, most permanent loss. At a rate of 2 pounds per week, your total program will last 5 weeks.

Or let's say you want to improve your muscle endurance. You'd love to be able to do five pushups at a time, but right now you can barely make one. If you added one pushup a week—a completely doable number when you're also doing other arm- and chest-strengthening exercises—in 5 weeks you'll have achieved your goal.

Now do your calculations and set your timeline to achieve your Main Fit Not Fat Plan Goal. Write it down on the same page or sheet of paper for safekeeping until this Sunday, when you will have your first Fit Not Fat Master Plan strategy session.

Devising Your Weekly Master Plan

Researchers have consistently shown that keeping track of your efforts to be healthy is the best method of ensuring you continue good habits—it keeps you accountable, and seeing your progress in black and white is very motivating.

Most people tend to organize their lives around their work and weekend schedules. That trait in mind, the Master Plan was designed to operate on a weekly agenda as well.

Turn to the Master Plan chart, page 76. You can either photocopy this chart or duplicate it in that handy notebook or journal you carry with you. Or, if you already have a weekly planner that you like, think of a way of incorporating the Master Plan chart's major components into each day's recording space.

Pick 1 day a week when you're likely to have a few minutes of rest—for most women, it's usually Sunday. Find a quiet space for yourself where you'll have 20 minutes of uninterrupted time when you can set your goals for the coming week. Be sure to let your family know this is not a onetime thing—you'll be taking these moments to evaluate your progress and set your goals every week. (Setting this habit is also good practice for your 20 minutes of mandatory "me" time per day!)

Every week, you'll look back over the past week's chart before you start your new one. Congratulate yourself on areas where you did well, and evaluate why other areas were a challenge for you. Weigh and measure yourself, then note certain information in your new Master Plan chart.

▶ The dates of the upcoming week (for example, "February 5 to February 12")

▶ The week number in your plan (the first week is "Week 1")

▶ Your Main Fit Not Fat Plan Goal (to keep it in the forefront of your mind)

▶ Your waist measurement (to keep track as you shed inches)

(continued on page 78)

YOUR WEEKLY FIT NOT FAT MASTER PLAN

Week of: _____
Week #: _____

My Main FNF Plan Goal is: _____

Waist measurement: _____

Begin weight: _____

End weight: _____

Total lbs lost to date: _____

	SUNDAY	MONDAY	TUESDAY
	TODAY'S BIG EVENT:	TODAY'S BIG EVENT:	TODAY'S BIG EVENT:

FNF FOOD PLAN

This week's daily calorie goal _____

Last week I found step _____ **challenging**

This week I'll focus on step ____ **with this strategy** _____

Food I want to try: _____

	TODAY'S FOCUS	TODAY'S FOCUS	TODAY'S FOCUS
	STEP 1: Eat More Often	**STEP 2: Keep Good Records**	**STEP 3: Sneak In Extra Fiber**

FNF EXERCISE PLAN

This week, my goals are:

____ **Calorie-burning units**

____ **Muscle-toning sessions**

____ **Flexibility and balance routines**

Exercise I want to try: _____

FNF RELAX & RECHARGE PLAN

This week, my goal is:

____ **"Me" time minutes every day**

Stress reliever I want to try: _____

WEDNESDAY	**THURSDAY**	**FRIDAY**	**SATURDAY**
TODAY'S BIG EVENT:	TODAY'S BIG EVENT:	TODAY'S BIG EVENT:	TODAY'S BIG EVENT:
TODAY'S FOCUS	TODAY'S FOCUS	TODAY'S FOCUS	TODAY'S FOCUS
STEP 4: Master Plate Power	**STEP 5: Savor Good Fats**	**STEP 6: Flush Out Pounds with Water**	**STEP 7: Boost Your Metabolism 'Round the Clock**

▶ Your begin weight (the weight you are on the Sunday beginning that week)

▶ Your end weight (the weight you are at the end of that week—so you can note your progress each week)

▶ The total pounds lost to date (to keep you motivated for the long haul!)

At the top of each day, note any big events that might throw you off your plan—maybe you have a big deadline coming up, or a family birthday party that's certain to throw a wrench into your weight-loss plans. Drawing attention to these events on your Master Plan weekly strategy will help you see where the potential traps are lurking, so you can plan your exercise sessions around your evening plans or make extra leftovers before a hectic work-week. After you've accumulated a few charts, you'll also see that every week has at least one or two of these big events; instead of seeing them as "special exceptions," you'll learn to negotiate them as part of your normal life, a part that needn't hamstring your best intentions.

Now you're ready to set the eating, exercise, and relaxation goals for the coming week.

The Fit Not Fat Food Plan

The first of the three Fit Not Fat Plan components—the Food Plan—is organized into seven steps, one for each day. During your

first week on the Fit Not Fat Plan, you'll adopt one new step every day until, by the end of the week, you'll have incorporated all seven steps, without having to change all at once. During your second week and beyond, these steps will serve as motivating reminders each day. (Read more about the Food Plan on page 82.)

During your weekly goal-setting session, try to remember which step gave you the biggest challenge in the preceding week. When you write that step in the left-hand column under "Last week I found step _____ challenging," try to devise a way of giving just a little extra attention to that step in the up-coming week.

One quick, no mix-up way to start your food program is to follow the Fit Not Fat 14-Day Menu Planner, page 391. Each of the 14 days automatically includes all seven steps—with no extra planning. Don't forget to consult the results of your daily calorie goal chart from chapter 5, which tells you your targets for safe weight loss. Enter that number in the "This week's daily calorie goal" space in the left-hand column.

The Fit Not Fat Exercise Plan

The second component of the Fit Not Fat Plan, your exercise plan, offers you tremendous flexibility. Choose from each of the Fit Not Fat Basics groups to design your weekly plan, keeping in mind the following targets for the week.

▶ Beginners: 15 units* of calorie-burning exercises, two or three 20-minute muscle-toning sessions, and three or four flexibility and balance routines

▶ Intermediate: 23 units* of calorie-burning exercises, two or three 25-minute muscle-toning sessions, and four or five flexibility and balance routines

▶ Advanced: 30 units* of calorie-burning exercises, two or three 30-minute muscle-toning sessions, and five or six flexibility and balance routines

Note: One "unit" of calorie-burning exercise is equal to 15 minutes of brisk walking. (See chapter 9 for a detailed explanation.)

Once you've written these objectives down in your Master Plan, turn to part 4, a giant smorgasbord of exercise options. Use chapter 8 to help you pick the style of exercise that's best suited to your temperament and tastes. And remember, what might not appeal to you now could become very interesting as you get fitter, and keeping your workout varied is the key to faster, more efficient results. Use the space under the day headings to note the times you plan to go to the gym or walk outside or attend a yoga class.

You can tailor your workout to your own circumstances even further with the "Customizing Your Workout" chapters. Take a look at chapter 14 to keep active when you're strapped for time. Or, if you're contending with a troublesome injury or a long-term condition—such as asthma, diabetes, or fibromyalgia—just look for your specific ailment in chapters 12 and 13, read about special considerations and suggestions, and find out how to make working out safe, effective, and fun again.

The Fit Not Fat Relax and Recharge Plan

You may be tempted to skip the third component of the Fit Not Fat Plan—to relax and recharge—but that would be a big mistake! Research shows that stress management may help keep belly fat from settling in, and nutritionists and fitness trainers agree that motivation is the key to long-term success.

"Setting goals to relax and recharge?" you wonder. It may sound a little counterintuitive. But until you make relaxation as much of a priority as other important meetings on your schedule, you will constantly be tempted to put it off.

Start by looking back at the results of your stress resistance test in chapter 5. Which statements did you mark "false"? Those are good places to look for your Relax and Recharge Goals. Take the statements that you've marked "false" and write them as positive statements on your Master Plan strategy. For example, if you wrote "false" for number 2, "I sleep at least 7 hours each night," then on your Master Plan, in the space "Stress reliever I want to try," write, "Sleep 7 hours a night." During the rest of the week's spaces, you can write in strategies that will support that goal, such as turning off the evening news, getting your work clothes ready at night, or telling your husband it's *his* turn to let the dog out in the morning.

In addition, the Fit Not Fat Master Plan also requires scheduling a *minimum* of 20 minutes of "me" time every day. Spend this any way you like—reading a good book, soaking in the tub, painting your toenails red—or choose from any number of the dozens of tension tamers in chapter 16. If you're feeling your resolve slip a little bit, turn to the 1-minute motivators in chapter 17 to recharge your motivation batteries.

Remember—the Relax and Recharge Plan is not optional! Think of it as preventive care just as you would brushing your teeth—skip that for a few days, and you know what happens. Don't let your soul get gunked up with the emotional equivalent of bad breath and plaque—take time for yourself.

Your map is now in hand, and you're about to embark on a voyage that will bring you face-to-face with the one goal that you've promised yourself, the one goal you know will make you happiest. In setting this week's Master Plan strategy, you've prepared yourself for anything the world can throw at you—nothing can stand in your way. Remember, the journey of 1,000 steps begins with just one—and the time to take that first step is *now*. To your success!

PART 3

THE
40-PLUS
EATING
PLAN

CHAPTER 7

THE FIT NOT FAT FOOD PLAN

If you're like most women, you probably think of a "diet" as a list of foods you "can't" eat—no fried foods, no chips, no fat, no fun. With all the dieting performance pressure we put on ourselves, you'd think we were a competing with a rival rather than feeding our bodies good, wholesome fuel.

Relax. Your tastebuds are not the enemy. Instead of obsessing about what to avoid, the Fit Not Fat Food Plan helps you focus on what to embrace. You eat to lose weight, working with your body's natural instincts and metabolism to turn that deprivation mentality on its ear.

This is your new credo: "Everything I put in my mouth helps me get thin."

Your best weight-loss ally? Awareness. Learning when your body needs food most, what a portion really looks like, and how good it can feel to eat healthfully are powerful tools and potent motivation. This chapter looks at the Fit Not Fat Food Plan, the last weight-loss plan you'll ever need.

Eat to Beat Fat

Aside from helping you feel fit and strong, shedding pounds is your best defense against one of the biggest health threats that face American women today: diabetes. Women with a body mass index (BMI) above 25 are three times more likely to develop type 2 diabetes.

The basic aim of the eating plan for people with diabetes—blood sugar control—can boost the effectiveness of any woman's weight-loss plan. Because their bodies have trouble processing too much or too little food at once, frequent small meals and snacks help people with diabetes avoid rapid shifts in blood sugar. Blood sugar balance translates to less hunger, fewer cravings, and more variety and choice—all of which sound pretty appealing no matter what your health status.

Keeping balance, variety, and choice in mind, we've developed a food plan that can be used by people with diabetes, those with the symptoms of syndrome X (see page 40), or even people who want just to shed a few pounds. Working with the natural tendencies of your post-40 body, the plan ensures that you get the perfect balance of protein and unsaturated fat—both keys to food's "staying power"—as well sustained energy from complex carbohydrates. When a group of 522 overweight people followed a plan with similar aims as the Fit Not Fat Food and Exercise Plans—reduce weight, total intake of fat, and saturated fat, and increase fiber and physical activity—they reduced their risk of diabetes by 58 percent.

The Fit Not Fat Plan at a Glance

SERVINGS

1+ green tea

2 lean proteins (fish, beans, eggs, lean meats)

2 or **3** calcium-rich foods

4 fruits

5 vegetables

3 to **6** whole grains

7 (10-ounce) glasses of water

The Fit Not Fat Food Plan was developed with Amy Campbell, R.D., a certified diabetes educator and program coordinator of the Fit and Healthy weight-loss program of the Joslin Diabetes Center at Harvard University. The plan's seven steps will help you not only efficiently, safely, and permanently attain your weight-loss goals but also defend against heart disease, diabetes, osteoporosis, and several kinds of cancer.

Beginning Your Fit Not Fat Food Plan

The idea behind the Fit Not Fat Food Plan is to change the way you eat, step-by-step, until healthier, leaner choices become second nature to you. Each step represents a day of the week: On the first day of your plan, Sunday, you'll adopt step 1; on the second day, Monday, you'll add step 2; and so on, until by the end of the first week, you will have adopted all seven steps.

You may have noticed that the seven steps are included as a permanent part of your Master Plan (page 76). After your first week on the program, the seven steps serve as useful daily reminders to help keep you on your program. On Thursdays, for example, your Master Plan will remind you to focus on step 5, incorporating "good" fats into your diet; on Fridays, your goal will be to think more consciously about step 6, drinking eight glasses of water. These daily reminders will reinforce your new habits and help to train your brain to remember the seven steps throughout the rest of the week.

One easy way to get a quick jump in learning the Fit Not Fat Food Plan is to follow the 14-day menu planner in chapter 19. Each day of the menu planner offers delicious, balanced eating options that adhere perfectly to the Fit Not Fat Food Plan. By eating according to the menu plan, you'll automatically be following the Fit Not Fat Food Plan's seven steps.

While the Fit Not Fat Food Plan is designed to keep you chomping away happily and healthfully for the rest of your life, it's also flexible and satisfying enough to help speed you to your weight-loss goals. If you're trying to lose weight, use the "Your Daily Calorie Goal" chart in chapter 5 to determine your optimal daily calorie level. Write that number in "This week's daily calorie goal" space on your Master Plan at the beginning of the week. Then, as you plan your daily meals, flip to the 14-day menu planner to use as a menu-planning blueprint. Each daily menu plan listed is calculated to include a total of 1,500 calories (add extra snacks as necessary, if your calorie goal is higher). Mix and match any of the planner's breakfasts, lunches, dinners, or snacks to get the most appealing meal plan for you—no matter how you shuffle them, they all add up to a thinner, fitter you!

Now, are you ready to learn the seven steps that will prevent cravings, provide sustained energy, and help blast away those unwanted pounds? Any one of these steps is a surefire weight-loss strategy—but in this combination they're unbeatable.

SUNDAY, STEP 1 Eat More Often

Our best weight-loss intentions are often foiled by very real, very physical symptoms: hunger pangs. Traditional weight-loss plans had you wear hunger like a badge of honor—but also set you up to devour the next calorie-

laden snack put in front of you, the first slip on a rebound slope to weight gain.

The Fit Not Fat Food Plan recognizes that good intentions won't keep your belly full. Eating a small snack or meal, averaging 300 to

400 calories each, every 3 to 4 hours will keep you satisfied and wipe out diet deprivation. Eating often will also:

Automatically reduce calories and boost nutrition. People who spread their food intake over the course of the day tend to take in fewer calories overall and eat more nutritious foods. In one study, a group of obese men were fed a specially prepared meal, and another group were served the same food split into five minimeals throughout the day. When permitted to eat whatever they liked at a later meal, researchers found, the men who had eaten the minimeals throughout the day continued to eat smaller portions and consumed 27 percent fewer calories than the men who hadn't.

TRY THIS: Start step 1 by cutting your meals by one-third and shifting that food to two snacks, eating them whenever you'd like them. Wrap your sandwich in two pieces, and eat one half at lunchtime and the other during the midafternoon energy slump.

Tame appetite. Your stomach is naturally the size of a clenched fist, but when you regularly eat a larger volume, you leave extra space that growls to be filled up. Eating more often allows you to head off hunger before it starts and to quickly shrink your appetite— while it can take months for your stomach to stretch, it takes only a week or two to shrink back to its natural size.

TRY THIS: When you're planning your next meal or snack, look for low-calorie-density, high-water-content foods. Veggies, for

example, are primarily water and low in calories, while meat and cheese are very dense and higher in calories. A huge salad, a bowl of minestrone soup, and one slice of pizza squeezes down to the same amount of space as two slices of pizza.

Prevent perimenopausal metabolism slowdown. One study found that older women burned about 30 percent fewer calories after eating a 1,000-calorie meal than did younger women, yet their ability to burn calories was equally powerful when eating 250- or 500-calorie meals. Spreading your calories out, instead of lumping them in three squares, could spare you 6 extra pounds a year.

TRY THIS: Stock your desk and refrigerator at work with preportioned 250- to 300-calorie snacks, like instant cups of lentil or pea soup and containers of low-fat yogurt. Well-timed snacks will keep your metabolism revving all day.

Decrease cravings and binges. When large meals dump huge amounts of sugar into your system, your pancreas has to work overtime to produce enough insulin to counteract it. It usually produces too much, and you end up even hungrier before your next meal. Repeated intense fluctuations like this can lead to insulin resistance, the precursor to diabetes, and also intensify sugar cravings. We reach for sweets because our bodies instinctively know sugar is processed quickly. By keeping blood sugar levels on an even keel, eating often wipes out cravings.

TRY THIS: Most people find that abstaining from refined sugar for 1 month cuts their cravings for candy entirely. Satisfy your sweet tooth with a midafternoon snack—eat an apple or pile ½ cup of fresh strawberries and blueberries into a cup of fat-free cottage cheese.

Increase flavor and variety. Eating more snacks means more opportunities to get a variety of foods, which studies show is the most important consideration in getting the maximum disease-fighting power from food.

TRY THIS: Choose from the same kinds of food that make up your meals—veggies, whole grains, dairy products—but in smaller portions. Shoot for 15 grams to 20 grams of carbohydrates per snack, along with low-fat protein to make them more substantial: skim milk string cheese and five baby carrots, or reduced-fat peanut butter spread on a chunk of banana.

Naturally heighten energy. Your body needs glucose for fuel, and that includes your brain. When you don't eat for long periods, your mental energy and stamina dip, primarily because your brain isn't getting nourishment.

TRY THIS: Many people need snacks most midafternoons to boost lagging spirits and tide them over until dinner; others like to crunch down a bowl of air-popped popcorn in front of prime-time TV. There's no "right" time, as long as you eat something about every 3 to 4 hours.

MONDAY, STEP 2 Keep Good Records

Now that you're in the habit of eating regularly, you've probably trimmed your calories without even trying. Time to capitalize on that and reward yourself at the same time.

You're already armed with your written Master Plan. Tracking your specific food intake gives you additional visual, as well as psychological, feedback—which is important for motivation before the pounds start flying off. After a few days of charting your meals, you're also liable to learn when you're most likely to need snacks, so you can plan accordingly and not be held hostage by the vending machine.

Perhaps the biggest surprise of tracking food intake is what it can teach about portions. One of the most notorious diet saboteurs is unmonitored amounts—some 35 to 40 percent of us have made the mistake of cutting fat without paying attention to portion sizes, which may lead to our consuming even more calories than before. The physical act of writing makes us conscious of what we're eating.

Whether you use a food diary, like the one shown on page 88, or keep a small notebook with you or write it in your day planner or plug the information in to a handheld computer or personal digital assistant (PDA), such as a Palm, tracking your eating can help weight loss for several reasons.

Teaches portion control. In order to write them down, first you have to know what portions are. Measuring portion sizes, at least for 2 weeks, will give you an eye for sizes. This skill is especially critical in restaurants—one dish at an Italian restaurant might include eight 1-cup portions of pasta!

TRY THIS: In order to develop your eye, use a portable measuring tool you'll always have with you: your hand.

- ▶ Closed fist: 1 cup of pasta, rice, or potatoes

- ▶ Thumb: 1 ounce of cheese

- ▶ Palm: 3 ounces of meat, chicken, or fish

- ▶ Tip of your thumb: 1 teaspoon of butter

- ▶ Cupped hand: 1-ounce serving of nuts

- ▶ Two cupped hands: 1 ounce of chips or pretzels

Increases label reading. The food label is a girl's best friend—a quick glance at grams of fiber, calories, and grain sources can teach you a lot about your favorite foods. Beware: A candy bar that appears to contain 220 calories could actually be two or more servings—and twice the calories—so be sure to check how many servings the package contains. The bigger the package, the more you're likely to eat—up to 44 percent more, according to one study.

TRY THIS: Pour a real portion (using a measuring cup) of your favorite cereal into a small dessert bowl or coffee mug, and try to use the same cup or bowl every morning. Do the same for frozen yogurt, popcorn, pretzels, juice—especially the things you're tempted to eat in greater quantities.

Balances nutrients. Some key nutrients, like calcium, are best to get from milk and dairy products—but did you count that latte? Food diaries help you see whether you're meeting all your nutrition goals.

TRY THIS: Our food diary (see page 88) has a place for you to keep track of servings using check marks. So even on busy days when you can't write down the specifics, you can still tally up your major groups and tell at a glance whether you're hitting your targets.

Improves motivation. Keeping a record is like giving yourself a gold star every day. But even if you slip up, be honest—keeping accurate records puts *you*, not the cheeseburger, in control.

TRY THIS: Make writing in your food diary a ritual—keep your small notebook and pen or your handheld computer with you and enter your food as soon as you're done with the meal. After you lose weight, keep a diary at least 1 day a week. People who keep food records lose more weight and keep it off longer than people who don't.

FOOD DIARY

Date: _____

MORNING

AM

Total calories: _____
Fiber grams: _____
Fat grams: _____

AFTERNOON

PM

Total calories: _____
Fiber grams: _____
Fat grams: _____

EVENING

PM

Total calories: _____
Fiber grams: _____
Fat grams: _____

Green tea (**1** or more) ◯ ◯

Lean proteins (**2**) ◯ ◯

Calcium-rich foods (**2** or **3**) ◯ ◯ ◯

Fruits (**4**) ◯ ◯ ◯ ◯

Vegetables (**5**) ◯ ◯ ◯ ◯ ◯

Whole grains (3 to **6**) ◯ ◯ ◯ ◯ ◯ ◯

Water (**seven** 10-ounce glasses) ◯ ◯ ◯ ◯ ◯ ◯ ◯

DAILY TOTALS

Calories: _____

Fiber grams: _____

Fat grams: _____

Date:_____

MORNING

Total calories:_____
Fiber grams:_____
Fat grams:_____

AM

AFTERNOON

Total calories:_____
Fiber grams:_____
Fat grams:_____

PM

EVENING

Total calories:_____
Fiber grams:_____
Fat grams:_____

PM

Green tea (**1** or more) ◯ ◯

Lean proteins (**2**) ◯ ◯

Calcium-rich foods (2 or **3**) ◯ ◯ ◯

Fruits (**4**) ◯ ◯ ◯ ◯

Vegetables (**5**) ◯ ◯ ◯ ◯ ◯

Whole grains (3 to **6**) ◯ ◯ ◯ ◯ ◯ ◯

Water (**seven** 10-ounce glasses) ◯ ◯ ◯ ◯ ◯ ◯ ◯

DAILY TOTALS

Calories:_____

Fiber grams:_____

Fat grams:_____

TUESDAY, STEP 3 Sneak In Extra Fiber

Eating more often and tracking your intake give out-of-control cravings the one-two punch—you rule your appetite instead of it ruling you. Now, how about a weight-loss secret agent, a sneaky ingredient that automatically cuts your calorie intake by 10 percent without your even realizing it? Enter fiber.

In addition to helping prevent heart disease, diabetes, and certain types of cancer, eating 30 to 35 grams of fiber a day is a time-tested weight-loss friend—but many of us don't get even half that amount. Start by reaching for fruits and veggies like zucchini, beans, apples, and blackberries, and whole grains like whole wheat, brown rice, oatmeal, and popcorn. Get to crunching—fiber battles pounds on many fronts.

Fights hunger. Fiber takes up a lot of room in your stomach, so when you start to eat more fiber, you'll get full more quickly. After your stomach signals to your brain that you're full, your appetite drops off dramatically, regardless of how good the meal tastes.

TRY THIS: If you're starving before dinner, reach for a whole grain cracker, like Wasa, with a slice of fat-free cheese. This clicks on your satiation cycle, the period of time it takes for your stomach to signal your brain that it's full. Like a stopwatch, it clicks off 20 minutes later, and when you start with fiber, you prevent more calorie-dense food from sneaking in under the wire.

Decreases calorie consumption. Fiber itself doesn't have any calories, but it takes a lot of time and effort to eat. An international study of more than 12,000 men found that the two most important determining factors in weight management were the amount of activity participants did and the amount of fiber they ate, not how much fat they consumed. Researchers believe the high fiber of low-energy-density foods, like vegetables and whole grains, rather than their lower fat content, was a strong force in weight control.

TRY THIS: Defend the fiber content of your favorite foods—keep skins on potatoes, shred unpeeled carrots into salads, resist the urge to trim all the white strings off your orange or grapefruit. Every little bit helps—fiber's rewards keep increasing the more you add to your diet.

TRY THIS: Next time you go to the movies, smuggle in a small bag of air-popped popcorn spritzed lightly with imitation butter spray. For an equal number of calories, you'll get four times the fiber and one-fifth the fat of movie popcorn, with much less sodium.

Boosts food's "staying power." Fiber not only fills you up fast; it also sticks around a long time. A study conducted at the New York Obesity Research Center in New York City found when people ate high-fiber oatmeal for breakfast, instead of low-fiber cornflakes, they slashed their lunch calories by one-third.

TRY THIS: Stay away from flavored instant oatmeal packages—most provide only 2 grams of fiber per 140-calorie serving, with a tablespoon of added sugar per packet. Buy a big container of instant oats—it's cheaper pound for pound, with no added sugar.

Helps regulate blood sugar. While we also need insoluble fiber, the kind found in many whole grain breads, cereals, and vegetables, for bowel regularity, researchers suspect that soluble fiber—found in oats, beans, and fruits such as oranges, cantaloupes, and strawberries—plays an important role in controlling blood sugar. Soluble fiber slows the movement of your food through the small intestine, tempering spikes in blood sugar. Some studies have found people that with type 2 diabetes who ate a high-fiber diet improved their blood sugar control by an average of 95 percent.

TRY THIS: Take 1 teaspoon of a powdered fiber supplement, like Metamucil, in 1 cup of water before each meal. Doing so can drop blood sugar levels from 210 to 140 milligrams per deciliter—enough for certain people with type 2 diabetes to reduce their medication. While you'd have to do this every day to achieve these results, this tactic can help anyone headed to a decadent buffet who wants to take the edge off her hunger. Keep a packet or two in your purse for high-fat emergencies. Just remember: Always speak with your doctor or health team before adjusting any diabetes medication you may be taking.

FIT
FLASH

Calcium Aids Weight Loss

With all the hubbub about getting enough calcium, you'd think it does more than protect our bones. You'd be right.

Although 99 percent of your body's calcium is stored in your skeleton, every nerve and muscle cell in your body needs calcium to function properly. Research now tells us it can help prevent weight gain, too.

People who take in the most calcium from food (about 1,300 milligrams per day) reduce their chances of becoming overweight by 80 percent, compared with those who eat only 255 milligrams daily. In fact, several studies on perimenopausal and older women found that the higher a woman's intake of calcium, the lower her body mass index (BMI). Researchers believe low calcium intake may raise parathyroid hormone and vitamin D levels, causing fat cells to switch from fat burning to fat storage.

Shoot for at least 1,500 milligrams of calcium a day, preferably from foods. Besides dairy, other good food sources include green leafy vegetables like broccoli, kale, and bok choy; soybeans and tofu made with calcium; and canned salmon with bones.

Displaces other calories. Fiber is found only in plant foods, so if you eat a lot of fiber, you're making better food choices automatically. Experts estimate that for each gram of fiber you eat instead of simple carbohydrates, like candy or white bread, you drop 7 calories from your diet. That means if you tripled your fiber intake from 13 grams per day to 40 grams, you'd displace 200 calories—that's 20 pounds of weight loss waiting at the bottom of your cereal bowl in the course of a year.

TRY THIS: Build fiber into your restaurant appetizer—instead of nibbling on Italian bread or tortilla chips, both of which are loaded with simple carbohydrates, start with a cup of pasta fagioli or black bean soup. In one study, when 24 women ate three forms of snacks, each with the same ingredients and calories, soup curbed appetite the most, trimming 80 calories from their next meal—2 hours later!

Helps keep weight off. A study in the *Journal of the American Medical Association* followed young men and women over 10 years to study the effect of fiber on weight maintenance. All calories being equal, those who ate at least 21 grams of fiber a day gained 8 pounds less than those who took in less than 12 grams per day.

TRY THIS: Fiber should not be a fair-weather friend. Even after you've nailed your weight-loss goal (and you will!), remember to choose fiber at every possible opportunity: Have baked beans instead of macaroni salad, raisin bran instead of cornflakes, hummus instead of onion dip.

WEDNESDAY, STEP 4 Master Plate Power

As helpful as it is, fiber gets us only so far. For a balanced, healthy weight-loss diet, you need to get a handle on the calories, carbohydrates, protein, fat, calcium, sodium, and other essential vitamins and minerals you're getting.

So how do you get all the foods you need, and leave room for all the foods you want, without doing crazy calculations or memorizing values? A simple tool called Plate Power.

When planning your meals and snacks, use this easy visualization: On a round dinner plate, mentally draw a line down the center, and pile one side with at least two kinds of veggies and one kind of fruit—the more variety, the better. On the other side, make one-quarter of the plate a serving of protein—beans, fish, tofu, chicken, or very lean

Calcium-rich food

Fruits and vegetables

Lean protein

Whole grains

beef. In the remaining quarter, put a serving of whole grain, such as whole wheat couscous or pasta, or brown rice pilaf. Now, to the side of the plate, visualize a cup of calcium-rich food—low-fat milk, calcium-enriched soy milk, or a small container of yogurt. This mental picture represents a perfectly balanced meal.

Getting all these food groups in any one meal, let alone one snack, can be a challenge. But as long as your general daily consumption meets this image, you're on track. Master step 4, and you'll never need to look at another diet plan.

ONE-HALF • Veggies and Fruit

Youthful skin, stronger bones, fewer colds, more energy, a longer life—what *don't* fruits and veggies give us? Yet somehow, we still find it a challenge to get five veggies and four fruits a day. Why is it so darn hard?

Perhaps with all this talk about cancer and disease prevention, you may not realize that vegetables can help you lose weight *today*. Your stomach demands that you feed it volume, not calories. On a day-to-day basis, your stomach expects the same volume of food, so you lose weight by eating more low-energy-dense, high-water-content foods: fruits and veggies. Eating more vegetable-based meals and snacks can automatically reduce the number of calories you eat by up to 20 percent, without making you feel hungry.

Sadly, the cancer-fighting antioxidants contained in fruits and vegetables last only 4 to 6 hours in the body. In order to get the long-term effects you're hoping for—lower blood pressure, cholesterol, and blood sugar and less risk of cancer, heart disease, and diabetes—you need a quick plant food infusion almost every time you eat. Now, how can you do that?

Consider veggies to be free! Vegetables contain only 5 grams of carbohydrates per serving and very few calories, so they have practically no effect on blood sugar. The Mayo Clinic Healthy Weight Pyramid even advocates eating unlimited quantities, words not often heard in conjunction with weight loss. Crunch all day on veggies like string beans, broccoli, cauliflower, tomatoes, spinach, and cabbage—they keep your mouth busy, fill up your stomach, and never show up on the scale.

Don't be daunted. If the idea of unlimited portions of anything green leaves you cold, don't worry—getting five servings of veggies doesn't mean you'll be wolfing down spinach like Popeye. One lightbulb-size portion (or about 1 cup) of broccoli counts as two of your five veggies for the day.

Camouflage your cauliflower. Frozen veggies can find their way into any soup, chili, casserole, pasta sauce, or stir-fry. Shred carrots into coleslaw, meat loaf mix, or banana bread. You (and your family) won't even notice they're there.

Shop for convenience. The prep time is often the problem—given a perpetually stocked salad bar, we'd snack on veggies all day. Stock your own with prechopped broccoli spears, cucumbers, and cauliflower from the in-store salad bar. Choose grape tomatoes and prewashed celery stalks and baby carrots in 1-pound bags for easy transport in the car, at work, and at the mall.

Go part-time vegetarian. Pick two meals a week that you'll have a bean-based meal, like vegetarian chili, black beans and rice, or veggie enchiladas with refried beans. When you go out to eat, make it a habit to ask yourself, "Is there a veggie-based option?" Probably the only veggie-based dish more fattening than a meat-based one is deep-fried zucchini!

Chunk it. Cutting carrots, celery, zucchini, cucumbers, red and green peppers, and other veggies in generous chunks, instead of shredding or slicing thinly, will give you the sensation of eating more because it takes more effort to eat them. The longer it takes to eat, the closer you get to that 20-minute satiation signal.

Make them weeknight ready. After you get your groceries into the kitchen, put all the veggies on the kitchen counter to be washed and chopped before they go in the fridge. Slice red and green peppers, wash cherry tomatoes, and chop broccoli and cauliflower for ready-to-eat dishes in the fridge. You can also bag meal-size portions for the freezer, ready to be dumped into a stir-fry, soup, or a pasta dish.

Buy in bulk. When your favorite summer berries go on their yearly I-can't-believe-how-cheap-this-is sale, buy as many pints as can fit in your cart (well, almost), freeze them in a thin layer on cookie sheets, and store them in individual-size resealable bags for midwinter smoothies. Zap them in the microwave for 30 seconds and add them to plain fat-free yogurt—you'll get more nutrition than regular fruit yogurt, without the added sugar and high-fructose corn syrup of sweetened yogurts.

ONE-QUARTER • Whole Grains

The Nurses' Health Study, involving almost 90,000 women, found that those who ate more than 5 grams of fiber from whole grains—like barley, bulgur, cornmeal, and whole rye—cut their diabetes risk, compared with those who ate less. Yet most Americans average just one serving of whole grains per day. How can we get more?

Scout the label. Some "wheat" bread is actually heavily processed white bread with a caramel-color tan. To be a true whole grain bread, "whole wheat" or a combination of whole grain ingredients should be the first items on the list of ingredients. One sandwich with true whole wheat bread gets you one-third of the way to your six daily servings of whole grains.

Barter some faves. Substitute 1 cup of whole wheat pasta for regular semolina—it pushes you 4 grams closer to your daily fiber goal, and wheat pasta's fewer calories and extra protein help make it a satisfying trade-off.

Prepare ahead. Some whole grains, like whole wheat couscous and tabbouleh, taste even better when they're prepared ahead and have time to "set" in the fridge. Sprinkle parsley and lemon juice over the top for extra tang.

ONE-QUARTER • Protein

For part of the last decade, protein has been the much ballyhooed king of weight loss. But while protein is a necessary part of our diet, the one thing a lot of the high-protein/low-carbohydrate diets do is simply cut options.

When kept to its quarter-plate status, protein plays a critical role in weight loss. A small Yale University study found that women who ate a mix of carbohydrate and protein at lunch ate 20 percent less at dinner than those who had eaten pure-carbohydrate meals. Researchers pointed to protein's effect on satiety hormones to blunt appetite and decrease food intake.

In the final quarter of your powerful plate, shoot for two daily portions of 2 to 3 ounces of lean protein from beans, tofu, fish, eggs, or meat.

BEANS: THE PERFECT WEIGHT-LOSS FOOD

Beans have protein, carbohydrate, calcium, B vitamins, and a little bit of unsaturated fat—almost everything we need to live. They're also the highest fiber foods you can find, with the single exception of breakfast cereals made with wheat bran. They are digested slowly, help regulate blood sugar, reduce the risk of cardiovascular disease, and even protect our bones. One study of more than 1,000 women over age 65 found that the higher the ratio of animal to veggie protein, the greater the risk of bone loss and broken hips. Researchers believe meat may have an acidic effect on bone, whereas vegetable protein acts more as a base.

Handy canned beans have the same nutritional benefits as dried, but be sure to rinse them to remove their excess sodium. Plan meals that feature beans or legumes as the main ingredient, like vegetarian chili, Tuscan white bean salad, or spicy curried lentil soup. Slip cannellini beans or chickpeas into pasta dishes and marinara sauce. Double the portions from a can of vegetable soup with an extra can of kidney beans. Spread hummus onto a thick wedge of ripe tomato inside a whole wheat tortilla or pita.

SOY: LOWER CHOLESTEROL AND DEFEND AGAINST CANCER

Gone are the days when people would turn their noses up at soy products, probably because we now know what a superfood soy truly is. Low in saturated fat, soy contains no cholesterol, and its isoflavones may directly lower blood cholesterol and help prevent certain kinds of cancer. The protein

BESTBET

14 Ways to Save 100 Calories

Are there foods you eat every day or several times a week? Each of these simple substitutions could save you 100 calories right out of the starting gate. Try:

- 1¾ cup of onion dip made with fat-free yogurt instead of 1 cup of onion dip made with reduced-fat sour cream
- 2¼ cups of oatmeal instead of ¾ cup of granola
- One container of fat-free yogurt with 1 teaspoon maple syrup instead of one container of low-fat yogurt with fruit
- 16 ounces of brewed iced tea with two packets of sugar instead of one 12-ounce can of cola
- 1 cup of black bean soup with eight baby carrots instead of 1 cup of cream of mushroom soup with six saltine crackers
- 2-second spritz with Misto instead of 3 teaspoons of olive oil
- Medium portion of french fries instead of a large portion of french fries
- 10 celery sticks with 4 tablespoons of fat-free hummus instead of five celery sticks with 2 tablespoons of cream cheese
- ¾ cup of soft frozen yogurt instead of ¾ cup of soft ice cream
- 4 cups of air-popped popcorn instead of 10 pretzel twists
- Two grilled veggie burgers with two slices of fat-free cheese instead of one plain grilled beef burger
- A grilled portobello mushroom instead of a grilled turkey burger
- 2 ounces of smoked salmon instead of 3 ounces of tuna salad
- Unlimited glasses of sparkling water with lime instead of one 5-ounce glass of white wine

from soy is easier on the kidneys than animal protein—a very serious concern for people with diabetes.

But until you grow to love the taste of tofu (will that ever happen?), your best bet is to sneak soy into foods you already love. Start by mixing onion dip mix with silken tofu (instead of sour cream) or chopping up firm tofu and smuggling it into stews and chunky vegetable soups. For snacks, try replacing pretzels or rye crackers with soy nuts, or crunch on edamame, fresh soy bean pods with a satisfying snap. Look for veggie burgers with textured soy protein.

FISH: PROTECT YOUR HEART AND WAISTLINE

In a study of almost 70 overweight people, adding one serving of fish a day helped participants lose more weight and increase their good cholesterol (HDL) more than those who ate fish once a week or less. Although replacing meat with fish can decrease total fat and saturated fat, what may be at work here are powerful fats, in some fish, called omega-3 fatty acids.

Omega-3s are being credited with everything from preventing irregular heartbeats to improving mood and memory. Although more research needs to be done, animal studies suggest omega-3s may even help the body use more energy to burn the same number of calories. To get the most omega-3s out of your fish, stick with 3-ounce portions of oily deep-water ocean fish instead of nonoily "white" fish. Try salmon, white albacore tuna, mackerel, or herring.

EGGS: NATURE'S PERFECT FAST FOOD

Long maligned as a source of evil dietary cholesterol, eggs are getting their just due these days, and for good reason. They're inexpensive, individually portioned, portable, and completely satisfying. Egg protein is also one of the most complete and digestible of all proteins.

While most women can have up to seven eggs a week, people who have diabetes or who are overweight should stick to four, just to be on the safe side cholesterol-wise. With its 75 calories and 6 grams of protein, one egg's staying power can stem the mightiest midafternoon hunger attack. Boil a dozen at once and store them on the top shelf of the fridge for a quick breakfast on the run or

hunger-blasting counterpart to whole wheat crackers. They can last a week and are an easy protein addition to your diet.

CHICKEN AND TURKEY: TRIM THE FAT AND VARY THE FLAVOR

Poultry is a great protein compromise between burgers and beans—low in fat and calories, high in complete protein, and boasting some of the most versatile meat around. Broiled, grilled, sautéed, baked, ground and pounded into patties, or crumbled into chili, chicken and turkey make nice accompaniments to almost every grain and veggie on the planet.

Skinless cuts help you avoid most of chicken's fat, but breasts can be pricey—buy an economy pack and portion it out into individual bags when you get home. (One quarter of a breast is a 3-ounce portion.) Ground turkey makes an excellent stand-in for ground beef. If you like the stronger flavor of beef, brown the turkey with a tablespoon of beef stock, and then drain it before adding it to your spaghetti sauce or lasagna.

BEEF: THE SPECIAL OCCASION TREAT

While the aroma of a steak sizzling on the grill has to be one of life's top 10 smells, the sad fact is beef is a mixed blessing. True, it is high in complete protein, iron, zinc, and niacin—but it's also very high in saturated fat and cholesterol. In a 10-year study of nearly 80,000 people, women who ate more than

HOW THEY DID IT

She Traded Candy for Charity Work—And Lost 120 Pounds

Twenty-nine-year-old Norma Jewell Bellissemo of Cincinnati was overweight and miserable, and her job was on the line. She prayed for strength, traded in her candy for charity—and lost 120 pounds. In the 20 years since, she's truly been living the sweet life.

One day in 1980, my boss at the beauty salon read me the riot act. At 5 feet 2 inches, I tipped the scale at 240. I was sullen and full of self-loathing, and my attitude and appearance were affecting my work.

I panicked. If I lost this job, who would hire me, a high school dropout? So I made a deal with God: "Help me lose weight, and the money I save from giving up junk food, I'll donate to charity. And the time I'd spend watching TV, I'll spend doing volunteer work instead."

A few days later I joined a program for people with compulsive eating. My first step? I gave up sweets. A modest change to some, but for me it was a titanic shift.

For years, my life had revolved around candy and fatty foods. If I awoke in the middle of the night, I'd eat four or five candy bars. I'd have one for breakfast. I'd sneak them in the restroom at work. Lunch was fried chicken, biscuits and gravy, mashed potatoes, and apple pie—topped off by more candy. Dinner was a gallon of ice cream.

So I started paying more attention to my meals—no more fried foods, between-meal snacks, or convenience store dinners. I stocked up on fruits and vegetables and grilled or broiled fish or chicken. With the help of prayer, my support group, inspirational tapes, and walking, I slowly and steadily shed 30 pounds the first year.

As the pounds slipped away, I remembered my bargain. My extra money and time went to causes that I believed in: a shelter for battered women, tutoring kids, counseling women with low self-esteem, and my church. Community service helped me realize I have worthwhile gifts to share.

Each positive step that I took seemed to loosen food's hold over me. I earned my high school degree and enrolled in college. When I married in 1988, I was a beautiful 135-pound bride in a size 10 gown.

Even bumps in the road often open up opportunities. After I regained 25 pounds from the grief of losing my parents in 1990, I took up things I'd always wanted to do, like playing the flute and horseback riding. I started working in child care. These activities gave me great joy—and took my mind off food. I slimmed down to 120 pounds.

Fear of losing her job spurred Norma to action.

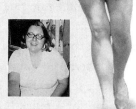

Now that I'm 51, I can see that the frustrations of my past are my greatest possession because they help me empathize with others. Twenty years—and 120 lost pounds—later, I feel my sweet life is just beginning.

seven servings of meat a week were 1½ times more likely to gain weight than woman who ate two or less.

The trouble we have with beef is that we get it mostly from hamburgers, but even ground beef labeled 80 percent lean still gets 70 percent of its calories from fat.

Save beef for special occasions and make it a great cut, like a 3-ounce sirloin steak or a few slices of fresh lean roast beef from the deli. Or substitute ground turkey or brown rice for half the ground beef in meat loaf, and add shredded carrots and chopped broccoli stems for extra fiber. Limiting yourself to one serving of meat every 2 or 3 days (or less!) and making up the difference in fruits or vegetables will help you shed pounds quickly.

ON THE SIDE • Calcium-Rich Foods

Standing proudly off to the side of your plate is a frosty glass of milk—or calcium-enriched soy milk or orange juice. You probably know that calcium is essential for women over 40 for the preservation of bone health—but did you also know that your daily three servings of calcium-rich foods also help to build muscle, and some may even deflect fat?

In a 2-year study, a group of women who ate at least 1,000 milligrams of calcium per day lost up to 6 pounds more than women who ate less.

The best sources of calcium are fat-free or low-fat dairy foods, but if you have trouble drinking it straight, sneak milk into foods where you won't notice it—whipped mashed potatoes, hot oatmeal, tomato soup, or instant hot chocolate.

As an alternative, look for orange or grapefruit juice and soy milk fortified with calcium, with at least 30 percent of the Daily Value for calcium per 1-cup serving. If those options don't appeal to you, move on to the third group of calcium foods—low-fat cheese, tofu, or fortified breakfast cereals. Bringing up the rear are dark green leafy veggies, like frozen spinach, which has 139 milligrams of calcium per ½ cup.

Between food and calcium supplements, just make sure each day you clear the 1,000-milligram mark if you're under 50; 1,500 if you're over.

THURSDAY, STEP 5 Savor Good Fats

Two weeks into the plan, and you're starting to think, "The name of this program is the Fit Not Fat Food Plan—when do I start cutting fat?"

In spite of the fat-free mantra spouted for years, fat may not be the pound-packing devil it was once suspected of being. A little unsaturated fat from olive or canola oil can help increase our level of satiety, food's "staying power," making us less likely to overeat later.

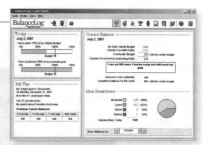

Personal Digital Assistant with BalanceLog

Need help keeping track of what you're eating on the Fit Not Fat Food Plan? Consider a handheld computer known as a personal digital assistant (PDA). BalanceLog is a Palm-compatible software program for PDAs that tracks food intake, nutrition content, menus, dietary goals, and your progress in meeting those goals.

WHAT THE EXPERT SAYS: Used correctly, this kind of tool can make a difference in your diet, says Franca Alphin, R.D., M.P.H., a licensed dietitian and clinical associate with the Department of Community and Family Medicine at Duke University in Durham, North Carolina.

"The sole purpose of keeping a food log is to increase awareness of habits and accountability for your actions," she says. "If you look at using the journal as a helpful tool to accomplish your goals, it can help you adopt a healthier diet."

However, she doesn't suggest using food logs to track calories and grams of fat. "Typically this makes everything more obsessive and takes some of the learning out of it. No one is going to remember calories and fat for everything, but they can learn about their habits," she says.

Just being aware of your eating habits, combined with proper motivation, can foster weight loss, she says.

"People often say that they know what they're eating and don't need to keep a log," she says. "But once they do it, they find they are surprised at what they eat."

PURCHASING INFO: The BalanceLog program costs about $50 and installs on a Palm handheld computer, which you can tuck into a pocket or purse.

That doesn't mean it's open season on french fries and nachos grande. On the contrary, saturated and hydrogenated fats, found in animal products as well as baked and fried processed foods, may be even more dangerous than previously believed. There is some evidence that changes in blood triglyceride levels from just one high-fat meal could increase your chance of having a heart attack for 8 to 12 hours afterward. And hydrogenated oils are being linked to everything from high cholesterol to immune system malfunction. However, by slightly increasing "good," unsaturated and polyunsaturated fats—like canola, olive, flaxseed, and fish oils—to 30 percent of our calories while drastically decreasing "bad," saturated and hydrogenated fats, we can reap many compelling benefits for weight loss.

Prevent "mystery" pounds. Many of today's saturated and trans fats are hidden, snuck into fast-food burritos or baked goods, unlike yesteryear's more visible fats, like butter and gristle on steak. These hidden fats are what makes eating out such a weight-loss trap—rather than give us healthier (and more expensive) ingredients, restaurants aim to make us feel "stuffed" with cheaper saturated and hydrogenated fats.

TRY THIS: When dining out, look for veggies and fruits in season—the fresher the ingredients, the less likely the chef will try to mask it with extra fat. If you're craving a high-saturated-fat appetizer like chicken wings, start with a meal-size salad (with nutrient-rich greens) and dressing on the side. Then order just two wings, enough to satisfy your craving without doing too much damage.

Increase food's staying power. Unsaturated fat can help food stick around longer, a primary Achilles' heel of fat-free foods. Fat replacer ingredients such as cellulose, polydextrose, maltodextrins, gums, and starches have carbohydrates and can affect blood glucose levels, and many fat-free foods have more sugar for taste. Some fat-free foods are actually higher in calories than their regular-fat versions.

TRY THIS: Instead of a snack of fat-free cookies that will just leave you hungrier, reach for nuts. A small handful of shelled walnuts or cashews will easily stem your hunger, and studies show that people who regularly eat nuts have less heart disease. Limit yourself to 2 tablespoons of nuts a day or five servings a week—they're high in calories and can quickly get out of hand.

Decrease calories automatically. In one study, when overweight people ate a high-fat meal before going to a buffet meal, they ate 56 percent more than lean people. But when they ate a low-fat meal ahead of time, neither group overate. Your body may take longer to detect fat than other nutrients, so if you begin your meal with fat, you could easily eat more calories than you intended—fat's 9 calories per gram add up quickly.

TRY THIS: Save the unsaturated fat for later in the meal, when you can enjoy it for the taste and its ability to help keep you satisfied longer. Drizzle a teaspoon of olive oil over roasted peppers or sprinkle 1 ounce of slivered almonds over sautéed spinach.

Thwart cravings. When you cut down on fat, you lose your taste for it. When you eat fat after having avoided it, certain enzymes and hormones that metabolize the fat aren't released as readily, so you end up feeling sick and nauseated after a heavy meal.

TRY THIS: Blotting fat from two slices of pizza will save you a teaspoon of oil—that's 40 calories and 4.5 grams of fat. Use an olive oil sprayer like Misto—a 2-second spray evenly distributes about ½ teaspoon of oil, compared with the 2 to 3 teaspoons you might get while pouring.

Prevent diabetes. A recent review of the Nurses' Health Study estimated that replacing just 2 percent of your trans fatty acids with polyunsaturated fats could reduce your chance of developing diabetes by 40 percent.

TRY THIS: Reduce your overall intake of ingredients high in trans fatty acids, especially hydrogenated oils like margarine and shortening. Don't stop there—aim to replace most of your saturated fat with unsaturated.

Maintain weight loss. In a study at Brigham and Women's Hospital in Boston, 101 overweight people were divided into two groups. One group limited fat to a very low 20 percent of calories. The other group ate mostly unsaturated fats from foods such as peanut butter, nuts, olive oil, and avocados, for 35 percent of their calories. Both groups got the same overall number of calories, and both lost weight, but twice as many people on the 35 percent diet stuck it out and maintained their weight for 18 months.

TRY THIS: Spread out your fat over the day—a little helps you absorb fat-soluble nutrients—such as vitamins A, D, E, and K, carotenoids, and essential fatty acids—from vegetables and fruit. Foods high in saturated fat are firm at room temp; use liquid oils instead of margarine, shortening, or butter whenever you can.

FITNESS MYSTERIES

Why can some women eat anything they want and not gain weight?

Because they are favored children of the gods? Actually, many of these women are more active, or have more muscle, which burns a higher number of calories per pound than fat. Yet some women exercise barely at all, eat whatever they want, and still are very lean. We attribute most of that to their genes. (That's the unfair part.)

But environmental factors also play a part. For example, how a person eats when she's a child may affect her metabolism for life. Consuming too many fatty foods or overeating can increase the number and size of the fat cells in a woman's body and predispose her to gain weight in the future. That freshman 15 you gained in college could be your current metabolic albatross.

Extreme dieting, or losing weight faster than 1 to 2 pounds per week, also decreases your metabolism, by shrinking your muscle mass. The hormones of fasting slow down metabolism even further, setting you up for rebound weight gain.

Often when we see women who eat candy and ice cream, they're actually treating themselves. When they get home, they'll compensate with a light dinner, healthier snacks, and more time on the treadmill. They may "eat to live" rather than "live to eat."

FRIDAY, STEP 6 **Flush Out Pounds with Water** ⎯⎯⎯⎯⎯⎯⎯⎯⎯●

The beauty of step 6 of the Fit Not Fat Food Plan is that it emphasizes something you've done every day, instinctively, since the first day of your life: drink. But this step isn't just scooping up a mouthful of water while you brush your teeth. Deliberately making sure you get eight 8-ounce glasses of water a day—almost the amount in a 2-liter bottle—can help you look and feel thinner immediately, as well as speed long-term weight loss, for many reasons.

Stokes your metabolism and prevents dehydration hunger. We lose up to 10 cups of water every day, so unless your urine is clear or very light straw-colored, you're not drinking enough water. When cells gets dehydrated, the body seeks water from other sources, including fat cells. After your fat cells give up their water, their ability to turn fat into energy is hampered, leaving you feeling hungry. Overall, dehydration can slow your metabolism by 3 percent. At a weight of 150 pounds, that would be 45 fewer calories a day—5 extra pounds a year.

TRY THIS: Pick club soda or seltzer as your first drink at a restaurant or bar so you can savor your next drink (alcoholic or not), instead of sucking it down to relieve dehydration.

Fills your stomach with no calories. Water can help fill up space during your stomach's transition back to its natural size. Water also helps your intestinal tract adapt to a high-fiber diet.

TRY THIS: If water tastes better, you'll be tempted to drink more. Invest in a water filter pitcher or consider renting a water cooler. Drink a full glass of water as soon as you wake up and before each meal, and sip water between bites.

Increases energy and fat breakdown. Without water, your kidneys can't remove toxic wastes and salt from the blood, and your liver is forced to pitch in with the kidneys' work, preventing them from metabolizing as much fat as they should. Your body also will have trouble transporting nutrients to your brain, leaving you dizzy, confused, and irritable—definitely not the state for energizing workouts.

TRY THIS: Make water a refreshing treat by squeezing cut limes into your glass of water or seltzer for extra flavor. Keep a bowl of the limes on the top shelf of your fridge to remind you to keep drinking.

Reduces "empty" calories. Added-sugar juice drinks and sodas, as well as alcoholic beverages, are a tremendous source of extra calories for Americans, primarily because liquid calories don't seem to "count" for our bodies. One study found that when 15 people drank an extra 450 calories a day, they gained weight; when they consumed the same number of additional calories from candy, they made up for the extra calories by eating less throughout the day, and their weight remained stable.

TRY THIS: Combine half of your normal amount of cranberry or orange juice with seltzer to cut up to 85 calories per glass,

The Glycemic Index—Mixed News from the Lab

These days you can't pass a bookshelf or magazine rack without seeing something about the glycemic index (GI), the "revolutionary" new way to control blood sugar and weight. So what is the GI, other than a phrase that sounds eerily reminiscent of 11th-grade chemistry?

The real definition isn't so far removed from the classroom. Designed as a diagnostic tool to be used in controlled laboratory experiments, the GI is a list that ranks foods according to how they may affect your blood sugar levels. Foods on the higher end (pretzels, 83; French bread, 95) cause your blood sugar to spike quickly and then plummet, leaving you hungrier than before; foods on the lower end (peanuts, 14; soy milk, 31) cause a more gradual affect, keeping blood sugar levels more stable.

That kind of list sounds pretty useful, huh? But how about this: Foods like potato chips and M&Ms have a lower GI than bananas and brown rice. "Taking it literally, people might assume the GI says to avoid brown rice and bananas but go crazy with chips and candy," says Amy Campbell, R.D., certified diabetes educator and program coordinator of the Fit and Healthy weight-loss program of the Joslin Diabetes Center at Harvard University. Many aspects of the glycemic index are confounding and defy what nutritionists believed about food properties until the 1996 study on which it was based was published. Campbell also avoids teaching the GI to her patients because of several unavoidable variables that affect it:

STATE IN WHICH FOOD IS EATEN. Whether a food is eaten whole, cut up, or mashed affects its GI. Fat slows down digestion, so any fat used in cooking or seasoning also affects a food's GI.

---

which adds up to 5 pounds or more per year. To get the flavor without sugar, try seltzer waters with essence of cherry or mandarin orange.

Prevents water retention. While you're getting used to the splendor of fresh veggies, you may add extra salt to jazz up the flavor. But added salt can make cells retain water, which can make motivation-busting pounds appear on the scale. Flushing your system with extra water will coax cells to give up their water, relieving some puffiness and bloating.

TRY THIS: Invest in one special beautiful glass for work and one for home, both soul-soothing inspiration and a visual reminder to drink water constantly. Get a sports bottle with a water filter for your walks, and keep a case of small water bottles in your trunk for emergencies, picnics, and soccer games.

ACCOMPANYING FOODS. In contrast to the way they're categorized in the GI, foods are rarely eaten in isolation. The various levels of the foods in a certain dish can make it impossible to gauge your meal's actual GI.

CURRENT BLOOD SUGAR LEVEL. If you have high blood sugar, food may take longer to empty from your stomach. Depending on your individual blood sugar level, a specific food may affect you completely differently than is suggested by the GI.

EMOTIONAL STRESS. When you're under stress, your body releases adrenaline and cortisol, hormones that can affect the rate at which food is absorbed by your body and your resulting blood sugar levels. Therefore, the *true* GI of your food may be totally dependent on your mood, which suggests the GI is not an absolute measure.

PHYSICAL ACTIVITY. Ups and downs in your metabolism over the course of exercise and afterward can change the effect a food has on your blood sugar.

As an alternative, Campbell recommends developing your own GI. Observe how your body reacts to certain foods—do you find that you get ravenously hungry or light-headed shortly after eating a specific food, like pretzels or French bread? "Over time, you may find that pasta is a tough food for you, but you do better with rice," says Campbell.

Foods are given a GI rating based on fixed amounts—say, one apple or ½ cup of whole wheat pasta. But if you eat more of a lower-GI food—three apples or 2 cups of whole wheat pasta—it will still have a significant impact on your blood sugar and total calories, regardless of how low it is on the GI scale. Portion control is always more important than the GI, says Campbell.

"Basically, the suggestion to 'eat according to the glycemic index' is just another way of advising we eat nutritious, high-fiber, whole grain foods," says Campbell.

Unless you're trying to turn yourself into a lab rat, the GI may end up being more hassle than it's worth.

SATURDAY, STEP 7 Boost Your Metabolism 'Round the Clock

It's the weekend, and you've earned the right to relax. Fittingly, the last step in the Fit Not Fat Food Plan is a snap, making the most of little-known metabolism boosters to give you that extra edge. If you've been diligent about the first six steps of the program, step 7's quick hints can help turn your earlier efforts into big results. Here are six more ways to turn on your body's natural calorie burners.

Keep nibbling. In evolutionary times, when hunts were long and berry pickings were slim, our bodies became pros at conserving energy. If you go 4 or 5 hours without eating, your body kicks into starvation mode, but every time you eat and digest food, you reboot your metabolism and thermogenesis, the rate at which your body burns calories. If you've been limiting yourself to two snacks a day, try adding a third—you may that find your appetite decreases while your metabolism increases.

Crunch through breakfast. Never skip the most important meal of the day—your body's been conserving energy for 8 hours, so the day's efficient metabolism depends on your morning repast. Stop at the store and buy the highest fiber breakfast cereal on the shelf, and have a bowl first thing in the morning. Fiber One, for example, boasts a whopping 14 grams of fiber and modest 1 gram of fat per 1/2-cup serving.

Or drink it instead. If you have trouble eating solid food early, try a Choco-Banana Smoothie (see page 397). You may feel like you're starting the day with a sinful treat when in fact you're getting your metabolism revved up with extra fiber and calcium.

Down a low-fat latte before walking the dog. You know that exercise boosts your metabolism, but drinking a cup of coffee before you take a stroll around the neighborhood can boost your metabolism even higher. Caffeine even helps to free stored fat so your body can burn it more easily.

Steer clear of coffee first thing in the morning, though—the hot water fills your stomach, and the caffeine could blunt your appetite before you get some critical nutrients. Also, because caffeine increases heart rate and blood pressure, people with high blood pressure, a history of heart disease or stroke, or abnormal heart rhythms (known as cardiac arrhythmia) should avoid it.

Pop a piece of sugarless gum in your mouth—and keep chewing. Researchers at the Mayo Clinic found that volunteers who chewed sugar-free gum at the rate of 100 chomps per minute burned significantly more calories than they did at rest.

Spice up your meals with hot red pepper. Early studies show that capsaicin, the active ingredient in hot peppers, may increase the body's fat-burning abilities, boost metabolic rate, and even cut appetite. In one study, Japanese women who ate red pepper with a high-carbohydrate breakfast decreased their desire to eat before lunch. What's more, they ate less fat at their midday meal.

Congratulations! It's the end of the week, and you've mastered all seven steps of the Fit Not Fat Food Plan. You're now armed with a weight-loss eating plan that can help you navigate the most hectic (or tempting) of weeks. To keep that momentum going, take a minute to read through your past week's food diary. Notice where your strongest and weakest points tend to be, and use that information to plan your eating strategy in the coming week's Master Plan. Above all, take time to savor and enjoy your food. Bread—whole grain or otherwise—is the staff of life!

PART 4

THE 40-PLUS EXERCISE PLAN

CHAPTER 8

WHAT'S THE BEST EXERCISE FOR YOU?

If only exercise were as fun for grown women as it is for little girls. Fitness centers would be filled with bubbly patrons eagerly climbing on a StairMaster machine and weight machines as if they were swing sets and jungle gyms.

While your gym probably won't be shipping in sliding boards or dodge balls anytime soon, you *can* have as much fun with exercise as you did as a kid. Just find something you love to do.

"Exercise doesn't have to be grueling to do you some good," says Michele Olson, Ph.D., professor of health and human performance at Auburn University in Montgomery, Alabama. "Research shows it's the *accumulation* of movement that counts—whether you walk the dog or do yoga, regular activity is more important than the specific activity."

One study conducted at the Cooper Institute for Aerobics Research in Dallas, for example, tested 235 formerly inactive men and women for 2 years; participants followed either a lifestyle activities program or a structured exercise program. Both programs produced the same improvements in fitness, heart health, and reduction of body fat percentage, indicating that an overall increase in lifestyle activity is just as effective as a structured exercise program.

Choose activities that mesh well with your personality and lifestyle, and you'll be more likely to stick to them. Plus, the mental relaxation and enjoyment you'll receive are as good for you as the physical activity itself.

Maybe you need a change from your current exercise routine, or you could be ready to tackle exercise for the first time. The following quiz will help you identify activities you will enjoy and stick with, based on your personality, schedule, and workout goals. Take each section of the quiz and combine the results of the three parts to get your total fitness personality. Then read chapter 9 for further descriptions of the best activities for you, including the number of calories they burn and how often you should do them.

If you've been an exercise dropout in the past, try an activity for 6 to 8 weeks. "At that point, either stick to it or switch to something else if you don't like it; but don't just say, 'Exercise isn't for me,' because there are so many activities from which to choose," says Dr. Olson. (Before you embark on any exercise program, be sure to talk to your doctor.)

PART I: **Personality and Hobbies**

1. As a kid, the activities I liked best were:

a) Gymnastics, cheerleading, jump rope, or dance classes

b) Playing outside—building forts, and lemonade stands, climbing trees, exploring the woods, etc.

c) Competitive sports

d) Playing with dolls, reading, coloring, or art projects

e) Parties, playing with my friends

2. My favorite hobbies today are:

a) Anything new and challenging

b) Outside activities: gardening, walking the dog, watching the stars, etc.

c) Tennis, card or board games, team and/or spectator sports

d) Reading, movies, needle craft, painting, or anything that provides an escape

e) Group activities with friends—anything from a walking or book group to just talking

3. I get motivated to exercise if:

a) I get a new exercise video or piece of equipment, or I try a totally new class

b) I get a new piece of exercise equipment I can use outside, I discover a new walking or jogging path, or the weather is nice

c) I'm challenged with some competition

d) I find an exercise that I get really into to the point that I forget my surroundings

e) I exercise in a group

4. I prefer to exercise:

a) Indoors, in a gym or at home

b) Outdoors

c) Wherever there's a chance to win

d) Wherever I'm not the center of attention

e) In a gym or fitness center

INTERPRETING YOUR SCORE FOR PART I

MOSTLY As OR A MIXTURE OF LETTERS: **The Learner:** "You're always trying something new—today you're painting, a few years ago you did photography," says Dr. Olson. You welcome physical and mental challenges.

You are most likely an "associative exerciser," meaning you focus on the way your body moves and feels when you exercise.

Choose activities that help you explore new moves. Try: aerobics classes, African dance (or any form of dance), Pilates, Tae-Bo, tai chi, seated aerobics, inline skating, skipping rope, fencing, or rebounding (aerobics on a minitrampoline).

MOSTLY Bs: **The Outdoorswoman:** Fresh air is your energizer. So why not include nature in your exercise routine? Try hiking, biking, nature walking, gardening, lap swimming, or cross-country skiing. If you have a piece of home exercise equipment you love, drag it out to the patio on a nice day. Or sit and do yoga on your back porch.

MOSTLY Cs: **The Competitor:** "You naturally like one-on-one, competitive types of activities," says Dr. Olson. Try fencing, cardio kickboxing, Tae-Bo, tai chi, and Spinning classes.

If you excelled in or enjoyed a sport when you were younger, take it up again. "If you can't play anymore due to injuries, consider coaching—you'll stay active by demonstrating the drills and exercises, and you'll help others learn to play," says Dr. Olson.

MOSTLY Ds: **The Thoughtful Gal:** You're a "disassociative exerciser," meaning you fantasize or think of events in your life when you exercise, rather than the exercise itself.

"Because you enjoy activities like reading, where you get lost in a story and forget your surroundings, you will like mind/body activities like yoga and Pilates," says Dr. Olson.

Also try nature walking or hiking. "You'll probably prefer walking in a beautiful place out in the country or on a neat nature trail to treadmill walking," Dr. Olson says.

Surprisingly enough, you will also probably love exercise classes. "Most introverts want to be part of a group, but they're content being in the back row of the class," says Dr. Olson. Try some classes, like aerobics, cardio kickboxing, seated aerobics, Spinning, step aerobics, Tae-Bo, tai chi, and water aerobics.

MOSTLY Es: **The Social Butterfly:** As a people person, you tend to prefer the gym to exercising in your living room.

Try aerobics classes, kickboxing, seated aerobics, yoga, Spinning classes, step classes, water aerobics, Tae-Bo, and tai chi classes. For weight lifting, find a buddy or two and do circuit training.

PART II: Workout Style and Exercise Goals

5. My primary exercise goal is:
  a) To lose weight/tone up
  b) To relax and/or relieve stress

The Best Exercises for Your Worst Problem Area

If you're like most women, you have at least one body area that you'd like to improve. Here are some exercises that will home in on those troublesome spots, with notes on where to find them in this book.

THIGHS

- ▶ Treadmill workouts (see page 164)
- ▶ Elliptical training (see page 130)
- ▶ Stairclimbing or step workouts (see page 153 or page 157)
- ▶ Inner- and outer-thigh lifts with 3-, 5-, or 7-pound ankle weights (see page 193)
- ▶ Squats with dumbbells (see page 221)

ARMS

- ▶ Aerobic machines that work your arms, like cross-country skiers or elliptical machines
- ▶ Biceps curls with dumbbells (see page 213)
- ▶ Triceps kickbacks with dumbbell (see page 214)
- ▶ Lat pulldowns (see page 203)
- ▶ Overhead presses with dumbbells (see page 211)
- ▶ Good old-fashioned pushups

ABS

- ▶ Using a rotary torso machine to work your oblique muscles (see page 179)
- ▶ Single-knee lifts (see page 180)
- ▶ Aerobic exercise (see chapter 9)

BUTT

- ▶ Squats with dumbbells (see page 221)
- ▶ Stairclimbing or step workouts (see page 153 or page 157)
- ▶ Adduction and abduction cable pull (see page 194)
- ▶ Elliptical training on a machine with pedals that adjust so you can operate it on an incline (see page 130)
- ▶ Spinning (see page 151)

c) To have fun

d) Depends on how I feel

6. I prefer:

a) A lot of structure in my workout

b) Some structure, but not too much

c) No structure

d) Depends on my mood

7. I prefer to exercise:

a) Alone

b) With one other person

c) In a group

d) Depends on my mood

INTERPRETING YOUR SCORE FOR PART II

MOSTLY As: **The Gung-Ho Exerciser:** You don't mess around when you work out. "You'll benefit most from doing what I call 'volume-based' exercise, where you spend an extended amount of time doing a specific activity, like cycling, aerobics, using elliptical machines, treadmills, stair climbers, etc., at a moderate intensity," says Dr. Olson. For optimal weight-loss benefits, you should burn 2,000 calories a week. One way to achieve this would be to perform 30 minutes of aerobic-based exercise daily and combine this with three sessions of weight training a week.

MOSTLY Bs: **The Leisurely Exerciser:** Your main exercise objectives are to relax and de-stress. To relax, try yoga because it teaches various relaxation methods, says Dr. Olson.

Studies have shown a direct relationship between physical activity and stress reduction. "If you're stressed and you have energy to burn, research has shown that interval workouts work well," says Dr. Olson. Hop on the treadmill or head outside and walk for 5 minutes, run slowly for 30 seconds, then run fast for 30 seconds, repeating this sequence for about 30 minutes.

Circuit weight training is another great interval workout. You do all your reps, then you rest, then you do a few more, and then you rest. "When you do intervals, your stress hormones go up and down. This helps lower overall stress hormone levels and, therefore, that stressed feeling," she says.

MOSTLY Cs: **The Fun-Loving Exerciser:** Fifty straight minutes on the treadmill is not your bag—there's no room in your fun-filled life. You'll be most likely to stick to activities that are already an integral part of your schedule. "Instead of leaving your dog crying in the house while you head to the gym, run around with him in the backyard," says Dr. Olson. Grab your inline skates and circle the neighborhood. Put on your favorite music CD and dance around the living room. And you can make your weight routine more amusing by doing circuit weight training.

MOSTLY Ds: **The Flexible Exerciser:** Exercise turns you on, but routine doesn't. You'd rather fly by the seat of your gym shorts—which is fine. "If you don't want to lift weights one day, go ahead and take a leisurely walk or yoga class instead," says Dr. Olson.

To add variety, use the elliptical machine one day, the treadmill the next, and the cross-country skiing machine the next. "Don't think just because you use the elliptical machine regularly that you have to use it every day—if you like a machine, chances are you'll like several different ones," she says.

PART III: **Lifestyle/Schedule**

One of the biggest exercise issues for many people is *when?!* The answer is whenever you can fit it in. "You get so much benefit from exercise, regardless of the time of day you do it; if you have a time that works for you, go with that," says Dr. Olson. Here's how to tell which time might be best for you.

8. I have the most energy:
  a) In the morning
  b) In the middle of the day
  c) In the evening or at night
  d) My energy level fluctuates

9. I have the most time:
  a) In the morning
  b) In the middle of the day
  c) In the evening
  d) Depends on the day

10. I:
  a) Go to bed early and get up early
  b) Go to bed and get up at the same time every day, but not particularly early or late
  c) Go to bed late and get up late
  d) Depends on the day

INTERPRETING YOUR SCORE FOR PART III

MOSTLY As: **The Morning Dove:** You like to get chores out of the way as soon as you get up because that's when you have the most energy. "Exercising in the morning will fit better with your whole psyche," she says. Whether you go to the gym before you start your day or you head outside for a dawn walk, you'll have an extra edge over those who hit the snooze button a few more times.

MOSTLY Bs: **The Midday Duck:** You'd rather plop down on an exercise bike than in front of a sandwich when noon rolls around. Fine. Whether you're at home or work, exercise is a great way to break up your day.

MOSTLY Cs: **The Night Owl:** You haven't seen a sunrise since that all-night party in 1974. If you have more energy at night, exercise then. Just don't do it too close to bedtime, or you'll have trouble sleeping.

MOSTLY Ds OR AN EVEN MIXTURE OF LETTERS: **The Flexible Bird:** The best time of day for you to exercise varies with your schedule. Just go with it. "In the summer, when I'm not teaching classes, I do all my exercise in the morning. But when my schedule changes in the fall, I do it in the afternoon—my body has to make a little transition, but it adjusts," says Dr. Olson.

Now that you know your unique fitness style, you can move on to chapters 9, 10, and 11, the Fit Not Fat Basics, to plan your three-part exercise program. Be sure you take a sampling from each chapter in order to get a balanced exercise diet of calorie burning, muscle toning, and flexibility and balance enhancement. The instructions in the beginning of each chapter will help you set up your Master Plan for the week.

CHAPTER 9

FIT NOT FAT BASICS:

BLAST CALORIES AND BURN FAT

The first basic component of the Fit Not Fat Exercise Plan is all about burning calories—the more you burn, the faster you lose weight. But before you swoon with visions of hours spent on the treadmill, read on—this chapter will make you rethink everything you thought you knew about aerobics. From now on, "working out" doesn't have to be work.

Taking the quiz in chapter 8 should give you a pretty good idea of which exercise (or exercises) best suits your schedule and preferences, and therefore give you the best shot at sticking with it. You now know whether you like exercising outdoors or indoors, solo or in a group, structured or unstructured. Use that knowledge as you peruse this chapter's wide selection of fun, effective, calorie-burning activities. Because when it comes to aerobic exercise, chances are, more than one type will suit your needs. And that's perfect.

"When it comes to sticking with an exercise program, and staying injury-free, the old saying 'variety is the spice of life' is a good rule to live by," says Philip Clifford, Ph.D., professor of anesthesiology and physiology and researcher in exercise physiology at the Medical College of Wisconsin in Milwaukee.

Walking, bicycling, yoga, kickboxing, swimming, and gardening can all have a place in your fitness regimen.

"Doing a variety of activities minimizes the strain on specific joints or any specific weaknesses that your body type may have," says Dr. Clifford. "It also helps maintain interest over the long run." The more activities you enjoy, the more you're apt to find something that suits your particular mood on any given day.

Get Your Exercise 15 Minutes at a Time

Just how much exercise is enough when it comes to boosting weight-loss efforts? Research conducted jointly at Brown University and the University of Pittsburgh indicates that you should aim to burn 2,000 calories a week via some combination of activities. That works out to the equivalent of an hour of brisk walking a day—or 45 minutes, if you work at a higher intensity.

But even a half hour is a great start, according to John Jakicic, Ph.D., assistant professor of behavioral medicine at Brown University in Providence, Rhode Island, one of the researchers who conducted the study.

BESTBET

Warm Up First, Stretch Afterward

Professional athletes who prepare for competition by "going through their sport motions" before a game or match are using those movements to get blood flowing to their muscles, which improves performance and prevents stiffness.

The same principle applies if you're working out to get in shape and/or lose weight. You should always start a workout with a few minutes of a slow, easy version of the exercise you're going to do. Most aerobics classes and exercise tapes begin with a warmup—or if they don't, they should. If you're exercising on your own, don't neglect this important step.

When you head out for a bike ride, for example, start cycling in an easy gear on flat terrain. If you're going on a hike, start walking on easy terrain at an easy pace.

When you're finished exercising, do some stretches to keep your muscles loose and flexible, maintain range of motion, and prevent future injury.

To make it easier to plan and track regular exercise, choose from the activities discussed in the following pages. Each entry describes how the activity can be adjusted to suit your individual fitness level, and each activity has been converted into a specific number of "exercise units" based on the

Sports Bras for Real Women

Wearing a fashion bra for exercise isn't a good idea—you won't get the support you need. Underwires and lacy fabrics may be attractive, but they aren't comfortable during exercise.

Browse athletic wear stores and catalogs or even intimate apparel racks at department stores, and you're more likely than ever before to find a sports bra that suits your individual physique and exercise needs. As with athletic footwear, many manufacturers rate bras for specific activities.

Yet even among the bras suited for certain types of activities, there are differences. Do you need a bra that compresses your breasts so they don't move at all, or will a bra that provides a more natural silhouette do the trick? It depends.

If you have fairly large breasts, you should always wear sports bras suited for high-impact activities because of the extra support they provide, notes Michele Olson, Ph.D., professor of health and human performance at Auburn University in Montgomery, Alabama. "Smaller-breasted women can wear bras with less support, but they still should wear sports bras," she says.

So how do you find the right size and level of support? You'll have to spend some time in the dressing room, trying on different bras and testing them out. Further, don't assume that your size will be the same for all bra styles. Actual sizes vary among manufacturers and styles.

Alice Lee, a buyer for Title 9 Sports, which specializes in women's sports bras and apparel, recommends giving a bra the "bounce test." Try it on, then hop up and down and simulate some of the moves you usually do when you work out.

"If you're not used to wearing a sports bra, it may feel tight," says Dr. Olson. "That's part of getting the support that you need. Obviously, a bra shouldn't be so tight that it leaves indentations in your shoulders, back, or rib cage, but it may feel tighter than your regular bra." She also notes that bras with wider straps provide better support.

number of calories you'll burn in 15 minutes. By mixing and matching various activities, you can design a complete program that will help you reach your overall fitness goals.

▶ If you're a beginner, shoot for 1,000 calories, or 15 units, a week (the equivalent of 30 minutes of brisk walking per day)

▶ If you're an intermediate-level exerciser, aim for 1,500 calories, or 23 units, a week (the equivalent of 45 minutes of brisk walking per day)

▶ For maximum benefit, burn 2,000 calories, or 30 units, a week (the equivalent of one hour of brisk walking per day)

Here's a rundown of the different types of bras and their characteristics.

COMPRESSION: This bra stops virtually all movement by compressing your breasts tightly against your chest. It can take some getting used to, but it does provide excellent support. Title 9 sells a Frog Bra for large-breasted women that earned its name because it "lets you leap without bouncing." This type of bra is good for all breast sizes, but it can be uncomfortable if you're not used to being constricted.

ENCAPSULATION: This bra cups each breast, providing a more natural silhouette. In the past few years, major improvements have been made in their performance and support. They're good for all breast sizes.

X/Y-BACK: Also called a racer-back bra, this type features either crisscrossing straps or a single wide band that runs down between the shoulders to the back band. This type provides the best all-around support but includes many pullover bras, which may not be the easiest for large-breasted women to put on and take off.

BRA TOPS, HALTERS, AND CAMISOLES: These often feature built-in shelf bras and are good for smaller-breasted women and for low-impact activities such as rowing, weight training, or yoga.

As with other athletic apparel, look for a bra made of "wicking" materials, often called technical fabrics, that pull moisture away from the body so it can evaporate, keeping you cool and dry. Most technical fabrics, such as DuPont's CoolMax and Nike's Dri-FIT, include a synthetic blend.

If you experience chafing under or between your breasts, your bra may be trapping moisture, so try switching to one made of wicking fabric. Also, your bra may cause discomfort if it is too large. "The less the bra moves on your body, the less friction and chafing there will be," says Lee. Double-check your bra and cup size each time you buy a new one, especially if you're losing weight. If you exercise regularly, you may need to replace your sports bras every 6 months or so as they tend to lose elasticity. As with regular bras, sports bras will last longer if you let them air-dry rather than put them in the dryer.

To prevent muscle injury, it's also important that you warm up for 5 minutes at the beginning of each workout and stretch afterward. (For details on stretching, see page 225.) To be sure you're working hard enough to burn calories but not too hard for your fitness level, monitor your pulse rate at rest and use the Karvonen Theory, also known as the heart rate reserve method, to determine your training zone.

To determine your heart rate reserve target zones, first find your resting heart rate by taking your pulse for a full minute first thing in the morning, before you get out of bed. Record that number and set it aside.

Next, subtract your age from 220, and subtract your resting heart rate from that number. Multiply that result by 0.5, and again by 0.85, then add your resting heart rate to each figure to get your lower and upper limits, or your training zone. For instance, a 45-year-old woman with a resting heart rate of 75 would have a lower limit of 125 and an upper limit of 160.

If you've been sedentary, keep your heart rate in the lower end of your range during your workouts. As you gain fitness, you can work harder.

To get the most aerobic benefit from your workouts, consider purchasing a heart rate monitor so you can be sure you're working in your aerobic zone. There are several types of monitors on the market; some strap around your chest, while others, like the Pulse PRO watch, simply slip around your wrist.

Finally, you shouldn't try to cram all your exercise units into 2 days of hard exercise—nor should you work hard day in and day out. Instead, pace yourself. "It's important to make sure your body gets enough rest and recovery time between workouts," says Michele Olson, Ph.D., professor of health and human performance at Auburn University in Montgomery, Alabama. If you work out hard one day, take the next day off or do a light workout so you don't run the risk of overtraining and being injured.

Aerobics Classes

If your answers in the exercise preference quiz in chapter 8 indicate that you would benefit from working out with other people, aerobics classes are for you.

"Aerobics classes can be loads and loads of fun, with lots of camaraderie," says Reebok master instructor Joy Prouty of Palm Beach, Florida, who is certified by the American College of Sports Medicine and the American Council on Exercise and a featured instructor on Healthy Learning exercise videos. "It's a great social environment as well as a great workout," she says.

It's not necessary or even advisable to jump, perform high kicks, or otherwise pound your joints to get a good workout during classes, says exercise physiologist Gwen Hyatt, a spokesperson for the American Council on Exercise and president of Desert Southwest Fitness in Tucson, a company that provides educational materials for fitness professionals. "Low impact is gentle on the legs and provides a good total-body workout," she says.

If you're a beginner, ease into aerobics. Make sure you warm up thoroughly, work out hard enough to break a sweat, and cool down adequately. "At the end of the workout, you should feel like you can do more," Hyatt says.

If you feel like marching in place while everyone else in class is doing jumping jacks, that's perfectly acceptable. And if you want to leave early, be sure to cool down and stretch out on your own.

YOUR AEROBICS WORKOUT PRESCRIPTION

Beginner: 10 to 20 minutes, 3 days a week, slowly working up to 30 minutes at 60 percent of maximum heart rate

Intermediate: 30 minutes, 3 to 5 days a week, at 65 to 75 percent of maximum heart rate

Advanced: A minimum of 30 minutes and optimum of 45 minutes, 3 to 5 days a week, with a target heart rate of 75 to 90 percent of maximum

Calorie burn per 15 minutes: 120
Exercise units per 15 minutes: 2

FIRST DO THIS

Preview classes before signing up so you know what you're getting into. Speak with the instructor before your first class so she knows you're a newcomer, and let her know about any concerns you may have. "Instructors should accommodate the class, not the other way around," says Prouty.

Also, the right instructor will make you feel comfortable in class and show you modifications for every move, based on your level of fitness.

MAXIMIZING CALORIE BURN

The secret to getting the most fat-burning potential out of each class, especially a low-impact class, is to perform every move with perfect form, extending your arms and legs as far as you comfortably can, says Prouty.

CUSTOMIZE YOUR WORKOUT AND MAKE IT FUN

Do you feel like a klutz trying to mambo, cha-cha, and grapevine? Or do you love the challenge of learning new fancy footwork? Either way, there's a class out there that will meet your needs.

If you consider yourself choreographically challenged, sign up for a class that offers more basic footwork. "If you spend your whole time trying to figure out the footwork while trying to see and hear the teacher, you won't enjoy it at all," says Prouty.

WORKOUT ESSENTIALS

▶ A good support bra, preferably made of material that "breathes" or wicks away moisture from your skin, is a must for aerobics classes.

▶ Wear loose, comfortable clothing that also allows sweat to evaporate so you don't overheat.

▶ Wear aerobics shoes or cross-trainers. When you're purchasing new shoes, try out some moves—jumping up and down, running in place, hopping from one foot to the other—to be sure the shoes fit correctly, are comfortable, and provide adequate support.

▶ Take a bottle of water and a towel to class so you can stay hydrated and wipe away sweat.

EXERCISE SENSE AND ETIQUETTE

Try to find a spot near the front of the class but on the side, so you can see and hear the instructor but won't create a distraction if you decide to leave early.

African Dance ●

If you prefer exercise with some structure but not strict footwork, and you feel motivated by exercising to music, try African dance. As you follow the beat of the drum, both your mind and body will get a superior workout. Your inhibitions will melt away as you tune in to the rhythm of the drum, your fellow dancers, and ultimately your own body.

Sound liberating? It is, says Michelle Bach-Coulibaly, instructor, senior lecturer, and director of the Mande Dance and Theater program at Brown University in Providence, Rhode Island. "You use muscles that you never knew you had. The drums let your mind soar to wherever your imagination will go."

African dance embraces what Bach-Coulibaly calls the Africanist sensibility, which celebrates the power of the mind, the heart, and the pelvis, or the source of life. This dance form is a great outlet for women because it isn't about attaining perfection or getting each step just right. "This is why older women can do this beautifully," she says. "The most beautiful dancers I've seen are women in their sixties and seventies—they have such grace, eloquence, and flow."

YOUR AFRICAN DANCE WORKOUT PRESCRIPTION

All levels: Two or three classes a week, generally 90 minutes. Pace yourself according to your level of fitness, incorporating more range of motion and footwork as you get in better shape.

Calorie burn per 15 minutes: 82
Exercise units per 15 minutes: 2

FIRST DO THIS

Start by learning the footwork, following the beat of the bass, or lowest-pitched, drum. As you become more comfortable, add some more moves, until you start coming up with your own version of the choreography. Bach-Coulibaly says that for those people who grew up too inhibited to let their bodies express themselves through free movement, letting them move freely through space can be difficult—but when it happens, it's an addictive feeling.

When you enter class, try to flex your joints and relax. Move your knees and pelvis so that you feel centered and balanced.

MAXIMIZING CALORIE BURN

Once you let go and feel the drum in an African dance class, you'll "break through the wall" and find your whole body moving in time with the beat, says Bach-Coulibaly, who advises newcomers to feel as if their bodies are "swimming in space."

"Anybody who steps into an African class is immediately drawn in by the music," she says. "If taught correctly, the tradition, at its core, is about the drum and the communicative nature of movement."

CUSTOMIZE YOUR WORKOUT AND MAKE IT FUN

Don't feel intimidated in an African dance class. The idea isn't to do every move perfectly. Instead, it's about hearing and feeling the rhythm of the drum. "You get fatigued, and then the drumming sort of takes over and propels you, allowing you to continue," notes Bach-Coulibaly.

For even more fun, recruit a friend to go with you.

WORKOUT ESSENTIALS

▶ African dance is usually performed in bare feet.

▶ Ask your instructor about appropriate clothing. In many classes women wear wraparound skirts, but in others, T-shirts and leggings are acceptable.

▶ Take plenty of water because you'll definitely work up a sweat.

EXERCISE SENSE AND ETIQUETTE

To get an idea if this is really for you before making a commitment, talk to the instructor and observe a class before you enroll.

Bicycling

If you liked to bicycle as a kid, road or trail cycling could be the perfect way for you to go from fat to fit as an adult. It's a great no-impact to low-impact activity to help burn calories, as long as you do it long enough and intensely enough to keep your heart rate in the fat-burning zone.

"Any fitness activity that gets you into the great outdoors is wonderful," says Prouty.

Whether you take to the road or the trail is up to you. Riding on the roads will give you a more predictable, steady workout with few bumps or unexpected turns, but you will probably have to deal with traffic. Trail riding can mean bumps and uneven terrain and might require your upper body to work harder, depending on how and where you ride, says fitness instructor Suzanne Nottingham, a spokesperson for the American Council on Exercise and president of Sports Energy, a fitness education company in Mammoth Lakes, California.

YOUR BICYCLING WORKOUT PRESCRIPTION

Beginner: 20 to 30 minutes, 3 days a week

Intermediate: 30 to 45 minutes, 3 to 5 days a week

Advanced: 45 minutes or more, 5 days a week, allowing adequate time for rest and recovery

Calorie burn per 15 minutes: road biking, 136; trail or mountain biking, 145

Exercise units per 15 minutes: 2

FIRST DO THIS

Be a little cautious your first time out: Don't venture miles away from your home or car unless you're absolutely sure you can make it back. Except for a sudden lightning storm, nothing ruins a ride more than getting out on the bike and then having your body rebel a few miles from home.

To avoid stiffness when cycling, regularly arch and round your back as you ride and be sure you don't lock your elbows when gripping the handlebar. Also, loosen your grip a bit so you don't end up with tingling hands.

MAXIMIZING CALORIE BURN

Casually riding a bicycle down the road for a mile or two may not be enough to qualify as a workout, Dr. Olson. Instead, she says you should bicycle four or five times as long as you would walk, run, or jog.

"If you jogged a mile, you would need to cycle about 5 miles to get an equivalent benefit," she explains. "If you use bicycling as your primary means of conditioning, you will get faster results if you follow that simple rule of thumb."

In order to burn the most calories during your ride, be sure you stay in a gear low enough to let you pedal at a steady but fairly fast cadence. If you coast for long periods, your heart rate will drop out of your target zone. Most experts recommend pedaling at about 90 revolutions per minute.

When you're pedaling, pretend that you're a dog digging in the dirt. Your feet shouldn't remain parallel to the ground; instead, point them slightly downward when you're at the bottom of your stroke, then pull back and up. This will help you gain more power from each pedal revolution.

CUSTOMIZE YOUR WORKOUT AND MAKE IT FUN

Bicycles are sleeker and more lightweight than ever. Road bikes are designed for maximum efficiency and speed, while mountain bikes are slightly heavier and stabler and built to take a pounding. Whichever you choose, have a technician make sure that the bike is set up to fit your body.

Bicycling can get you outdoors and allow you to explore your neighborhood and area parks. It's also a great way to get around when you're on vacation. Many cities feature bicycle trails that take you off the roads and away from traffic.

If riding the roads isn't your style, you may enjoy mountain or trail riding. It's a great back-to-nature activity, but stay on trails for safety. If you've never ridden on dirt before, Nottingham suggests getting started on dirt roads so you can become accustomed to the difference in traction. Once you get comfortable, move to a trail.

WORKOUT ESSENTIALS

▶ If you have a bicycle that's been sitting in the garage for a while, take it to a repair shop for a tune-up.

▶ Be sure to wear a well-fitting helmet.

▶ Carry a full bottle of water so you can drink often.

▶ Wear a loose, comfortable top that lets perspiration evaporate from your skin.

▶ You may want to wear special padded bicycling shorts to cushion your bottom on the saddle. A gel seat cover is another option. If you still end up with a sore bottom after your first few rides, hang in there: It won't take long for your body to adjust, says Nottingham.

EXERCISE SENSE AND ETIQUETTE

It's a good idea to have spare tubes and a tire pump with you in case you get a flat tire when you are miles from your car or home. And always carry some money and identification (such as your driver's license and insurance card) with you.

Cardio Kickboxing ————●

Looking for a fun way to relieve fat-generating stress *and* get a great workout that not only burns calories at an astonishing pace but also tones all of your major muscles? Give cardio kickboxing a try.

"Cardio kickboxing can help you release tension and aggression in a positive format. It can easily be modified because it's not about kicking higher or punching harder than everyone else," says Kevin Burns, a fitness instructor in Mankato, Minnesota, who is certified by the American Council on Exercise. "Cardio kickboxing doesn't have to involve high-impact movement at all. The old adage of 'no pain, no gain'

simply does not apply. You should finish the class feeling better both mentally and physically."

YOUR CARDIO KICKBOXING WORKOUT PRESCRIPTION

Beginner: 10 to 20 minutes, 3 days a week
Intermediate: 20 to 40 minutes, 3 to 5 days a week
Advanced: 30 to 45 minutes, 5 days a week

Calorie burn per 15 minutes: 170
Exercise units per 15 minutes: 3

FIRST DO THIS

Even if you're a seasoned exerciser, don't push yourself too hard during your first couple of classes. Give your body a chance to get used to the movements. "Keep your kicks low, and don't punch with a lot of intensity," says Burns. "Listen to your body. If you are tired, take a break. If you get thirsty, drink some water. If you feel discomfort, stop. You should pace yourself but also challenge yourself during the workout." And if you leave class early, remember to cool down and stretch on your own.

MAXIMIZING CALORIE BURN

Performing each move with perfect form and pacing yourself are the keys to getting the most out of a workout.

Focus on posture and holding in your midsection during workouts to help tone your muscles, protect your back, and maintain good form.

"It definitely gets you very fit, and it strengthens your abs, legs, and hips, but it is very explosive, which can cause problems with your joints," says Keli Roberts, a Los Angeles–based personal trainer and fitness instructor certified by the American Council on Exercise and the Aerobics and Fitness Association of America, who is featured in several fitness videos. She suggests that you proceed with caution in class and always keep your elbows and knees slightly bent because most cardio kickboxing injuries occur when people hyperextend their joints.

CUSTOMIZE YOUR WORKOUT AND MAKE IT FUN

Most kickboxing classes include a warmup with a stretch and then 20 to 40 minutes of cardio work that includes kicking and punching drills. Some instructors also incorporate running and skipping into their classes, which can be modified by marching in place.

Because music is a driving force in many cardio kickboxing workouts, Burns says not to be afraid to suggest songs or certain styles of music to the instructor. "When a favorite song comes on, let the music take you somewhere else," he says.

Customizing kickboxing is easy: If you want to work your lower body, focus on the kicking drills. If you want an intense upper-body workout, emphasize the punching drills. Caution is the watchword, however. Stay within a comfortable range of motion.

WORKOUT ESSENTIALS

▶ Clothing varies from class to class and ranges from traditional T-shirts and shorts to funkier outfits, including colorful bra tops and leggings. Whether you go for a modest look or more daring attire, be sure your clothes are made of fabric that allows your body to breathe by wicking moisture away from your skin.

▶ Dress in layers, but not in bulky clothes that can restrict movement or make you overheat, says Burns.

▶ Wear a good support bra.

▶ Well-fitting shoes that provide plenty of lateral support and cushioning are also important. Burns suggests using cross-training shoes that you wear only in the fitness studio. "If you wear the shoes outside, not only might they ruin the studio floor, but they may also lose traction," he says.

EXERCISE SENSE AND ETIQUETTE

"Hiding out" in the back of the class is okay in cardio kickboxing class. It may even be helpful because you can follow along with your classmates if you get lost during the routine.

Circuit Training

If you have trouble finding enough time to exercise, you want to see results fast, or you've hit a weight-loss plateau, circuit training may be your answer. There are many ways to implement a circuit-training regimen, says Jennifer Carman, a personal trainer in Columbia, South Carolina, who is certified by the American Council on Exercise and featured in several exercise videos produced by the Firm.

"I use circuit training for nearly all of my clients because it's so fast and effective," says Carman. "It's amazing what doing a circuit of weight training followed by cardio intervals will do for you."

Here's how it works: You perform a series of strength-training exercises without stopping, immediately do 3 to 5 minutes of cardio work, and then start the cycle over again. Here's an example of a circuit that targets the whole body: doing pushups, lunges, squats, overhead presses, biceps curls, and triceps extensions without stopping between exercises; hopping on a stationary bicycle for 3 to 5 minutes of challenging pedaling; then starting the circuit again.

You can also perform circuit training to target specific body parts, such as your legs or upper body. And there's a bonus: Because the workouts move quickly, there's little time for boredom.

YOUR CIRCUIT TRAINING WORKOUT PRESCRIPTION

Beginner: 2 days a week, one exercise per body part, one set of 12 to 15 reps. Work your chest, back, shoulders, hamstrings, quadriceps, and calves, with 30- to 60-second rest intervals between strength exercises.

Intermediate: 2 days a week, one exercise per body part, two to three sets of 12 to 15 reps. May increase cardio to 70 percent to 90 percent of heart rate reserve, or time can be increased 2 to 3 minutes per week or intensity by no more than 10 percent a week.

Advanced: 2 or 3 days a week. Include exercises for your biceps and triceps, and begin to include more exercises for specific body parts that you want to target. Increase cardio intensity, and aim for 80 percent to 90 percent of heart rate reserve for 20 minutes at least once a week.

Calorie burn per 15 minutes: 136
Exercise units per 15 minutes: 2

FIRST DO THIS

"If you're new to circuit training or working out, you may want to cut the cardio portion to just 1 minute or simply march in place," suggests Carman.

"During the weights portion of a circuit, you should start with a light weight and perform the move at a pace that's comfortable for you. Lifting the weight deliberately protects your joints and prevents you from using momentum to help you lift," advises Hyatt.

MAXIMIZING CALORIE BURN

Lifting weights with proper form and moving quickly from activity to activity are the keys to getting the most out of circuit training. But be sure that you don't lift the weight so fast that momentum assists you and also that the weight isn't so heavy that you recruit other muscles to help complete the movement. If burning the most calories during the workout is your goal, perform longer or more intense aerobic activities between the weight circuits.

"It's not a race," cautions Hyatt. "You should feel like you can do a couple more repetitions at the end."

"It should be a challenge for those two or three reps," says Shari Tomasetti, an exercise physiologist at the Pentagon and personal trainer in Washington, D.C., who is certified as a health and fitness instructor by the American Council on Exercise. But, she says, once your body is used to weight training, during your last set of a particular exercise, you should lift until "failure," the point at which your muscles can't perform the move again. You should always use good form.

You should wait at least 48 hours between circuit-training workouts so your muscles can recover. Muscle building occurs not during the actual workout but during the recovery process. That doesn't mean, however, that you can't cross-train with other aerobic activities on your off days.

CUSTOMIZE YOUR WORKOUT AND MAKE IT FUN

You can do circuit training on machines or with free weights—it's up to you. You can include any cardio activity that gets your heart rate up, such as marching in place, skipping rope, riding a bike, or even dancing.

No matter what form of circuit training you do, says Tomasetti, you should work your largest muscles first, starting with your legs, chest, and back.

WORKOUT ESSENTIALS

▸ Get good cross-training shoes that provide plenty of lateral support for the weight-training portion of the circuit as well as cushioning for the cardio portions.

▸ Wear comfortable clothing that's neither baggy nor constricting.

EXERCISE SENSE AND ETIQUETTE

If you are circuit training at a gym, move away from the equipment quickly after you've finished your reps so others can use the machines; don't linger to chat with other exercisers.

Cross-Country Skiing and Ski Machines

It's easy to see why cross-country skiers are among the fittest athletes in the world. The fluid skiing motion requires all of the muscles of the body to work together, which not only conditions them but also gives the cardiovascular system an unbeatable workout.

"Cross-country skiing, or using a machine that simulates cross-country skiing, is one of the most aerobically challenging activities you can do," says Prouty. Also called Nordic skiing, cross-country skiing requires balance and coordination since your arms and legs need to work in concert.

"There is definitely a learning curve, and it takes some practice to do it correctly," notes Dr. Olson.

Don't let the challenging nature of cross-country ski machines put you off, however. Both machine workouts and actual Nordic skiing provide a great low-impact and joint-friendly workout that can help encourage weight loss as well as boost endurance and stamina.

YOUR CROSS-COUNTRY SKIING WORKOUT PRESCRIPTION

Beginner: 20 to 30 minutes, 3 days a week

Intermediate: 30 to 45 minutes, 3 to 5 days a week

Advanced: 45 minutes or more, 5 days a week, allowing adequate time for rest and recovery

Calorie burn per 15 minutes: 120
Exercise units per 15 minutes: 2

FIRST DO THIS

The movements required by a cross-country ski machine might feel awkward at first. To get comfortable, set up the machine so that you move only your legs, and then, after you've mastered that, add the arm movements. Once you get accustomed to the motion, the fun (and fat burning) really begins.

The key to mastering the machine is practice. Don't pressure yourself to get the motion exactly right during your first several workouts. Take it slowly and gently.

"Also, don't feel that you're a failure if you don't go for a whole hour," says Prouty. "When you're starting a program, think of yourself as taking baby steps."

MAXIMIZING CALORIE BURN

After you work up to being able to use the machine for 30 consecutive minutes, try incorporating interval workouts, which are occasional bursts of speed followed by short periods of slower skiing. Don't do interval workouts more than twice a week, or 2 days in a row, however, because they can be very intense, and your body needs time to recover.

If you're cross-country skiing outdoors and you want a challenge, try skate skis, which have edges that prevent them from sliding sideways as you begin to incorporate "skating" motions into your stride, pushing the skis out to the side as if you were speed skating. You can rent skate skis at some skiing places or at a local sporting goods shop; call ahead to be sure.

CUSTOMIZE YOUR WORKOUT AND MAKE IT FUN

Don't feel that you need to ski for 45 minutes nonstop. If you can do it for only 10 or 15 minutes and want to extend your workout beyond the time you can comfortably spend on the machine, combine cross-country ski exercise with another activity, such as jumping rope, walking on a treadmill, or riding a stationary bicycle.

Providing plenty of distractions may be the key to making a ski machine workout fun. "Put on some of your favorite music, or put the machine in front of the TV," suggests Prouty.

WORKOUT ESSENTIALS

▶ The type of shoe you wear when using a cross-country ski machine isn't critical since the exercise is very low impact. For outdoor skiing, wear boots designed for use with cross-country skis.

▶ For indoor cross-country ski workouts, wear comfortable, nonconstricting clothing that breathes and won't get in the way of the works of the machine. Outdoors, dress in layers of clothing made of moisture-wicking material so sweat can move away from your body.

EXERCISE SENSE AND ETIQUETTE

If you're thinking of buying a cross-country ski machine, try one first to see if you like it. There are several types on the market. With some, the arm levers automatically move with the foot pedals, while with others the movements are independent and more closely simulate Nordic skiing, providing more of an upper-body workout. Try both to see which suits you.

If you're buying skis, work with a qualified salesperson to get well-fitting equipment and boots. It's also a good idea to rent equipment before buying to make sure that skiing is an activity you will enjoy doing often. Also, it helps to take a lesson and learn the "rules of the road" for trail use.

Dancing

If you love to dance the night away, you'll probably be pleasantly surprised to learn that you burn 75 or more calories for every 15 minutes you do the cha-cha or the bump.

"Dance is a universal art form," says Ann Cowlin, assistant clinical professor at Yale University School of Nursing, dance/movement specialist in the Yale athletic department, and founder of Dancing through Pregnancy. "There's something for everyone."

Cowlin suggests picking a style—ballet, ballroom, modern, tap, or whatever appeals to you—then giving yourself at least a month to decide whether it's really for you. "If you don't like it after that amount of time, try a different teacher or a different style," she says.

If you're considering dance classes strictly for exercise, be aware that some forms burn more calories than others. For instance, slower ballroom dances such as the samba or waltz burn upward of 50 calories per 15 minutes, while jazz dancing can burn more than 80 calories during the same time span—a difference of more than 100 calories over the course of an hour.

Whatever style you choose, dancing can be a great stress reliever because you focus on your body and the music. It's difficult to worry about what's for dinner or next week's presentation when you're trying to master a new dance step.

YOUR DANCING WORKOUT PRESCRIPTION

If you are new to dance and have been sedentary for some time, start with whatever amount of activity makes you comfortable. Find a spot in the back of the class, follow along, and do the moves that feel best for you. Gradually increase the amount of time you dance and the size of your movements.

Calorie burn per 15 minutes: jitterbug and tap, 80; country and western, disco, Irish step, line, flamenco, and swing, 75; cha-cha, 50

Exercise units per 15 minutes: 1 or 2, depending on intensity

FIRST DO THIS

To get the most enjoyment out of your dance class, try to find an instructor with whom you click, someone who is familiar with teaching adults and encourages a nurturing atmosphere. Observe a class or two before you sign up for a series of lessons.

If you're worried about not being able to follow along with the rest of the class, it's fine to just stand in back and watch.

"Standing behind someone who seems to know what they're doing is a great trick. In a dance class, you're very dependent on the people who are a little more advanced than you," notes Cowlin.

"It takes time to become proficient at most dance styles, so work on one or two steps at a time, slowly putting things together, and once you have a small vocabulary of movements, you can begin to practice on your own," she says.

Before you begin to dance, try to feel "centered" within yourself. Stand up straight; rock your weight from side to side to ensure that your weight is evenly distributed on both feet and that your body is moving in balance. Breathe deeply and shrug off the worries of the day. "Take a deep breath and bring your mind inside your body," says Cowlin.

MAXIMIZING CALORIE BURN

Dancing burns calories whether you're a novice or an experienced dancer. The act of learning a new dance step can burn quite a few calories because your body isn't working efficiently. As you become more proficient, you'll be able to move more quickly and with more range of motion, automatically boosting the calorie burn.

In a dance class, you can sometimes become so focused on what you're doing that you don't even notice that you're getting a great workout.

CUSTOMIZE YOUR WORKOUT AND MAKE IT FUN

Once you master the moves, the real fun begins. "That can lead to improvisation, creating movements, or what I would consider your own particular version of choreography. It can be very expressive," says Cowlin.

The sky's the limit when it comes to picking a dance style that feels right for you. Dance is universal, with numerous ethnic styles in addition to the more traditional forms.

WORKOUT ESSENTIALS

The type of clothing you need depends on the style of dance you're planning to study. The best bet is to ask your instructor what kinds of shoes and clothing are most appropriate.

▶ *Ballet:* Some teachers require leotards, pink tights, and ballet slippers. If you've never taken a ballet class, find an adult beginner class that permits you to wear a shirt, leggings, and socks.

▶ *Ballroom:* Hard-soled shoes are a must in this class—no sneakers allowed. You can check with your instructor, but generally women wear skirts and low-heeled shoes.

▶ *Jazz:* Depending on the custom of the teacher, you'll either go barefoot or wear jazz shoes or sneakers. Leggings and a shirt are customary attire.

▶ *Middle Eastern:* A loose, flowing skirt and a comfortable top are normal costumes, and the dances are performed barefoot.

▶ *Modern:* Leggings or tights and a comfortable top are good clothing options, and the class is generally conducted in bare feet.

▶ *Tap:* Before investing in tap shoes, ask the instructor whether you can work in hard-soled shoes. Normal attire includes leggings and a top.

EXERCISE SENSE AND ETIQUETTE

Each instructor has a particular flow or routine for each class. If you get lost, follow along with the more experienced students.

Elliptical Training

Elliptical trainers offer a workout as intense as running or cross-country skiing but without any of the impact. "It's a fantastic workout. It's not weight-bearing, so it's gentle on the joints and provides a very fluid movement," says Hyatt.

The fluidity happens because the machine forces your legs to make slightly circular—or elliptical—motions, similar to those of running or bicycling. There are several types of elliptical machines. Some have arm levers that move in opposition to the pedals to help provide an upper-body workout, while others have pedals that you can adjust to operate on an incline, letting you increase the intensity or target your buttocks muscles.

YOUR ELLIPTICAL TRAINING WORKOUT PRESCRIPTION

Beginner: 10 to 20 minutes, 3 days a week, in the lower end of your target heart rate range

Intermediate: 30 minutes, 3 to 5 days a week

Advanced: 45 minutes or more, up to 5 days a week

Calorie burn per 15 minutes: 138
Exercise units per 15 minutes: 2

FIRST DO THIS

If it's been a while since you've worked out regularly, Tomasetti recommends letting your body slowly adjust to using the elliptical trainer. "It's pretty intense," she says. "If the machine has arm levers, don't use them, and don't use the incline function."

MAXIMIZING CALORIE BURN

Once you work up to spending 30 minutes on the trainer, you can vary your workouts to boost your calorie burn. On some days, work out longer at a lower intensity; on others, pick up the pace by doing intervals, which consist of working hard for a short period of time, then resting briefly before repeating. The bursts of hard work can include going faster, raising the incline, or increasing the resistance. "You should shock your muscles every once in a while by changing the way you work them," says Tomasetti.

CUSTOMIZE YOUR WORKOUT AND MAKE IT FUN

Some elliptical trainers come with preprogrammed workouts that you can choose from a computerized control panel. Punch a couple of buttons, and the machine automatically increases resistance or simulates a hill-climbing workout by increasing and decreasing the incline. Thus, you can not only boost cardiovascular fitness and calorie burn but also help target your thighs and glutes. "This can contribute to your overall strength level because the load is greater and the cadence is slower," says Hyatt.

WORKOUT ESSENTIALS

▸ Wear comfortable clothing that "breathes" to allow moisture to evaporate.

▸ Because elliptical training is low-impact, either walking or running shoes will do.

▸ Keep a water bottle and towel nearby so you can stay hydrated and wipe away the sweat as you work out.

EXERCISE SENSE AND ETIQUETTE

Elliptical trainers come in a number of different configurations. Try several to see which features suit you. If you want to simulate walking or running up hills, a machine that has an incline option may be your best bet.

If the trainer you use has handrails, don't lean on them. You'll get the best workout if you keep your full weight on the pedals. Also, be sure to maintain good posture, with your abs contracted to protect your lower back.

Exercise Video Workouts ———•

Instructional videos are perfect for women who feel self-conscious, hate outdoor exercise, or have a hard time getting to the gym. With exercise videos, you can work out whenever you want and however you want, all in the comfort of your home. "There are so many different videos on the market that you're bound to find something that interests you," says Carman.

You can find instructional videos for a number of exercises in this book, including yoga, weight training, step aerobics, kickboxing, high-impact aerobics, low-impact aerobics, tai chi, and Pilates. "For every form of exercise, it seems there are videos to go with them," says Carman.

Choosing the right video for your interests and level of fitness takes a little research. Online, www.videofitness.com offers a wide array of video reviews written by home exercisers. Mail-order companies, such as Collage Video, offer detailed descriptions of hundreds of videos. Check that the instructor is ACE-certified and/or certified in that particular exercise.

Another good way to tell whether a video may be right for you is to look at the cover, says Prouty. "Look at the photos of people in the video," she says. "Is everyone 20 years old and lean and mean and fit? That may be great for somebody who wants to be challenged, but it may not be the best choice for you if you are 40, 50, or 60 years old and just beginning to exercise."

YOUR EXERCISE VIDEO WORKOUT PRESCRIPTION

Beginner: 30 minutes, 3 days a week, with a beginner-level video

Intermediate: 45 minutes, 3 to 5 days a week, with a slightly advanced program of higher intensity

Advanced: 45 to 60 minutes, up to 5 days a week

Calorie burn per 15 minutes: Varies from 110 for aerobic dancing to 145 for step aerobics, depending on intensity. (For calorie burn information on specific types of exercise, refer to the individual discussions in this chapter.)

Exercise units per 15 minutes: 2 to 3, depending on impact type

FIRST DO THIS

Hang an inexpensive mirror on a wall or door in your workout area so you can check your form and make sure your posture is correct. Plus, says Carman, it's motivating to see your body change as your workouts progress.

MAXIMIZING CALORIE BURN

Videos that provide pointers on proper form help you get the most out of your workouts, especially if you haven't exercised regularly for a while. If you don't do the exercises correctly, you won't get the most benefit from them, says Carman.

To get the most out of your workouts, you can get free online assistance from companies such as TheFIRM (www.firmdirect.com or www.firmbelievers.com) and Collage Video (www.collagevideo.com). Take advantage of those services, urges Carman.

CUSTOMIZE YOUR WORKOUT AND MAKE IT FUN

There's almost no end to the variety if you pick exercise videos that meet your particular interests. For instance, if you love to dance, choose a ballet-oriented video. If you want to sculpt your muscles, try a weight-training video.

"Don't pick something that doesn't interest you just because you think it'll be a good workout, because it won't be fun," advises Carman.

Doing the same routine day after day can get boring, too. To get the most variety in your regimen, try using different videos.

WORKOUT ESSENTIALS

▶ While one of the joys of working out at home is that you don't have to wear fancy workout clothes, don't skimp on your shoes. If you want shoes for a variety of workouts, get cross-trainers that provide plenty of support. Replace them every couple of months to ensure that you have the most cushioning possible.

▶ Also, don't neglect necessary equipment just because you're working out at home. "If the video requires weights, you could start out with soup cans, but if you really want to progress, you should buy an inexpensive set of weights," advises Prouty.

EXERCISE SENSE AND ETIQUETTE

If you live in an apartment, be sure that music from the tapes or the noise from your jumping around on the floor doesn't bother your neighbors, especially if you exercise first thing in the morning.

Fencing

If you like your fitness pursuit served up with camaraderie, strategy, and plenty of action, consider fencing, suggests Nat Goodhartz, Ph.D., an exercise physiologist and fencing coach in Rochester, New York. Once you're used to the moves and footwork, you may get so wrapped up in the action—or the game, as Dr. Goodhartz calls it—that you don't even notice you're getting a workout.

"Fencing is a very forgiving sport for a variety of age groups, for both genders, and for different body types," says Dr. Goodhartz. Fencing uses blunt-tipped instruments—the épée, foil, and saber—in a way that simulates swordplay. You get points for making contact with your opponent.

HOW THEY DID IT

She Eased into Exercise and Escaped a Bad Marriage

Years of physical and verbal abuse left LisaKay Wojcik of Romulus, Michigan, with a battered body, shattered self-esteem, and hundreds of extra pounds. She lost 230 pounds once she realized that she could change—and that she deserved to be thin.

I grew up feeling like a nobody. No wonder, then, that at age 18—and a healthy 100 pounds—I married the first boyfriend who came along. Soon he started beating me at least three times a week. Later, he would cry apologetically but imply that it was all my fault. I believed that I needed to make the marriage work, no matter what.

Over the next 9 years, I ended up in the emergency room 27 times. The more I was beaten, the more I ate. Food felt like my only friend, the one thing that wouldn't hurt me. When I finally left my husband at age 27, I weighed 300 pounds.

Severely depressed, with no self-esteem, I went right into another bad marriage where the abuse was verbal, rather than physical. My new husband belittled me constantly and kept me feeling insecure. So I continued to eat away my pain. A miscarriage in 1995 finally woke me up. I saw that things needed to change. I didn't know how to fix my marriage or to leave my husband, but I realized that I could improve myself.

At 350 pounds, I'd never seriously tried to lose weight, so I started with an exercise video. At first, I immediately got out of breath, which was scary. After I learned to slowly ease into exercise, I was soon up to 10 minutes on the tape, then 15, then 20. And the pounds were going in the opposite direction: 340, 330, 320. I took my workouts outdoors, walking 2 miles to a friend's house. Every 10 days, I dropped a pound or two.

I drastically altered my diet, too. I swapped fried, fatty foods for lean chicken and fish, plus fresh fruits and vegetables. I also gradually downsized my portions. At my peak weight, I probably consumed 4,500 calories a day—enough for several people—so I cut down to 3,500, then 3,000, and so on.

One year later, I had lost 75 pounds and felt great. I joined a gym and started running on the treadmill and lifting weights 3 days a week. But my husband was unsupportive, insisting that my success was only temporary. What a motivator!

The next year, I reached my goal weight—117 pounds—and found the strength to leave my marriage. Today, I'm at a stable 125 pounds, a healthy weight for my 5-foot-2-inch frame. It's more of a struggle to stay in shape because I now have multiple sclerosis—but I work at it. My new husband—the most supportive man I've ever met—helps me on and off the treadmill when my flare-ups are bad.

LisaKay walked her way to greater self-esteem.

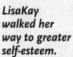

I've learned that I matter—and I want others to see that they do, too.

"A well-executed touch makes you feel like a million bucks," says Dr. Goodhartz.

First, you'll learn fencing footwork and how to use the "playing field," the long rectangular area where bouts occur. Then you'll receive instruction in using the weapons and the rules of the sport.

Many community recreation centers offer fencing classes. The U.S. Fencing Association (www.usfencing.org) is a great resource for finding a fencing center in your area.

YOUR FENCING WORKOUT PRESCRIPTION

Beginner: 60 minutes, 3 days a week

Intermediate: 60 to 90 minutes, 3 days a week

Advanced: 60 to 90 minutes, 2 or 3 days a week, with challenging drills and workouts

Calorie burn per 15 minutes: 102
Exercise units per 15 minutes: 2

FIRST DO THIS

If you've been sedentary for a while, start by riding a bike for a few weeks to get your legs ready for the footwork and stances you'll learn. "You don't need to be particularly strong or powerful, but it helps decrease the potential for injury or soreness if you already have some level of fitness," says Dr. Goodhartz.

When you're starting out, it's best to attend class at least three times a week so you can practice the new movements, which can seem awkward at first. "There are a lot of people who think of fencing as a very artistic endeavor, but it's really a sport, filled with athletic activity," he says.

MAXIMIZING CALORIE BURN

Although fencing is characterized by short, frequent bursts of action with rests in between, it's a great calorie burner because when you move, you work intensely. Once you know the basic techniques, the calorie burn increases because you're able to fence longer and move your feet more as you engage your opponent.

CUSTOMIZE YOUR WORKOUT AND MAKE IT FUN

Many people go to fencing classes and get hooked, then decide to begin a total-body regimen that includes strength and flexibility training and cardiovascular workouts to help get them in better shape to excel at fencing. "The better the fencer is, the more she can manipulate the level of the workout so she can derive different benefits from it," says Dr. Goodhartz.

It's important to practice the moves outside class, notes Peter Harmer, Ph.D., member of the medical commission of the International Fencing Federation and professor of exercise science at Willamette University in Salem, Oregon. "For example, practice the *en garde* stance for 5 minutes or so a couple of times a day," he says.

WORKOUT ESSENTIALS

▶ If you're new to fencing, all you'll probably need for your first class are a pair of cross-training shoes, sweat pants, and a T-shirt.

▶ Most clubs provide protective gear, such as a mask, jacket, and gloves.

▶ Although traditionally beginners started with the foil, newcomers frequently get to select the weapon they prefer—épée, foil, or saber.

EXERCISE SENSE AND ETIQUETTE

Because fencing an ancient sport filled with traditions and its own code of etiquette, the instructor will show you the correct behavior, such as the proper way to salute an opponent and how and when to shake hands.

Fitness Walking

Walking is so natural, it takes little or no training or special equipment, making it the most practical way of all to exercise. And because it's weight-bearing exercise, it can help prevent bone loss from osteoporosis.

"It's one of the best exercises, and almost everyone who doesn't have a physical disability can do it," says Prouty. "Walking can be a wonderful start for fitness, and it's a great social activity. You can walk almost anywhere—in your neighborhood, in parks, and even in malls."

You can choose to walk alone and have a chance to reflect on the day, or walk with a friend and socialize.

YOUR FITNESS WALKING WORKOUT PRESCRIPTION

Opposite is a step-by-step program for a month's worth of walking workouts.

Calorie burn per 15 minutes: 65
Exercise units per 15 minutes: 1

FIRST DO THIS

Shoes may be the only walking "equipment" you really need, but quality and fit are critically important. Before you take to the streets or treadmill, visit a good shoe store and try several different brands and styles to see which suits you best. Walk around for a while to be sure the shoes fit well and provide good cushioning and support. Don't expect to "break in" shoes that aren't comfortable from the start. For details, see "Exercise in Comfort with the Right Shoes," page 257.

MAXIMIZING CALORIE BURN

To burn more calories, you need to cover ground more quickly. But taking longer strides doesn't make you walk faster. Instead, shorten your stride slightly without letting your steps become choppy, then pick up the pace. After walking regularly for a few weeks, boost calorie burn by adding periods of fast walking followed by brief "rest periods" during which you slow the pace.

Fitness Walking Workout Sampler

	DAY 1 TEMPO	DAY 2 BUMP IT UP	DAY 3 LONG	DAY 4 TEMPO	DAY 5 1-MINUTE COUNT
Week 1	15 min	20 min	30 min	15 min	20 min
Week 2	20 min	25 min	30 min	20 min	25 min
Week 3	15 min	25 min	30 min	15 min	25 min
Week 4	20 min	25 min	35 min	20 min	25 min

Key

Tempo and Long: Walk at a moderate pace that's brisk enough to get your heart pumping but doesn't leave you out of breath.

Bump It Up: Walk for 5 minutes at a moderate pace, then speed up for 1 minute. Continue alternating for the total time.

1-Minute Count: Walk for 5 minutes at a moderate pace, then count the number of steps you take during 1 minute. Continue for the total time. (As you walk faster, the number of steps will increase.)

CUSTOMIZE YOUR WORKOUT AND MAKE IT FUN

One of the great things about walking is that—weather permitting—you can do it almost anywhere. "Many of the women I know love to walk in malls, where they are indoors and safe and the heat or other elements won't affect them. Plus, they get to window-shop," says Prouty.

If you have a tough time staying motivated to go on solo walking expeditions, enlist a friend or two and make your walks social events.

After you've been walking regularly for a while, you may want to challenge yourself by participating in a 5-K walk/run. Consult your local newspaper or runners' clubs for listings of 5-K walk/runs in your community.

WORKOUT ESSENTIALS

▶ Replace walking shoes regularly, even before they start to look worn-out. Depending on how often you walk, you may want get a new pair every 2 to 3 months.

▶ Wear loose, comfortable clothes that let your body breathe. Consider trying some of the fabrics that let moisture evaporate. Cotton shorts and a T-shirt may be comfortable, but if it's warm or you work up a sweat, they could weigh you down.

EXERCISE SENSE AND ETIQUETTE

For safety's sake, says Prouty, avoid walking in isolated areas, especially if you're alone. And if you wear a headset and listen to music

Turn Your Walk into an Ab-Solutely Amazing Tummy Workout

Getting a flatter, more toned tummy may be as simple as taking a walk. By standing tall and focusing on your abdominal muscles, you can help tighten them without doing a single crunch.

First, be sure you're standing erect, with your chest open and your shoulders back. To help you find the perfect stance, imagine how your body would react if you were drawn upward by the top of your head.

Next, get your abs into the action. Think of pulling your abdominal muscles up and back as if a seat belt were drawn low and tight across your lap, says Elizabeth Larkam, a Pilates instructor who is on the faculty of the exercise and sports science department of the University of San Francisco and a dance medicine specialist at the Centers for Sports Medicine at St. Francis Memorial Hospital in San Francisco. It's not enough to simply suck in your abdominal muscles; it's more effective to pull them up and back because it works them more deeply. In fact, Larkam suggests working the abs this way during regular daily activities to strengthen the body's "core muscles"—the abs, pelvis, and lower back.

Once your abs are in the right position, you're ready to engage all the major muscles of the body. As you begin to walk, pretend that you are pushing your body through chest-high water, which is resisting your movement. Don't swing your arms, but push them deliberately through the imaginary water (there's no need to push them too high—waist level is fine).

As you continue to walk, twist your torso and your arms to work the oblique muscles, at the sides of your waist.

When you work your abs, it's also effective to strengthen the opposing muscles—the gluteals, or buttocks muscles. To do that, squeeze and contract your glutes as if you were trying to hold a $50 bill between your buttocks. This move strengthens the lower back as well.

Repeat these actions every 5 or 10 minutes during the course of your walk to be sure that your abs stay controlled.

or other recordings, be sure the volume isn't so loud that you aren't aware of what's going on around you.

Gardening

If tending to your flowers, lawn, and vegetables sounds like the perfect workout, add gardening and working in the yard to your fitness regimen. And while weeding doesn't burn lots of calories, planting, mowing, and hoeing certainly do, according to Dr. Clifford.

"It's wonderful to be outdoors, and there is something spiritually restorative about digging in the dirt," says Dr. Clifford. "Most of us, however, don't spend our gardening time using large muscle masses, which is what you have to do to elevate your heart rate and burn calories."

So, what can you do to boost the fitness element of gardening? Don't just sit (or kneel) there—move! Getting your legs into the action will elevate your heart rate.

"If you are an avid gardener and spend your time digging and going great guns, you probably do build some good muscle strength and stamina," Dr. Olson.

YOUR GARDENING WORKOUT PRESCRIPTION

Beginner: 20 to 30 minutes, 3 days a week

Intermediate: 30 minutes, 3 to 5 days a week

Advanced: 45 minutes or more, 5 days a week

Calorie burn per 15 minutes: Planting and weeding, 75; tilling and digging, 85; mowing with a push mower, 100

Exercise units per 15 minutes: 1 or 2, depending on intensity

FIRST DO THIS

Plan your sessions to include some variety. For instance, start by doing some weeding as a warmup, then move on to more strenuous chores, such as pruning trees or shrubs and cutting up or disposing of the debris.

MAXIMIZING CALORIE BURN

Any gardening activity that elevates your heart rate or makes you breathe harder will burn more calories. Using a leaf blower or a weed trimmer won't increase calorie burn much, but activities that require making large movements—such as putting in a new garden plot, digging, and raking or hoeing an existing plot—will help boost your fitness.

Try to avoid sitting in one spot for long periods of time. More sedentary chores, such as planting and weeding, while necessary, probably won't burn fat at a very fast rate. "While they are pleasurable activities and are better than sitting down in front of the TV, I wouldn't classify them as much of a fitness activity," says Dr. Clifford.

He says one old-fashioned way to burn calories in the yard is to use a manually powered push mower. "I've seen more and more people going back to that kind of mower, and it certainly provides some exercise," he says.

One 40-year-old woman who was part of an exercise study in Great Britain burned 30 percent more calories (392 versus 306) while doing yard work than she did in an aerobics class. The hour-long session, which included sawing, carrying, and piling debris, kept her heart rate in her training zone for 44 minutes, while in step class it was in the target zone for only 24 minutes.

CUSTOMIZE YOUR WORKOUT AND MAKE IT FUN

"Gardening is a great holistic, rejuvenating activity," says Dr. Olson. "It allows you to express your creativity while getting some fresh air."

What you do is completely up to you: Plant a new flower bed or a patch of herbs, or grow enough tomatoes and zucchini to provide your family (and the neighbors) with a healthy supply for months.

WORKOUT ESSENTIALS

▶ In addition to gardening tools for the task at hand, a cushion or kneeling pad helps make it more comfortable to kneel or sit for extended periods.

▶ If you're going to do much digging, look for sneakers that provide side-to-side support, or try specially-made gardening clogs.

▶ Protect yourself from the sun with sunscreen and a hat.

EXERCISE SENSE AND ETIQUETTE

If the size of your property, or physical or time limitations, demand that you sometimes need to use noisy equipment such as a leaf blower or power mower, wait until a reasonable hour to tackle those chores. Your neighbors may not be early risers.

Hiking

For a workout that not only burns calories but also is soothing to the soul, hit the trail. When you're surrounded by trees and chirping birds, it's easy to forget that you're burning calories as you walk.

Hiking may also do your bones a favor, according to Dr. Olson. Research indicates that because of the varied terrain, hiking may be more effective than regular walking in combating osteoporosis that attacks the hip joints. Wearing a light backpack increases the benefits even more.

"What we've found is that to provide enough positive stress to develop the hip joint, you have to work against gravity. Walking uphills is one way to do that," she says.

YOUR HIKING WORKOUT PRESCRIPTION

Beginner: 20 to 30 minutes, 3 days a week
Intermediate: 30 to 45 minutes, 3 to 5 days a week
Advanced: 45 minutes or more, 5 days a week, allowing adequate time for rest and recovery

Calorie burn per 15 minutes: 120
Exercise units per 15 minutes: 2

FIRST DO THIS

If you're not used to hiking or haven't hit the trails for a while, stick to level terrain at first.

"I recommend starting on a well-groomed, level trail. Also, be sure to wear appropriate footwear," says Hyatt. "Carry a walking stick if you need to, wear a hat and sunscreen, and stretch when you're finished."

MAXIMIZING CALORIE BURN

When you think of boosting calorie burn, think of one word: *hills*! Trekking uphill increases your calorie burn exponentially.

The first studies pointing to the health benefits of regular activity were done on people who worked at mildly strenuous jobs, such as postal carriers who walked their routes and carried bags of mail—an activity that resembles hiking.

CUSTOMIZE YOUR WORKOUT AND MAKE IT FUN

Take along a picnic lunch and turn your hike into a special occasion. Whether you choose to go solo or invite a friend or family member to come along, enjoy the scenery and relax.

You can hike up mountains, along rivers, and even through city parks. Hiking is a staple in Nottingham's workout regimen. Although she used to push herself to make her hikes more intense, "once I gave myself permission not to kill myself every workout, I found I was naturally extending my hikes two or three times as long, and I was enjoying myself more," she says.

WORKOUT ESSENTIALS

▶ For short hikes on level ground, walking shoes are fine Otherwise, wear good hiking shoes that provide plenty of support and traction. To avoid blisters, be sure to break in your shoes before wearing them on the trail.

▶ The weather can change with little warning, especially if you're tackling a mountain, so dress in layers. Look for athletic wear in fabrics that allow moisture to evaporate from your body. Pack a windbreaker or wet-weather coat made of a water-repellent material that is also "breathable."

▶ Take extra water to be sure you stay hydrated—allow yourself 8 to 12 ounces per hour.

▶ Pack snacks, preferably complex carbohydrates such as granola bars, bananas, or bagels.

▶ A walking stick is helpful, but don't forget a hat and sunscreen.

EXERCISE SENSE AND ETIQUETTE

Don't skimp on stretching, especially if you're walking up and down hills. Your lower back, hamstrings, calves, and Achilles tendons will repay you with decreased soreness the next day. (For details, see chapter 11.)

Always leave the trail looking just as it did before you arrived. Don't leave any trash behind.

Inline Skating

If you like to cover a lot of ground fast, inline skating lets you zoom off calories *and* tone your trouble spots.

"It is an excellent thigh and butt shaper," says Carman. Once you master the technique, you can work up quite a sweat.

"In some respects, inline skating is like riding a bicycle because you are relying on equipment to help you do a lot of the work," says Dr. Olson. "It may be worthwhile to experiment with a heart rate monitor when you're skating so you can see at what cadence you need to skate and how much area you need to cover to remain in your target zone."

When you're just beginning, however, you don't need to worry about covering lots of ground to get a good workout. "Just learning how to use the skates is good exercise because when you're not good at something, it requires a lot of energy to do it correctly," notes Dr. Olson.

YOUR INLINE SKATING WORKOUT PRESCRIPTION

Beginner: 20 to 30 minutes, 3 days a week

Intermediate: 30 to 45 minutes, 3 to 5 days a week

Advanced: 45 minutes or more, 5 days a week, allowing adequate time for rest and recovery

Calorie burn per 15 minutes: 84 to 119, depending on intensity

Exercise units per 15 minutes: 1 to 2, depending on intensity

FIRST DO THIS

Before you zoom off on a pair of skates, you have to learn to stop. Take at least one half-hour lesson, and learn how to use the heel brakes on the skates, says Nottingham, coauthor of *Fitness In-Line Skating*. "Stopping an inline skate is a somewhat unnatural motion,

which is why people have such a hard time with it." To find a qualified instructor, Nottingham suggests consulting the International Inline Skating Association, which has an online database at its Web site, www.iisa.org.

For your first foray on skates, find an empty parking lot with a smooth, level surface. "Skating on neighborhood roads can be surprisingly bumpy, and I find that until you're used to them, bumps can make your shins hurt," says Carman.

MAXIMIZING CALORIE BURN

Once you master the fundamentals, try to skate in a "squatting" position, using long, graceful strides. The moves will really target your buttocks and thighs and dramatically boost the number of calories you'll burn.

"Think of inline skating as more like ice skating, not roller skating," says Carman.

As with riding a bike, the more you coast, the fewer calories you'll burn, so try to stay in motion, with few rests. "It's amazing how challenging it can be, especially if you're doing hills," says Carman. "It's also a lot of fun."

WORKOUT ESSENTIALS

▶ Be sure to get comfortable skates. Many sports equipment shops will let you rent them by the day, so it makes sense to try them out before you commit to buying a pair. Inline skates fit somewhat like ski boots and can take a while to break in, so do it slowly to avoid getting blisters. It's also a good idea to wear socks that won't make your feet sweat.

▶ Wear a helmet, as well as wrist, elbow, and knee pads. Nottingham says that wearing the pads will give you extra confidence when you're first starting because you won't be so worried about injuries from falls.

EXERCISE SENSE AND ETIQUETTE

Before you venture anywhere near traffic, be sure you know how to stop. Until you master the technique, stick to an empty parking lot.

Pilates

With its promise of lengthening and strengthening your body, it's no wonder that Pilates has grown in popularity over the past decade. The regimen was originally developed by Joseph Pilates in the 1920s to rehabilitate injured military personnel and later used to help train dancers. Pilates, which includes the use of clinical-looking equipment complete with pulleys and straps, can improve your posture, tone your muscles, and make you more flexible with minimal risk of injury.

"I think it's one of the ideal forms of exercise because it is so easily modified. It can be altered to meet the individual needs of the participant," says Elizabeth Larkam, a Pilates instructor who is on the faculty of the exercise and sports science department of the University of San Francisco and a dance medicine specialist at the Centers for Sports Medicine at St. Francis Memorial Hospital in San Francisco.

The key to Pilates is using perfect form, which can make it somewhat daunting for newcomers. "It's very instructor intensive," says James G. Garrick, M.D., head of the Centers for Sports Medicine at St. Francis Memorial Hospital in San Francisco. His rehabilitation centers have used Pilates-inspired workouts for the past 2 decades. "If you don't do it right, you don't get all the benefits of it," he adds.

While most Pilates regimens include using apparatus such as the Reformer, mat work is becoming more popular with home exercisers because it doesn't require expensive, complicated equipment. Despite its apparent simplicity, however, mat work is often tougher than workouts involving equipment. According to Larkam, apparatus such as the Reformer assist the muscles through moves, but with mat work, you move your body yourself.

Neither Larkam nor Dr. Garrick recommends relying on Pilates as your only fitness regimen, because it is not cardiovascular. Rather, it's excellent to use as a cross-training workout with cardio activities such as walking and cycling.

YOUR PILATES
WORKOUT PRESCRIPTION

Beginner: 20 to 30 minutes, 3 (nonconsecutive) days a week

Intermediate: 30 to 45 minutes, 3 (nonconsecutive) days a week

Advanced: 45 to 60 minutes, 3 (nonconsecutive) days a week

Calorie burn per 15 minutes: 45
Exercise units per 15 minutes: 1

FIRST DO THIS

Look for an instructor who has trained at an official Pilates studio. Both Dr. Garrick and Larkam stress that it's important to find a good Pilates instructor who has a lot of experience. Because of its recent boom in popularity and the fact that training and certification standards for Pilates are ongoing, it's vital for you to know your instructor's background. You can check with the Pilates Method Alliance at its Web site (www.pilatesmethodalliance.org), which has a listing of member studios, or call the group at its toll-free number: (866) 573-4945. A Pilates instructor should have a minimum of 400 hours of training with an already-certified Pilates instructor.

MAXIMIZING CALORIE BURN

Even though mat Pilates workouts are more demanding on the neck and back than machine-based workouts, you'll burn more calories on machines because they involve your arms and legs in full range of motion, says Larkam. Mat workouts tend to focus on what is called the powerhouse—the abs, hips, and pelvic girdle. By incorporating your legs and arms into the workout, you'll involve more muscles and boost fat burning.

An experienced instructor can make sure that you use correct form when performing the exercises, notes Dr. Garrick. If you decide to continue with Pilates at home, he suggests checking with an instructor regularly to make sure your form remains perfect. "A lot of people don't realize that they aren't doing the movements correctly," he says. "If you're supervised properly, you can't cheat, and you will activate more muscles."

CUSTOMIZE YOUR WORKOUT AND MAKE IT FUN

Although the right Pilates instructor is essential, you can get a good workout at home, says Larkam. The price of home equipment has dropped significantly over the past couple of years, and there are now many good Pilates videos on the market, such as Denise Austin's Mat Workout Based on the Work of Joseph Pilates from Artisan Entertainment, which is widely available where exercise videos are sold.

Several mail-order companies specialize in Pilates equipment and videos. Both Living Arts (www.livingarts.com or www.gaiam.com; toll-free, 877-989-6321) and Balanced Body (www.balancedbody.com or www.pilates.com) carry a wide range of Pilates and Pilates-inspired videos and equipment. Collage Video (www.collagevideo.com; 800-433-6769) also offers many videos.

Some instructors follow strict Pilates style, while others offer Pilates-inspired workouts that include hybrid moves using other equipment, such as exercise balls.

WORKOUT ESSENTIALS

▶ Wear loose but not bulky workout clothing. Because Pilates isn't a cardiovascular exercise, dress so that you won't feel too cool as you work out. Your muscles should be warm and pliable, says Larkam. "Leggings or sweat pants are just fine."

▶ You can wear slipperlike shoes or work out in bare feet, but most people favor socks.

▶ If you're doing floor work, it's best to have a mat to cushion your spine. If you want to splurge on a piece of home equipment, Larkam recommends the Pilates Reformer, available through Balanced Body, which she says is very versatile.

EXERCISE SENSE AND ETIQUETTE

When doing Pilates moves, draw your abs in and up toward the back of your head as you exhale. This will help ensure that your spine and torso are in proper alignment.

Rebounding ──────●

If you loved to bounce on the bed when you were a kid, try minitrampoline workouts, also called rebounding, You can now bounce to your heart's content with no threat of being scolded. In the process, you'll break a sweat and save your knees.

Good balance is helpful—but not essential. You can modify the moves and actually use rebounding to improve your balance, Dr. Olson.

"Standing on a minitrampoline while you are doing strength exercises such as biceps curls, triceps extensions, and shoulder exercises can help develop better balance," says Dr. Olson.

YOUR REBOUNDING WORKOUT PRESCRIPTION

Beginner: 20 to 30 minutes, 3 days a week

Intermediate: 30 to 45 minutes, 3 to 5 days a week

Advanced: 45 minutes and up, 5 days a week, allowing adequate time for rest and recovery

Calorie burn per 15 minutes: 75
Exercise units per 15 minutes: 1

FIRST DO THIS

If you're thinking of buying a minitrampoline to use at home, look for quality. Although there are low-cost models on the market, be sure that the one you buy has enough cushioning and "bounce" to protect your joints.

MAXIMIZING CALORIE BURN

You can get a good low-impact workout on a minitrampoline, but don't expect the same calorie burn that you'd get from something like jogging or aerobics since the trampoline "lifts" your body for you, reducing effort, says Dr. Olson.

If you're used to attending step class or cycling class and you decide to use a rebounder, you'll notice that it does so much of the work for you that it's hard to sustain an appropriate target heart rate for an extended period of time, says Dr. Olson.

"That said, rebounding is a fine component of an overall exercise routine," says Dr. Olson. "And with a doctor's approval, rebounding can be excellent for people who have knee or other joint problems. If you don't feel that you're getting much of a workout, try exaggerating the moves to use a greater range of motion."

CUSTOMIZE YOUR WORKOUT AND MAKE IT FUN

Pretend that you're jumping rope, running or kicking, or even bouncing on the bed. The motion itself is fun. If you've passed up regular aerobics classes because they stress your knees or feet, you'll be happy to find that you can do many of the same moves on the minitrampoline.

You can also use the rebounder as part of a circuit-training workout, in which you do a series of strength-training exercises alternated with aerobic activities. Many fitness clubs across the country feature Urban Rebounding classes, which involve jumping only a few inches and incorporate strength-training movements and cardiovascular work into the workout.

There are also many rebounding videos on the market, but if they don't interest you, just turn on some good music and bounce to your heart's content.

WORKOUT ESSENTIALS

▶ A sturdy minitrampoline is essential for a safe workout. The American Institute of Reboundology (toll-free, 888-464-5867; www.healthbounce.com) offers several models, as does Needak (800-232-5762; www.needakmfg.com). Prices range from $200 to $300. If you're worried about losing your balance, you can buy a stabilizing bar for about $65.

▶ You can simulate a health club rebounding class with videos, several of which are available through Collage Video (800-433-6769; www.collagevideo.com).

▶ Wear a good sports bra, to reduce excessive bounce.

If you're a beginner, or want to go right to other fitness activities without changing shoes, it's best to wear a low-profile fitness (not walking) shoe. Skilled rebounders usually jump barefoot because it gives them a better feel of the trampoline and range of motion in the foot area. Don't rebound in just socks, however, because they can be slippery.

EXERCISE SENSE AND ETIQUETTE

Until you feel confident of your footing when you're rebounding, it's a good idea to look down once in a while to be sure that you're not about to bounce off.

Rowing Machine Workouts ———•

If you've tried rowing before but abandoned your rowing machine out of frustration or boredom, you're missing out on the excellent cardiovascular workout and muscle toning that these workouts provide.

If you want to shape up your female physique, maybe it's time to dust off your rowing machine. Rowing uses the muscles of the back, shoulders, and arms, making it a great workout for women, who frequently spend time sitting in front of a computer or behind a steering wheel with not-so-great posture. "We're not used to using our upper-body muscles very much with exercise," points out Dr. Olson. Conditioning those muscles can help women maintain good posture during daily activities, she says.

YOUR ROWING WORKOUT PRESCRIPTION

To keep from getting bored, don't force yourself to do it for 30- or 45-minute sessions, like other exercises. Instead, combine rowing with other activities in the same workout. For instance, you could row for 10 minutes, then hop on the treadmill for a 20-minute power walk.

FIRST DO THIS

Start slowly, says Prouty. Take the time to learn proper rowing form, and don't push yourself too hard in the beginning.

MAXIMIZING CALORIE BURN

Because rowing involves so many muscles, it's a natural fat burner. The key to getting the most out of the machine may be to build endurance so that you can continue the workout for more than just a few minutes.

When you're a newcomer to rowing machine workouts, the movement—which involves grasping the bar or "oars" with your hands and using your arms to pull back the bar and your legs to push your body—can seem awkward. It's important not to hunch over and, at the end of your stroke, to remember to pull your shoulder blades back and toward each other.

"When we get on exercise machines that make us use our upper-body muscles, it's uncomfortable because we're not used to doing that," notes Dr. Olson. "We perceive the effort to be a little greater than what we're used to feeling on the treadmill at the same heart rate."

Spend only as much time on the rowing machine as is comfortable for you, then move on to another activity if you want to continue the workout, Dr. Olson suggests. Once you build up your strength and endurance, you can increase the resistance on the rowing machine to boost the intensity of your workout.

CUSTOMIZE YOUR WORKOUT AND MAKE IT FUN

If you want to work your upper body harder, concentrate on using only the arm pulleys; to get a better leg and buttocks workout, concentrate on the leg motions.

For a more enjoyable rowing workout, visualize yourself sculling along a coastline or listen to your favorite music.

You can also vary your workout by doing intervals, says Tomasetti. Row hard for 1 to 2 minutes, rest by decreasing the intensity for a couple of minutes, then continue to alternate.

WORKOUT ESSENTIALS

▶ If you're using an old home rowing machine, be sure it's in good working order. Some older machines have "oars" that operate independently of each other, and if they don't work correctly, they can cause shoulder strain.

▶ Because rowing requires a wide range of motion—leaning forward and pulling back—a baggy T-shirt can get in the way. Instead, wear a slightly loose top made of material that won't trap sweat next to your body. Choose shorts or leggings made of nonslippery material so there's no chance of your sliding off the seat as you row.

▶ On your feet, nearly anything goes: running, walking, or cross-training shoes will do just fine.

EXERCISE SENSE AND ETIQUETTE

Take the time to learn proper rowing form. While Olympic rowers make it look easy as they glide smoothly across the water, it can take a while to master the mechanics behind the stroke, notes Dr. Clifford.

Seated Aerobics

If you're injured, unfit, or very overweight, or you have other physical problems that limit participation in traditional forms of exercise, consider trying seated aerobics, which can burn calories and tone nearly all your muscles suggests Eva Montee, a fitness instructor certified by the American Council on Exercise and the Cooper Institute and coordinator for wellness and community health programs for Mountain View Hospital District in Madras, Oregon. Your fitness level will improve, and if your physical condition allows, you'll probably find that you can branch out into other activities before too long.

Seated aerobics classes are offered through hospitals and community centers, and videotapes are also available. "It's a safe, gentle activity that most people can manage," says Hyatt.

The classes can be an enjoyable alternative for people with physical limitations who are resistant to trying other forms of exercise, notes Jodi Stolove of Delmar, California, who developed "chair dancing," a form of seated aerobics, and is the instructor on several seated aerobics videos. "They take one look at what we're doing and say, 'That, I can do,'" she says.

Although you do the routines while seated, both your legs and arms get into the action as you march, kick, cha-cha, twist, and samba. Stolove even has one popular routine in which students pretend to ride a horse to the accompaniment of the William Tell Overture. "The routines are playful and fun because that's how I like to exercise," she says.

YOUR SEATED AEROBICS WORKOUT PRESCRIPTION

Beginner: 20 to 30 minutes, 3 days a week
Intermediate: 30 to 45 minutes, 3 to 5 days a week
Advanced: 30 to 45 minutes, 5 days a week

Calorie burn per 15 minutes: 45
Exercise units per 15 minutes: 1

MAXIMIZING CALORIE BURN

You get out of the workout what you put into it, comments Stolove. Her motto for those who want to boost the fat-burning quotient: "Do it bigger with more vigor."

Montee says that rather than making sure a student's heart beats at a certain rate during a class, she relies on perceived exertion as a good measure of whether students are working hard enough. They should be breathing harder than normal but not so hard that they're out of breath.

To help improve balance, which can decrease with age and make falls more likely, she also concentrates on developing strength, especially in the lower body. To this end, Montee sometimes has students sit on big inflatable exercise balls during classes.

One of her goals is to have students who are physically able progress to performing their workouts while standing instead of sitting. Some have improved their fitness to the point where they are not only participating in line dancing classes but actually teaching them, she says.

CUSTOMIZE YOUR WORKOUT AND MAKE IT FUN

Most seated aerobics classes include components that promote flexibility, strength, and balance, in addition to boosting the heart rate. But if you want to address a specific concern or trouble spot, there's probably a way to do it while sitting down.

Mary Ann Wilson, a Spokane, Washington, nurse and fitness instructor certified by the American Council on Exercise, is creator and host of the *Sit and Be Fit* exercise show broadcast on public television stations across the United States. Her programs include workouts aimed at a variety of conditions, including arthritis and multiple sclerosis. Her exercise show and classes include taking joints through their range of motion to increase flexibility and lubricate them, as well as strengthening muscles through the use of gravity, resistance bands, and light weights.

WORKOUT ESSENTIALS

▶ Seated aerobics workouts don't require special clothing or shoes. Just be sure that what you wear is loose and lets your skin breathe and that your shoes are comfortable. If you "graduate" to standing aerobics, you'll need shoes with more support.

▶ Keep a bottle of water handy so you can replace any fluids you lose through sweating.

EXERCISE SENSE AND ETIQUETTE

If your class includes drills for balance and upper-body strength, pay attention. Improving balance lessens the chance of a fall, and good upper-body strength increases the likelihood that you'll be able to catch yourself if you do fall.

Skipping Rope —————————•

Skipping rope was good exercise back in grade school, and it's still a good (and enjoyable) way to stay fit. And if done correctly, it's actually a low-impact activity.

"Most people think jumping rope is really hard on the feet and knees, and it can be if you're not skilled at it. But once you learn to do it correctly, it's an excellent low-impact activity," says Dr. Olson.

In fact, research shows that skipping rope is easier on the knees than running, yet it provides sufficient weight-bearing benefits to help prevent osteoporosis. It's also a super-efficient way to burn calories in a short amount of time.

YOUR ROPE-SKIPPING WORKOUT PRESCRIPTION

All levels: Start by skipping for as long as you comfortably can. Begin with 30 seconds of jumping followed by 1 minute of walking, and repeat this 5 to 10 times (for a total of about $7\frac{1}{2}$ to 15 total minutes). Then slowly increase the time to 15 to 20 minutes, about three times a week.

Calorie burn per 15 minutes: 170
Exercise units per 15 minutes: 3

FIRST DO THIS

If you can skip rope for only 30 seconds at first, don't give up. Jump for as long as you can, walk around and catch your breath, then jump some more, continuing for as long as you're comfortable. You'll quickly gain stamina.

MAXIMIZING CALORIE BURN

If you've ever tried to skip rope, you probably know that there's no need to make the exercise more intense. The trick is being able to keep jumping for more than a few minutes at a time.

Keep your jumps as close to the ground as possible. Don't jump with both feet. Instead, mimic a jogging motion by jumping on one foot at a time, keeping your knees slightly bent and making an effort to gently land on the balls of your feet (instead of the entire foot) so that your weight is distributed toward the heels. This jumping style helps not only to cushion your feet but also to keep you from tripping over the rope. "Instead of thinking 'jump, jump, jump,' think 'toe-ball-heel, toe-ball-heel, toe-ball-heel,'" suggests Dr. Olson.

CUSTOMIZE YOUR WORKOUT AND MAKE IT FUN

Skipping to the beat of your favorite lively music is much more fun than keeping your eye on the clock, waiting for an allotted time period to pass.

You can also skip rope along with other activities. In a circuit-training workout, skipping works well to keep you in your target heart rate zone between strength-training exercises. To boost endurance, cardio kickboxing instructors incorporate rope-skipping movements, sometimes without the rope.

Nottingham uses rope skipping in many of her sports conditioning classes. She says that it's fun to incorporate fancy footwork or even get assistance from some friends for a double-Dutch session. "Double-Dutch jumping is great, but obviously it requires more than one person because others have to swing the rope," she says.

To avoid excessive jarring, skip rope on a forgiving surface such as wood or a high-quality exercise mat. Avoid thick carpeting or grass, however, since the rope can get caught in them.

WORKOUT ESSENTIALS

There's no need to use weighted ropes—they increase the risk of injury to your shoulders or wrists. A regular, high-quality rope will do.

▶ Tangle-resistant beaded ropes or those with handles that allow the rope to spin freely are best and can be purchased for less than $15 at sporting goods stores.

▶ Wear a sports bra that provides good support.

▶ Dr. Olson suggests using court sneakers designed for tennis, racquetball, and squash because they provide the ankle support in all directions that skipping rope requires.

EXERCISE SENSE AND ETIQUETTE

When you're jumping rope, don't forget about your upper body. Turn the rope with your wrists, not your arms, and keep your elbows close to your sides. Relax your shoulders. And smile!

Spinning

After just one Spinning class, you'll never again look at stationary cycling as a one-dimensional, rather boring workout. Using music and visualization, Spinning instructors lead students on a heart-pumping, fat-blasting, leg- and butt-burning bicycle trip without leaving the gym or studio.

A Spinning bike is a specially designed stationary cycle with a weighted, fixed flywheel. During a typical class, you sprint, ride up hills, stand up, "jump," and spin the pedals at a cadence determined by the instructor.

It's non-weight-bearing, which means it's easy on the joints. And since students have control over their bikes, they can choose how hard they work by setting the bike's resistance to meet their specific needs.

YOUR SPINNING WORKOUT PRESCRIPTION

Beginner: Introductory classes 2 days a week; don't jump or stand up if it feels uncomfortable

Intermediate: Three days a week; start to spin the pedals faster and perform more jumps

Advanced: Three days a week; incorporate as many of the more intense moves, such as jumping, standing up, and sprinting, as you comfortably can. "Maintain form; don't let momentum carry you," says Burns.

Calorie burn per 15 minutes: 175
Exercise units per 15 minutes: 3

FIRST DO THIS

"Look for a beginner class to help you get acclimated to the bike and to the workout," says Burns, who has taught Spinning classes for about 6 years. Check for proper bike fit by sitting on the saddle and extending one leg as it would be at the bottom of the pedal stroke. In that position, your knee should be only slightly bent. On most bikes, you can adjust the seat height. If you're not sure the fit is right, ask the instructor to double-check it.

MAXIMIZING CALORIE BURN

It's not difficult to burn a lot of calories during a Spinning class, especially if you're sprinting, jumping, and standing while pedaling. "Work out aerobically, not anaerobically," advises Burns. "You don't want to work so hard that you are out of breath."

When you work out aerobically, you keep your heart rate within its target training zone. In terms of breathing, you can carry on a conversation but wouldn't be able to sing.

Prouty loves to attend Spinning classes. "You can control your individual cycle so that while the teacher might say to raise the intensity, you don't have to do that, and no one knows but you. That's what is so great," she says. "As you become more fit, you can increase the intensity."

CUSTOMIZE YOUR WORKOUT AND MAKE IT FUN

Listen to the instructor's cues and let visualization work for you: Imagine your legs powering you and your bike up a hill or see yourself riding through scenic countryside.

Let the beat of the music, an important part of Spinning classes, motivate you. "I encourage people to find a class, a format, a time, and particularly an instructor they are comfortable with," says Burns. If those criteria are met, you'll leave each class feeling great. Also, he says, "come to class prepared to ride to your favorite place."

WORKOUT ESSENTIALS

▶ You'll definitely work up a sweat during Spinning class, so clothes that let moisture evaporate are essential. Don't wear anything bulky that could hold moisture and become heavy and uncomfortable.

▶ Dress in layers, such as a sports bra under a T-shirt, so you can remove clothing if necessary during the class.

▶ Although specially padded shorts or a gel-cushioned seat isn't necessary for most Spinning classes, you may want to use one or the other for comfort. If you aren't thrilled about wearing tight, padded shorts, you can opt for the seat cushion, which slips over the bike seat.

▶ There are special shoes with clips that attach to the pedals, and some gyms supply them for classes. While the shoes are a nice accessory, they're not necessary, says Burns. Well-fitting, good-quality fitness shoes are all you really need.

▶ Make sure you have a full bottle of water so you can stay hydrated, as well as a towel to wipe away sweat during the workout.

EXERCISE SENSE AND ETIQUETTE

If possible, meet with the instructor before class and ask which bike would be best for you. Some Spinning students are protective of "their" bikes because fit is such an important part of avoiding injury.

Stairclimbing

Stairclimbing is a fast, effective way to burn calories and target the muscles of the thighs and buttocks, key problem areas for many women. It's a no-fuss workout that gets the job done, fast.

You can work out on a stairclimbing machine; use a stair mill, which features an escalator-like set of stairs that you walk up; or walk up actual stairs. Whatever you use, you'll burn calories and work your muscles, but when you are required to actually step up with your full body weight, such as on the stair mill or stairs, you boost the exercise's bone-saving benefits.

Research suggests that weight-bearing exercises that fight gravity, such as going up hills or stairs, may strengthen the bones of the hip more than walking on level ground, according to Dr. Olson.

YOUR STAIRCLIMBING WORKOUT PRESCRIPTION

Beginner: 20 to 30 minutes, 3 days a week
Intermediate: 30 to 45 minutes, 3 to 5 days a week

Advanced: 45 minutes or more, 5 days a week, allowing adequate time for rest and recovery

Calorie burn per 15 minutes: 153
Exercise units per 15 minutes: 2

FIRST DO THIS

The first time you do a stairclimbing workout, watch yourself in a mirror, if possible. Be sure that you're standing tall and not leaning on the handrails. Try not to touch the rails at all except to balance and keep yourself from falling. Also, don't step on the pedals with just the balls of your feet; use your entire foot and your full body weight. Good form will help prevent injury and ensure that you get the most out of your workout.

MAXIMIZING CALORIE BURN

Set the resistance at a comfortable level. If you find that you need to lean on the handrails, lower the resistance, says Tomasetti. Working at a lower resistance that lets you maintain good form is better than stepping with poor form at a higher resistance.

If you try a stair mill, don't be surprised if you find yourself sweating buckets at what seems to be a slow pace. You don't get "rest stops" on a stair mill as you do between floors when you climb successive flights of actual stairs.

If you want a challenging workout that targets your buttock muscles, try climbing flights of stairs by taking two steps at a time.

CUSTOMIZE YOUR WORKOUT AND MAKE IT FUN

If you get bored on the stairclimber, find something to distract you as you work out, such as reading, listening to music, or watching TV.

If you're at a health club and it's not too busy, it can be fun to do a circuit of cardio machines. Spend 10 to 15 minutes on each machine, keeping your heart rate in the target zone. If you include lots of variety, your workout will stay fresh and seem to fly by.

Some stairclimbers and stair mills have readouts that show how many steps you've climbed. Keep track and, who knows, maybe you'll do enough to equal the 1,860 steps that lead to the top of the 102-story Empire State Building.

WORKOUT ESSENTIALS

▶ If you use a stairclimbing machine, any athletic shoes will do, but if you use a stair mill or tackle actual flights of stairs, you'll need shoes with a bit of support and cushioning, such as walking shoes.

▶ Wear clothing that lets moisture evaporate from your skin.

▶ Be sure you have plenty of water handy.

EXERCISE SENSE AND ETIQUETTE

If you're using a stairclimber at a health club and there are people waiting to use it, observe the club's time limits. You can get a great workout in 20 to 30 minutes.

COOL
TOOL

Shoe Inserts and Insoles

Many women who exercise for fun and fitness turn to shoe inserts to ease the effects of repetitive impact on their feet, bones, and joints. They can choose simple, off-the-shelf inserts such as cushioned insoles or heel cushions or cups or custom-fitted orthotics made by a podiatrist from molds of their feet.

WHAT EXPERTS SAY: "Over-the-counter inserts are supportive and helpful in limiting pronation (the tendency of the feet to turn inward). They can also help limit the pain-associated problems we see most often in women—heel spur syndrome, plantar fasciitis, tendinitis, bursitis, and ankle and arch pain—which are often due to wearing high heels," says Jay LeBow, D.P.M., director of the foot center at Mercy Medical Center in Baltimore and team podiatrist for the Baltimore Orioles baseball team. "They don't cure the problem, but they will help." Podiatrists note that heel pain is especially common in middle-aged women who are overweight.

"If your feet get tired and sore, either from sports or just from being on your feet on the job, insoles provide additional shock absorption," says Joanne Gordon, N.D., a physical therapist in Portland, Oregon.

When researchers at UCLA School of Medicine studied the use of shoe inserts among 250 middle-aged people (168 of whom were women), they found that 80 to 95 percent of those who used over-the-counter inserts said that they relieved heel pain, compared with 72 percent who used custom-made orthotics.

One sign that you need orthotics: You wear down one side—either the inside or outside—of your shoes more quickly than the other. Try an over-the-counter insert first, says Dr. Gordon. If the pain doesn't go away, you may need custom orthotics.

Both Dr. LeBow and Dr. Gordon, as well as other experts, stress that shoe inserts are not a substitute for proper footwear, foot care, and regular stretching to prevent exercise-related injury.

PURCHASING TIPS: Off-the-shelf inserts, which are available at athletic shoe stores and sporting goods stores, sell for $10 to $40. Look for inserts with sorbethane gel, which provides shock absorption. Custom orthotics can cost $300 or more.

Stationary Cycling ─────●

It may not be included on your list of the most exciting workouts, but stationary cycling is tops as a safe cross-training activity, according to Dr. Garrick.

Stationary cycling not only provides a great aerobic workout but may also help prevent injury because it builds the quadriceps, the large muscles in the front of the thighs that help stabilize the knees.

There are many types of stationary cycles on the market. In addition to the old-fashioned stripped-down bicycle with a weighted flywheel, there are machines that include levers to work your arms, recumbent bicycles that let you sit in a slightly reclining position, and others that provide preprogrammed computerized workouts.

YOUR STATIONARY CYCLING WORKOUT PRESCRIPTION

Beginner: Up to 20 minutes, 3 days a week, using low resistance and a pedal cadence of 40 to 60 rpm

Intermediate: 30 minutes, 3 to 5 days a week, increasing cadence to 70 to 80 rpm

Advanced: 45 minutes or more, 5 days a week, increasing cadence to 90 to 100 rpm

Calorie burn per 15 minutes: 65 to 165, depending on cadence and intensity

Exercise units per 15 minutes: Leisurely pace: 1; moderate pace: 2; intense pace: 3

FIRST DO THIS

Whether you purchase an exercise bike or use one at the gym, check it for fit. When you're sitting on the saddle, your knee should be only slightly bent when your leg is fully extended at the bottom of a pedal stroke. Most bikes are adjustable, so you can raise or lower the seat as necessary.

MAXIMIZING CALORIE BURN

"Stationary cycling is a really good cardio workout," says Tomasetti. "It's good for cross-training because it's non-weight-bearing and can really help boost your endurance."

It's not necessary or even advisable to crank up the resistance so much that it's hard to move the pedals. Instead, aim for a consistent, fairly fast cadence. How fast depends on your fitness level. If it's been a while since you've ridden a bicycle, keep your cadence (measured in revolutions per minute, or rpm) at around 50, says Tomasetti. After a couple of weeks, increase it to 70 to 80 rpm.

If you want a more steadily paced fat-burning workout, you can keep the resistance fairly low and spin the pedals faster. If you consider yourself advanced and your exercise bike has preprogrammed workouts, try the hill-climbing or interval option to boost calorie burn. If your bike doesn't have that feature, you can simulate climbing a hill by manually increasing the resistance for a short while and then decreasing it. You can also create an interval workout by pedaling fast for a minute or two, then slowing down for a brief rest before repeating.

CUSTOMIZE YOUR WORKOUT AND MAKE IT FUN

If you get bored on a stationary bike, read, watch TV, listen to music, or try a stationary cycling workout video. The preprogrammed workouts available on some bikes help increase the variety factor, or you can concentrate on tracking your mileage and make a game of seeing how far you can go.

If you'd like to feel that you're not riding solo, find a video that provides a Spinning class atmosphere or simulates a group ride through scenic countryside.

WORKOUT ESSENTIALS

▶ You may want to consider either a padded seat or padded cycling shorts to ease any soreness from sitting on the saddle for extended periods. Your clothing should breathe, allowing moisture to wick away from your skin.

▶ You don't really need special shoes for stationary cycling, although some bike models come with an option for clip-on shoes.

EXERCISE SENSE AND ETIQUETTE

Many health clubs post time limits for equipment such as stationary bikes. If others are waiting to use your bike, observe the club's rules. Even if you're limited to 20 to 30 minutes, you can get in a good workout.

Step Workouts

Whether you love intricate footwork or prefer basic choreography, step workouts are a fun, efficient, and challenging way to burn calories. They're also a great alternative to joint-pounding, higher-impact aerobics because you simply step onto and off a sturdy, specially designed platform in time to music. There's no running or jumping required.

"It's a very natural movement," says Burns, who has taught step classes for more than a decade. "The whole key to enjoying a step class is comfort. It is not a matter of how high you can step. It's all about proper form."

You can take step classes at a health club or buy a step and work out at home with some exercise videos. Either way, be sure to check your form in a mirror to make sure you're standing tall as you step—and smile at yourself once in a while, says Burns.

YOUR STEP WORKOUT PRESCRIPTION

Beginner: 2 or 3 days a week, preferably in a beginner class; use just the step with no risers

Intermediate: 3 days a week; increase your range of motion to boost intensity

Advanced: 3 to 5 days a week; challenge yourself to maintain perfect form

Calorie burn per 15 minutes: 145 for 6- to 8-inch step, 170 for higher step

Exercise units per 15 minutes: 2 to 3, depending on step height

FIRST DO THIS

"Don't be intimidated by someone who grabs a high step," Burns says. "Use a step height that's comfortable for you. This is *your* workout." And to avoid straining your hips or knees, be sure to stand tall while stepping; don't lean forward or backward.

MAXIMIZING CALORIE BURN

Concentrate on using perfect form—rather than a higher step—to get a better workout. Step up with your whole foot, and move your limbs with purpose. "Don't let momentum do the work for you," advises Burns.

Being able to use a higher step doesn't necessarily mean that you're in better shape. "I find that if I go through a full range of motion, my workouts can be very intense," says fitness instructor Janis Saffell of Miami, who is certified by the American Council on Exercise and the Aerobics and Fitness Association of America and is featured in several workout videos. She notes that she is 5 feet 7 inches tall and uses only one step riser during her own workouts. "Do the moves in as controlled a way as possible. The more muscle you use, the more calories you burn," she adds.

CUSTOMIZE YOUR WORKOUT AND MAKE IT FUN

There are nearly as many types of step workouts as there are instructors. Some step classes are dance-oriented, and for those who like the challenge of learning new choreography, they're a great mental and physical workout.

For those who prefer a straightforward approach, many step instructors and videos feature more athletic or basic choreography. Before buying a video, read the box carefully for details about the type of choreography and music.

WORKOUT ESSENTIALS

▶ In addition to a sturdy step platform, good cross-training shoes that provide plenty of lateral support are vital. Wear your workout sneakers only indoors, advises Burns. If you wear them outside, they can lose traction and make it difficult to perform moves safely. He recommends replacing your shoes every few months, even before they show signs of wear.

▶ Burns recommends dressing in layers: close-fitting shorts and a good sports bra under a T-shirt. Your clothes should wick moisture away from your body.

EXERCISE SENSE AND ETIQUETTE

Staying in the back of the class is fine, provided that you can see the instructor, says Burns.

Swimming Laps

When it comes to providing a total-body workout, few activities beat swimming.

It works nearly every muscle in the body, including your heart, without stressing your joints. Swimming laps can also be a stress reducer because there are few distractions: It's just you, gliding through the water.

Swimming requires a higher skill level than many other fitness activities, but don't let that stop you, says Margot Putukian, M.D., associate professor in orthopedics at Hershey Medical Center in Hershey, Pennsylvania, and team physician and director of primary care sports medicine at Pennsylvania State University in University Park. If you take it slowly and build up over time, you'll increase both your strength and stamina.

"I recommend swimming especially for people who have conditions that might limit their ability to do weight-bearing activities, such as severe degenerative joint disease, or who have a degenerative disk disease in their lower backs," says Dr. Putukian.

Because swimming is not a weight-bearing sport, it doesn't have the osteoporosis-fighting benefits of activities such as walking. So if you're able, it's best to incorporate fitness walking or strength training into your regimen.

YOUR SWIMMING WORKOUT PRESCRIPTION

Beginner: 20 to 30 minutes, 3 days a week

Intermediate: 30 to 45 minutes, 3 to 5 days a week

Advanced: 45 minutes or more, 5 days a week, incorporating some interval workouts

Calorie burn per 15 minutes: 136
Exercise units per 15 minutes: 2

FIRST DO THIS

If you can do only one or two laps at first, don't be discouraged. Swim as long as you comfortably can, rest for a few minutes, then start swimming again. In time, you'll be able to swim farther and longer.

To find a pool near you, check out local Y's or community centers. Also, if you don't want to fight for lane space during your first few sessions, ask when the pool is least crowded.

MAXIMIZING CALORIE BURN

The longer you can swim continuously, the more calories you will burn while you're in the pool. But that doesn't mean that you're limited to just swimming back and forth in one lane. Many swimmers customize their workouts—and boost their endurance, speed, and strength—by incorporating interval training.

You don't have to be an advanced athlete to benefit from this type of training. In fact, many newcomers who begin by swimming a couple of laps, resting, and then swimming some more are basically doing intervals. With actual interval training, however, the swimming and resting are more intentional.

You warm up with a couple of laps, swim faster than normal for a set number of laps, then rest for 30 seconds to a minute before repeating the sequence.

To help make your stroke more efficient and create less drag in the water, try to hold your body parallel to the pool floor. One way to attain good alignment is to push your chest down slightly while you're swimming, which brings your legs closer to the surface.

CUSTOMIZE YOUR WORKOUT AND MAKE IT FUN

Variety—and pool accessories—can be the key to an enjoyable swimming workout. Since sticking to one stroke for lap after lap can get boring, incorporate different strokes into your regimen: Try the breaststroke, freestyle, backstroke, and even the sidestroke.

Swim fins can help you swim faster and give your legs a great workout. Or, if your arms get tired after a few laps, grab a kickboard and give them a rest. "I have always been a big fan of changing things to add variety. Using a kickboard is great," says Dr. Putukian.

Once your arms and shoulders become accustomed to swimming, you can focus on them during your laps by using a pull buoy, a floating device that you hold between your legs to keep them immobile, or wearing resistance paddles on your hands. "Be careful of doing too much too quickly when it comes to resistance, however," says Dr. Putukian. She suggests that you don't try more than one device at a time, and stop at the first sign of pain. You can build your time up gradually.

WORKOUT ESSENTIALS

▶ For fitness swimming, select a suit that performs well in the water and that you feel comfortable wearing. Try on several, checking for adequate coverage and ease of movement through a wide range of motion. Racer-back suits can be the most flattering and offer good freedom of movement.

▶ Wear a bathing cap to keep your hair under control and goggles to protect your eyes. (Hint: If you wet a bathing cap before putting it on, it won't pull your hair.)

EXERCISE SENSE AND ETIQUETTE

Some pools have a "stick to the right" policy when it comes to sharing lanes. Even so, it's a good idea to double-check before getting into a lane that's being used by another swimmer so you avoid a midlap collision.

Tae-Bo

You've probably seen the TV infomercials for videos featuring Tae-Bo founder Billy Blanks and a roomful of exercisers punching and kicking in time with the music. If you take a closer look, you'll notice that many of the videos feature people of all ages and shapes, and most of them have grins on their faces.

Tae-Bo instructor Michele Reber of Canton, Ohio, says that's because the workout, which is a blend of kickboxing, a little dancing, and some of Blanks's "you-can-do-it" approach, is fun and easily modified to meet specific needs.

"We have basic and advanced workouts. The basics are done at a very easy, slow pace that nearly everyone can do. We've even taken it to nursing homes and assisted-living centers, where people have done the workout while sitting in a chair," says Reber, who lost 92 pounds doing Tae-Bo workouts.

There is also a "gold" workout, aimed at exercisers over the age of 40, that is slightly lower in intensity than some of the more advanced workouts.

YOUR TAE-BO WORKOUT PRESCRIPTION

Beginner: Basic video, 3 days a week

Intermediate: Beginner or advanced video, 3 days a week, modifying moves to meet your fitness level

Advanced: Advanced video, 3 to 5 days a week

Calorie burn per 15 minutes: 170

Exercise units per 15 minutes: 3

FIRST DO THIS

Many newcomers don't bother to use the instructional videos that come with Tae-Bo kits, according to Reber. That's a mistake because failing to learn how to do the moves properly increases the chance of injury. Also, don't kick higher than the height that feels comfortable or natural, especially at first.

MAXIMIZING CALORIE BURN

Focus and *form* are two buzzwords for getting the most out of Tae-Bo. Contract your abdominal muscles when punching and kicking, and be careful not to fully extend your arms or legs, which could injure your joints. Don't just flail your limbs when performing moves. Instead, think about the point in space at which you're aiming a punch or kick.

"It's all about focus and how much you get into the workout. If you focus on the muscles you're working, you will get much better results," Reber says.

CUSTOMIZE YOUR WORKOUT AND MAKE IT FUN

With so many Tae-Bo tapes on the market, it's easy to keep your workouts fresh. Feel like doing a basic, no-frills workout? Try one of the Tae-Bo in-studio tapes. Want more company and spontaneity? Plug in one of the "Tae-Bo Live" videos.

If you want to tone specific body parts, the

Tae-Bo "focus" series includes workouts aimed at the abdominals, buttocks, and upper body. And for more variety, Blanks has released Tae-Bo "full-contact" video workouts, which include the use of a punching bag and gloves and incorporate more self-defense–type moves.

Reber says it's also fun to do some of the Tae-Bo moves in a swimming pool because the water increases the resistance against the muscles and boosts the toning benefits.

WORKOUT ESSENTIALS

▶ If you don't plan to do high-impact moves such as running or jumping, do the workout barefoot on a carpeted floor. Without shoes, your feet can grip the floor better and help you keep your balance. If you want to increase the intensity by adding more propulsion moves, light-weight shoes are best; heavy shoes can put stress on your joints.

EXERCISE SENSE AND ETIQUETTE

Once you've learned the basics, review your instructional video once a month or so to be sure that you're still using perfect form. "I do this and really take my time with it because it's easy to fall into bad habits," says Reber.

Tai Chi ————————————————•

What probably comes to mind when you think of a tai chi class is a group of people standing in a field, moving their arms and legs gracefully through space. That's one form of this low-impact, low-intensity regimen that devotees say helps them release tension and focus their minds.

The slow, flowing movements can help build strength and balance, says Dr. Harmer. "The way the program is structured is really important because it can very gently lead people into using their bodies, particularly those who haven't been doing that for a while," he says.

Although it seems like a slow dance, tai chi is actually a martial art. The latest trend in tai chi is a "harder" version that emphasizes more powerful movements and higher intensity but remains low-impact. "Tai chi can really get your heart rate up and work every muscle in your body," says Saffell, who is featured in an exercise video that focuses on tai chi.

Learning moves such as "repulse the monkey" and "embrace the tiger" also offers a mental challenge. "It's a study, a lifelong journey," says Saffell. "In any kind of study, consistency is important." She recommends using tai chi as a cross-training workout with other aerobic or strength-training activities.

Prouty likes tai chi's ability to both improve balance and teach students to focus on the power of the body.

YOUR TAI CHI WORKOUT PRESCRIPTION

Beginner: 15 to 30 minutes, 1 day a week
Intermediate: 30 to 45 minutes, 2 or 3 days a week

Advanced: Up to 60 minutes, 2 or 3 days a week

Calorie burn per 15 minutes: 68
Exercise units per 15 minutes: 1

FIRST DO THIS

"If you're new to tai chi, you should find an instructor you are comfortable with to teach you what to do and how to breathe," says Prouty. "You need to leave your troubles behind and focus on the workout because it requires a lot of mental concentration." Be sure to let the instructor know if you have neck, back, hip, or knee problems.

MAXIMIZING CALORIE BURN

To get the most fat-burning potential out of tai chi, remember that every move has a purpose. "Think about what you are doing, and concentrate on the muscle," says Saffell. "It's all about putting the mind into the muscle."

Be sure to follow the posture and form instructions recommended by the leader. Generally, in martial arts, you should keep your knees bent and your abs contracted in order to perform powerful moves safely.

CUSTOMIZE YOUR WORKOUT AND MAKE IT FUN

According to Saffell, thinking about what the individual moves represent helps keep tai chi workouts fresh. "Many of the movements represent how animals move in nature," she says. "Everything is about balance—masculine and feminine, hard and soft—and also about the elements—fire, water, metal, and earth."

Most tai chi workouts are highly choreographed. Try to clear your mind and focus on your body as one movement flows into the next.

WORKOUT ESSENTIALS

▶ It's best to ask your instructor what kind of shoes are recommended. If you're studying the "harder" form, cross-training shoes that provide support for lateral movements may be best. However, some instructors of traditional tai chi recommend slipperlike shoes, such as a ballet shoe, or any lightweight shoe with a smooth, flexible sole. Some people feel more comfortable in socks or bare feet. The instructor can give you additional information.

▶ Wear a top that lets you see your muscles move so you can be aware of your form, says Saffell. Loose, comfortable workout pants, shorts, or leggings are fine for the lower body.

EXERCISE SENSE AND ETIQUETTE

Don't feel that you need to stand in the front of the class. Often, even if you can't mimic the instructor's moves, you can still follow along with your classmates.

Treadmill Workouts

If you like to run but your joints rebel at the pounding, you may be surprised at the intensity of a walking workout on a treadmill. By programming the treadmill for an incline, you can burn as many calories as you could by running.

"I sometimes walk on the treadmill, and I'm constantly amazed at how difficult it can be," says Dr. Olson. "When I increase the incline, I use my abs, lower back, and glutes, and even though I'm walking, I'm putting out every bit as much energy as I do when I run."

Treadmills provide a wide variety of options and can be programmed to meet your particular needs, whether you're new to exercise or an elite athlete. If you're just starting out, you can walk at a slow pace on a level surface. As you become fitter, you can increase the pace, the incline, or both so that you can keep your heart rate in your target zone.

If you decide to pick up the pace and run on the treadmill, the cushioning provided by the treadmill track makes it slightly more forgiving than running on pavement.

YOUR TREADMILL WORKOUT PRESCRIPTION

Beginner: 20 to 30 minutes, 3 days a week

Intermediate: 30 to 45 minutes, 3 to 5 days a week

Advanced: 45 minutes or more, 5 days a week, allowing adequate time for rest and recovery

Calorie burn per 15 minutes: Walking at 3 mph, 55; walking at 4 mph, 85; walking/jogging at 5 mph, 136

Exercise units per 15 minutes: 1 to 2, depending on intensity

FIRST DO THIS

If you're used to walking or running outside, increase the incline on the treadmill to 1 to 2 percent to more closely simulate outdoor conditions.

MAXIMIZING CALORIE BURN

Many treadmills have programs that show your heart rate. If yours has this feature, use it to help stay within your target zone. If there's no readout on the treadmill, check your pulse occasionally or follow the perceived exertion rule: You should be breathing at a rate that allows you to carry on a conversation but not to sing.

If you attempt to walk too fast, in excess of the 4.5 mph range, you may find that you begin to feel awkward and somewhat out of control. Dr. Olson says that at that point, it can actually feel less awkward if you start to jog. If you're not used to jogging on a treadmill, take it slowly, adjusting the speed so that you alternate walking and jogging, and give yourself time to become comfortable.

Interval training can help boost the number of calories you burn on a treadmill. After warming up, walk fast or jog for a minute or two, slow down for a minute, and then pick up the pace again. If you enjoy challenging interval workouts, however, don't do them on consecutive days because your body needs extra time to recover. Instead, pick a more moderate activity for the day after an interval workout.

CUSTOMIZE YOUR WORKOUT AND MAKE IT FUN

Sometimes distraction is the key to sticking with a routine like treadmill workouts. If you can read while you're walking, try that, or turn on the TV or don some headphones and listen to music or a recorded book.

Some treadmills have lap counters so you can track your "progress," which can help motivate you.

If you run, be sure to pace yourself. Pushing too hard can lead to fatigue. "If it doesn't feel good, it's probably not something you'll want to keep doing. That doesn't mean don't push yourself, but you should listen to your body," says Tomasetti.

WORKOUT ESSENTIALS

▶ Even though you're not walking on pavement, you still need a pair of well-fitting walking or running shoes. Some stores that specialize in athletic shoes have trained salespeople who can analyze your walking or running gait and help you find the perfect shoes, which may help you avoid injury.

▶ A good sports bra and clothing that breathes are also important.

▶ Don't forget water. You need to drink while you're on the treadmill to stay hydrated during and after your workout.

EXERCISE SENSE AND ETIQUETTE

If you're used to running outdoors, it can take a while to get used to the sensation of a surface's moving under you rather than your moving over the ground. Jog for only as long as you feel comfortable, and use the handrails if that makes you feel safer.

Water Aerobics

Even if swimming is not your thing, you can still get a heart-pumping, joint-friendly workout in a pool. Aerobics performed in water will help you tone your muscles, burn calories, and, as a bonus, have a great time!

"Once they try water aerobics, women just love it—it's a lot of fun and doesn't feel like work at all, although it gives you a great workout," says Prouty.

Offered by community recreation centers, health clubs, and some senior centers, water aerobics classes are especially popular among people with joint pain because working out in water elevates the heart rate but is easy on the joints. Yet because the water provides resistance, the workouts help tone muscles.

HOW THEY DID IT

She Got a Treadmill and Lost 60 Pounds

Patricia Deener of Mason City, Illinois, was once so loath to climb on a scale that she relegated hers to the garage. Then something happened to make it clear that her excess weight could cut her life short. So she cast out her steady diet of junk food and lost 60 pounds, gaining a new self-image in the process.

In September 1997, we took my oldest son, Patrick, to college. His room was on the third floor of the dorm. After the final flight, I felt a funny feeling in my heart. And it wasn't the anxiety a mother feels when she leaves a child at college for the first time.

Climbing those stairs was a serious physical effort. I carried 167 pounds on my 5-foot-3-inch frame. I took a good, hard look at myself and realized that my eating habits were all wrong. I picked up some books on weight loss. I learned to set small, reasonable weight-loss goals. I knew losing weight wouldn't happen overnight.

In October, I started buying healthier snacks, like bananas, cereal, and popcorn. I started walking outdoors, too. After 1 week, I went into the garage to climb on the scale. I'd lost 2 pounds! I realized I did have what it takes to lose weight. I went from a cautious, intimidated woman to a rarin'-to-go super chick with the willpower, self-esteem, and desire to beat this thing. On the 1-month anniversary of the first weigh-in in my garage, I was elated to discover I'd lost 10 pounds.

Junk-food habits once saddled Patricia with painful extra weight.

Yet even greater challenges awaited me. On the morning of December 11, 1997, I answered the phone and heard the words "Dad died." Things would never be the same.

I don't know why, but something motivated me to ask for a treadmill for Christmas that year. Even though I'd walked outside for 3 months, that first day on the treadmill was a killer. But I stuck with it, and I saw constant improvement.

I kept on with the treadmill and eating healthier and, in the spring of 1998—8 months after my first garage weigh-in—I had lost 50 pounds. In the following weeks, I proceeded to lose 10 more pounds. I've gone from 167 to 107 pounds, and I've maintained my loss ever since!

By August 1998, I was able to walk on the treadmill for 3 miles at a pace of nearly 4 mph. And in May 2000, I added a light treadmill jog to my routine, another milestone.

Now, at age 47, I've kept the weight off for more than 3 years, and I feel better than I have since high school.

You can take classes or do workouts on your own by running, walking, marching, and kicking underwater while moving your arms. Some women even "run" laps through the water, with their feet never touching the bottom of the pool.

A new breed of water fitness classes is emerging, says Nottingham. She incorporates sports drills into her water classes, having the students toss balls, do sprints, and work on balance, agility, and endurance. "It's a tough workout, but it's also a lot of fun," she says.

YOUR WATER AEROBICS WORKOUT PRESCRIPTION

Beginner: 20 to 30 minutes, 3 days a week

Intermediate: 30 to 45 minutes, 3 to 5 days a week

Advanced: 45 minutes or more, 5 days a week, allowing adequate time for rest and recovery

Calorie burn per 15 minutes: 68 to 135, depending on intensity

Exercise units per 15 minutes: 1 or 2, depending on intensity

FIRST DO THIS

When you get into the pool for your first water aerobics class, be sure you're in water that's deep enough to suit your fitness level. The lower your body is in the water, the more resistance there is against your muscles.

"You can easily lose the challenge if your torso is out of the water," says Dr. Olson. She recommends keeping only your neck and head above water and, if you're comfortable doing so, working where your feet can't touch the bottom of the pool.

MAXIMIZING CALORIE BURN

Along with working out in deeper water, there are all sorts of gadgets to make water aerobics more challenging, including webbed gloves that increase resistance for your hands and arms in the water.

For a tough workout, try "running" laps in the pool. Strap on a foam flotation belt (many pools provide them) and head to the deep end. You'll get a workout that is surprisingly taxing to your legs and buttocks muscles.

CUSTOMIZE YOUR WORKOUT AND MAKE IT FUN

Water aerobics workouts are often enjoyable social gatherings performed to music. That doesn't mean that they're not hard workouts, but there's just something about working out in the water that makes you smile, says Prouty. The "toys" used in classes—kickboards, "noodles," gloves, and water dumbbells—add to the fun factor.

There are many water aerobics videos on the market, some of which even feature kickboxing moves. Many come packaged with instructional audiocassettes so that you can watch the moves on the video outside the pool and then play the accompanying cassette (some are just music; some are music and cues) at the pool and follow along. Collage Video (800-433-6769; www.collagevideo.com) carries a variety of water aerobics tapes.

WORKOUT ESSENTIALS

▶ A comfortable, well-fitting swimsuit is a must. If you're not comfortable in just a bathing suit, you can wear a T-shirt over it.

▶ For outdoor classes, slather on plenty of sunscreen, and if your instructor agrees, wear sunglasses that provide UV protection.

▶ If you're taking an organized class, ask your instructor if you need to take along a flotation or resistance device such as a noodle or a flotation belt.

EXERCISE SENSE AND ETIQUETTE

When you're in the pool, stand far enough away from your classmates so that you can move your arms and legs freely in all directions without hitting anyone.

Yoga ●

Yoga has become so popular lately that there's now a yoga workout available for nearly everyone. Whether your approach is strictly physical or you enjoy yoga's spir-

itual and stress-relieving benefits, there's an instructor, class, style, or video out there for you.

After a yoga class, you'll feel relaxed and balanced, with your muscles loose and strong. As you gain strength and progress through the movements, yoga can even offer some aerobic benefits. "Yoga builds awareness of your own body, your own rhythm, your own cycle—but not through rules or by forcing yourself. It helps you begin to adapt how you live to a healthier way of life," says John Schumacher, a certified Iyengar yoga instructor and founder of Unity Woods Yoga Centers near Washington, D.C.

YOUR YOGA WORKOUT PRESCRIPTION

Beginner: One or two classes a week, plus 20 minutes of practice on other days

Intermediate: One or two classes a week, plus 30 minutes of practice on other days

Advanced: One class a week, plus 60 minutes or more of practice on other days

Calorie burn per 15 minutes: 45
Exercise units per 15 minutes: $\frac{1}{2}$

FIRST DO THIS

Before you sign up for a class or purchase a video, it's a good idea to spend some time researching the various types of yoga and evaluating your level of strength and flexibility.

Some types of yoga are athletic and require quite of bit of strength.

When you're starting out, find a beginner-level class so that you learn the intricacies of proper posture, says Roberts. "If you can't do that, try an introductory-level video," she says. "When you're doing the video, try to be somewhere where you can see yourself in a mirror or, failing that, in the glass of a framed picture."

MAXIMIZING CALORIE BURN

Yoga exercises are commonly called poses, and the standing poses will burn the most calories. In Iyengar yoga, beginners start with standing poses and then, as they gain strength and flexibility, work toward more complex ones. This type of yoga encourages the use of blocks, straps, and other tools to help students maintain good form while in a pose.

Some yoga practices can raise your heart rate enough to be aerobic, but don't expect that during your first few months. Schumacher says that it takes time to build up to the point where you can perform yoga that vigorously. "To work at that level, you either have to be young and strong already, or you have to build up your strength to sustain that kind of action without injury," he says.

Some yoga purists believe that it's not necessary to cross-train with aerobic activi-

ties in order to gain fitness and promote weight loss. However, Dr. Olson recommends supplementing yoga a few days a week with exercises that elevate and maintain a higher heart rate for sustained periods of time.

CUSTOMIZE YOUR WORKOUT AND MAKE IT FUN

If you sign up for yoga classes, your instructor will help you design a practice that best suits your needs and abilities. For instance, if you can't bend over and touch the floor with your hands, the instructor will show you how to use a block so that you can get into the pose safely.

There are also many yoga videos on the market that target specific needs, such as toning a specific body part, reducing stress, increasing flexibility, or promoting weight loss.

Some forms of yoga include poses aimed at helping women through different stages of life, including menopause. "There are practices for the menstrual cycle, for premenopause, for menopause, and for postmenopause," says Schumacher. "Hormonally, women (and men, to a lesser extent) go through times when their body chemistry is different, and yoga practice recognizes this."

Schumacher also says that anything that lengthens and balances your spine is beneficial. Think of it as the channel for energy in your body.

WORKOUT ESSENTIALS

▶ Wear comfortable clothing that allows your instructor to see the outline of your body and determine whether you are in good alignment. If possible, wear some-thing that exposes your knees and elbows. Choose clothing made of natural fabrics that allow your skin to breathe.

EXERCISE SENSE AND ETIQUETTE

Arrive on time so you don't disturb a class in progress, and don't wear perfume or jewelry.

CHAPTER 10

FIT NOT FAT BASICS:
SCULPT AND STRENGTHEN MUSCLES

Shopping for bathing suits in front of three-way mirrors may give you the sense that gravity has it in for you. Now's your turn to make that law of nature work for you, not against you.

The second basic component of the Fit Not Fat Exercise Plan, weight and strength training, is the only type of exercise that can markedly increase muscle strength and tone and improve body composition—all helpful in counteracting gravity's post-40 pull. Although aerobic exercises can increase calories burned and help you lose weight, they don't effectively target your metabolism-boosting muscle.

At its essence, weight training couldn't be simpler. You pick up and lower weights, using your arms, legs, back, abdomen, and posterior. When a certain amount of weight becomes easy, you increase the challenge. As your sessions progress, your muscles prepare themselves for the extra demand. In the process, the muscles of your arms, legs, back, abdomen, and backside automatically become firmer, leaner, and stronger. You look and feel fit, not fat. Plus, weight training gives you the strength to enjoy your daily activities with less fatigue.

Exercising with weights (as well as other weight-bearing activities, like walking, running, and aerobics) also stimulates bone to generate new cells, preserving bone density and reducing your risk of hip fractures later in life. As a bonus, weight training improves your mood, self-esteem, and thinking ability.

BESTBET
Check with Your Doctor

Before starting a strength-training program, you should check with your health care provider to make sure you have no medical problems that prevent you from safely doing the exercises. He or she should check for erratic heartbeats, severe high blood pressure, or other cardiovascular ailments; uncontrolled diabetes; or muscle, joint, or bone conditions that would be worsened by lifting weights.

Slim Down without Bulking Up

The step-by-step weight-training routines in this chapter won't leave you looking muscle-bound and masculine. They're designed for women who want to increase strength and tone up. The workouts aren't nearly intense enough to create the heft achieved by people who work out for hours a day, several days a week, says the designer of this program, Arthur Weltman, Ph.D., director of the exercise physiology program at the University of Virginia in Charlottesville.

Plus, women secrete only small amounts of testosterone, the hormone that the body uses to make muscles bigger and that occurs in far larger amounts in men. So you'll be "toned and muscular, but you won't be hypertrophied (bulky) to the same degree that you'll see in male bodybuilders," says Dr. Weltman.

Be prepared, though. You may actually see the scales edge upward a bit after you start lifting weights since muscle is denser than fat and takes up less space than fat. As you add weight training to your program, you'll be better off tracking your progress by the way your clothes fit (more loosely) or by taking your waist measurement than by weighing yourself.

Guidelines for Your Muscle-Toning Sessions

On the Fit Not Fat Exercise Plan, shoot for at least 20 minutes of weight training two or three times a week. During your Master Plan goal-setting session, pick 2 or 3 days when you're most likely to hit the weights, either at the gym or in your own basement, and write them into your schedule. Check out routines that target common problem areas: your belly (page 175); or your legs, hips, and butt (page 185); or your arms and chest (page 197). Or tone your whole body (page 209). Try one, or mix and match a few through the week, and you'll see why so many women swear by weight training for fast, visible results.

If you can, you should work out at a gym, especially if you are a beginner. Your gym may have the benefit of a trainer who can guide you through the program the first few times and give you direction that can help you even when you can't make it to the gym. Also, gym equipment allows you to do a greater variety of exercises with more weights as your fitness level increases, says Dr. Weltman.

But some days, a trip to the gym may as well be a trip to the moon. So, many workouts include two exercises that provide similar benefits—one you can do at home, and one at the gym. Others require no special equipment and can be done at either place. Either way, doing the exercises consistently is more important than *where* you do them.

For most of these exercises, if you're a beginner, you should use a weight that you can lift 12 to 15 times. When you can easily lift it more than that, move up to a heavier weight that you can lift only 10 to 12 times, to give your muscles a new challenge. (While instructions accompany each photo, it's also a good idea to follow the directions printed on any particular machines you use, says Dr. Weltman. Even better, get assistance from a trained member of the gym staff.)

Setting Up a Home Gym

A home gym is a great way to work out without a big investment or to keep up with your workout sessions when the roads are icy or you can't get to the gym for some other reason. Any workout area that's safe, private, and well-ventilated will do. You don't have to spend a lot of money. You can assemble the following components for under $200.

A pair of handheld dumbbells. Depending on your beginning fitness level, pairs of 3-, 5-, or 10-pound weights will be most useful for working your upper body. *Cost:* About $10 for a pair of 3-pound weights to $16 for a pair of 10-pound weights.

Ankle weights. These come in a variety of weights and, used properly, give your legs a good workout. *Cost:* About $10 for a pair of 2-pound weights or about $17 for a pair of 5-pound weights.

A padded weight bench. Look for a sturdy, stable bench that's long enough to support you from head to butt. *Cost:* About $75 from sporting goods stores and catalogs.

A padded barbell. Equipment like the Body Bar is useful for chest presses and "good morning" exercises. *Cost:* Costs and weights vary, but a 9-pound bar is about $30.

A cushioned exercise mat. This will make crunches and other floor exercises more comfortable. *Cost:* It will set you back as little as $15. For more details on exercise mats, see "Cool Tool," page 235.

A sturdy armless chair. This comes in handy for a number of exercises.

A full-length mirror. This lets you check your form as you lift and train properly, helping to avoid injury. *Cost:* About $10.

Safety Tips for Women over 40

As more women have started lifting weights in the past few decades, more have injured themselves in the process. Injuries range from strains and sprains to cuts and bruises, fractures, or nerve damage.

Don't let that list scare you. *Do* practice safe lifting.

Warm up and stretch before each weight-training session. Do 5 minutes of easy aerobic activity—like walking and swinging your arms—followed by some simple stretches. For details on how to stretch safely, see page 225.

Work out with a buddy. Or make sure someone's around to offer help if necessary. The encouragement is useful, too.

Stay in control of the weights. If you jerk them up and down, you put more strain on your joints, tendons, and ligaments. Plus, that allows momentum to help propel the weights, instead of your working your mus-

cles. Instead, move the weights only as fast as you can control the movement, no faster. If it helps, count to four as you lower them and again as you raise them.

Breathe normally. If you hold your breath while raising and lowering a weight, you can trigger what's called a "Valsalva maneuver" in your body. This "drives your blood pressure through the roof," Dr. Weltman says. (Performed regularly, the Valsalva maneuver can increase the risk of a cardiovascular event—heart attack or stroke—in some people.) It's best to exhale when you curl the weight up and inhale when you lower it.

Track Your Progress

Once you add regular weight training to the Fit Not Fat Exercise Plan, you should start to see and feel the difference in as little as 2 weeks.

To chart your progress, write down which exercises you did during each workout, how much weight you lifted, how many repetitions you completed, how many sets of these repetitions you did, and how your body feels afterward.

Your training journal will show you how you're progressing, says Dr. Weltman. Some women may not think they see a high degree of muscle definition when they look in the mirror, but if they log the weights they use, they can say "Look at how much stronger I've gotten," he says.

Reclaim Your Waist and Flatten Your Abs

As discussed in chapter 1, even women who manage to maintain their weight may notice a thickening middle as they approach or pass the age of 40. And if you've ever been pregnant, the baby growing in your uterus pushed and stretched your abdominal muscles outward, leaving them less taut than before.

Stress, too, contributes to the accumulation of belly fat. The hormone cortisol makes you want to eat after stressful episodes, then promotes the accumulation of fat around your midsection.

Unfortunately, situps alone won't flatten your abs.

"You can do thousands of situps and not lose any fat," says Dr. Weltman. Situps strengthen your muscles but don't burn many calories. Furthermore, it's not possible to spot reduce.

Does that mean your midsection will persist for as long as the memory of that awful bridesmaid dress you had to wear in 1984? Not at all.

By combining the Fit Not Fat Food Plan in part 3 with some form of regular aerobic activity from chapter 9, you can shed fat all over your body, including your belly. The fol-lowing strength-training exercises, recommended by Dr. Weltman, will tone and tighten the muscles around your abdomen and lower back so that firmer muscles surrounding your midsection will become more noticeable. A stronger abdomen will also improve your posture and help you carry yourself more upright, further improving your appearance, Dr. Weltman points out.

The muscles you'll be working with these exercises include:

▶ The rectus abdominis, which runs up the center of your belly and gives a tight stomach the "washboard" look

▶ The obliques, which are at the sides of your abdomen

▶ The erector spinae muscles running up and down the center of your back; you need to work these back muscles to keep them balanced in strength with your abdominal muscles.

Do these exercises two or three times a week, alone or in combination with other workouts in this section.

MUSCLE TARGETED **RECTUS ABDOMINIS**

HOME EXERCISE • **Crunches**

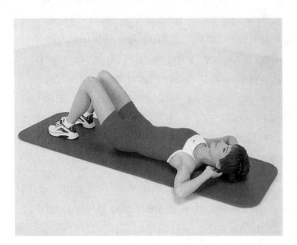

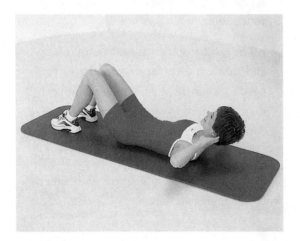

Lie on your back with your knees bent slightly so your feet are flat on the floor and spaced shoulder-width apart. Lightly support your head by placing your fingertips behind your ears, pointing your elbows out to the sides.

Lift your head, shoulders, and upper back off the floor, keeping your abdominal muscles tight and maintaining a fist-width space between your chin and chest. You don't need to sit all the way up—just lift your upper body a few inches. Hold for a moment and slowly lower yourself to complete the repetition.

For an advanced version, do your crunches while holding a 10-pound weight plate or dumbbell to your chest.

REPETITIONS

Beginner · 3 sets of 10 repetitions

Experienced · 3 sets of 10 repetitions while holding a weight for extra resistance

DO IT RIGHT

▶ Don't pull up on your head as you lift your torso.

▶ Press the small of your back into the floor as you lift yourself.

▶ Don't rest your head on the floor between repetitions.

▶ Raise and lower yourself in a controlled manner, without jerking your body or bouncing.

MUSCLE TARGETED **RECTUS ABDOMINIS**

GYM EXERCISE • **Ab machine**

Adjust the seat so it's the appropriate height, and choose the desired weight. You should be sitting straight up.

Place your chest against the padded bar. Lightly wrap your hands around the bar. Slowly lean forward, using your abdominal muscles to push yourself down and forward as far as you can comfortably go. Pause a moment, then slowly lean back to the beginning point.

REPETITIONS

Beginner • 12 to 15 repetitions at a weight you can do comfortably only that many times

Experienced • 10 to 12 repetitions at a higher weight

DO IT RIGHT

▶ Don't bend your head forward as you push your body down.

▶ Don't use your hands to pull the bar forward.

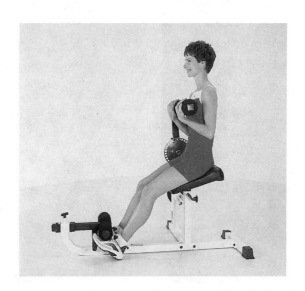

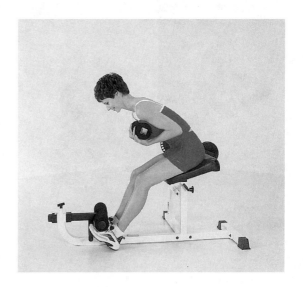

MUSCLES TARGETED

INTERNAL AND **EXTERNAL OBLIQUES** AND **RECTUS ABDOMINIS**

HOME EXERCISE • **Crossover crunches**

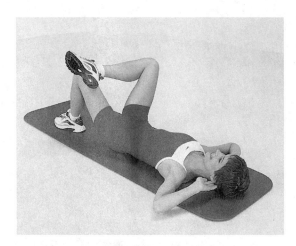

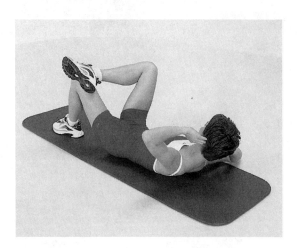

Lie on your back with your knees bent and your feet flat on the floor. Rest your right ankle on your left knee and your hands lightly behind your head with your fingertips behind your ears and your elbows pointing out to the sides.

Slowly lift your left shoulder toward your right knee, raising your upper back off the floor and twisting slightly. Be sure to keep your elbows out through the whole motion. Pause, then slowly lower yourself. Repeat until you've done all your repetitions, then switch to the other side.

REPETITIONS

Beginner · 3 sets of 10

Experienced · 3 sets of 10 with a 10-pound weight held to your chest

DO IT RIGHT

▸ Don't bounce up and down.

▸ Don't pull on your neck as you're lifting.

MUSCLES TARGETED
INTERNAL AND **EXTERNAL OBLIQUES** AND **RECTUS ABDOMINIS**

GYM EXERCISE • **Rotary torso machine** •

Sit in the seat and set the weight where you want it. It should be heavy enough to challenge your obliques, but not so heavy that you need to use your arms to help swivel the machine. Adjust the machine so it swivels your hips and legs all the way to the left, with your upper body still facing forward.

Grasp the handles, lean into the chest pads, and slowly rotate your lower body to the front, pulling with the muscles on the sides of your abdomen. Pause and slowly return. When you've done all your repetitions, adjust the machine so your lower body swivels the other way, and repeat.

REPETITIONS

Beginner · 12 to 15 repetitions

Experienced · 10 to 12 repetitions with increased weight

DO IT RIGHT

▶ Use your abdomen, not your arms, to pull yourself into position.

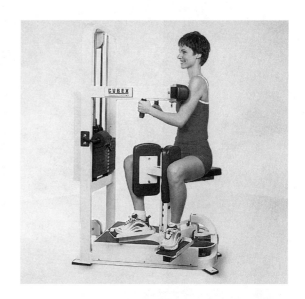

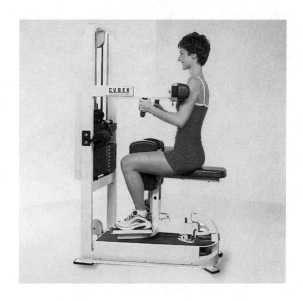

HOME EXERCISE • **Single-knee lifts**

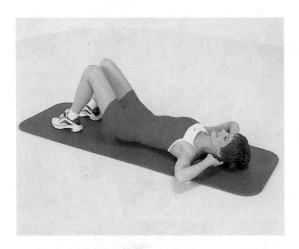

Lie on your back, placing your feet flat on the floor and your fingertips loosely behind your head. Lift your right knee and torso at the same time, bringing both elbows toward your knee. Pause at the top, then lower your torso and knee back to the starting position. Repeat with the opposite leg.

REPETITIONS

Beginner · 10 to 12 repetitions

Experienced · 12 to 15 repetitions

DO IT RIGHT

▶ Don't tug on your head with your hands.

▶ Move in a steady, controlled motion.

MUSCLES TARGETED
RECTUS ABDOMINIS, HIP FLEXORS, AND QUADRICEPS

GYM EXERCISE • **Hanging knee raises** •

This exercise is done on a device bearing two parallel, padded troughs at shoulder level with handles sticking up on the far end of each pad, called a "captain's chair." Stand between the pads, step up onto the foot rails, rest your forearms on the grooved pads, and grasp the upright handles at the front of the pads with your hands.

Step off the foot rails so your legs hang straight down and all your weight hangs from your forearms. Slowly lift your knees toward your chest, briefly pause when they're at their highest point, then slowly lower them until they're hanging straight.

REPETITIONS

Beginner · 8 to 10 repetitions

Experienced · 12 to 15 repetitions

DO IT RIGHT

▶ Don't swing your feet up and back. Stay in control of the movement the whole time.

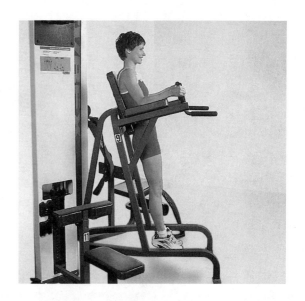

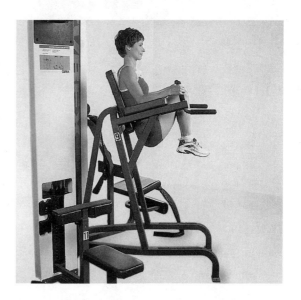

HOME EXERCISE • **Land swim**

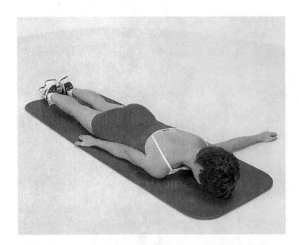

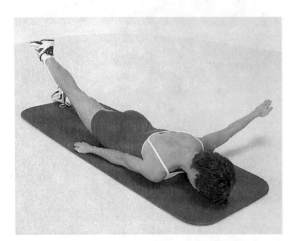

Lie facedown on a padded mat with your legs out straight and the tops of your feet against the floor. Keep your right arm down at your side, parallel to your body, and put your left arm out to your side at a 90-degree angle.

Slowly raise your right leg and left arm and shoulder into the air as high as you can. Keep your right leg straight as it rises. Pause momentarily, then lower your arm and leg. Do all the repetitions on that side and switch to your right arm and left leg.

REPETITIONS

Beginner · 10 to 12 repetitions

Experienced · 12 to 15 repetitions

DO IT RIGHT

▶ Don't tilt your head back.

▶ Keep your toes pointed away from your body.

▶ Lift in a controlled movement.

MUSCLES TARGETED **ERECTOR SPINAE**

GYM EXERCISE • **Back machine** •

Adjust the seat or foot platform so it's in the appropriate position for you, and set the weight to the desired amount. Sit on the seat and fasten yourself in with the seat belt, if it's provided.

Cross your arms in front of your chest. Lean back against the pads behind your back. Without arching your back, slowly press against the pads and push them down. Pause briefly at the bottom, then slowly lean forward to the starting point.

REPETITIONS

Beginner · 12 to 15
Experienced · 10 to 12 at a higher weight

DO IT RIGHT

▶ Move slowly, and don't bob up and down.
▶ Don't arch your back or neck during the movement.

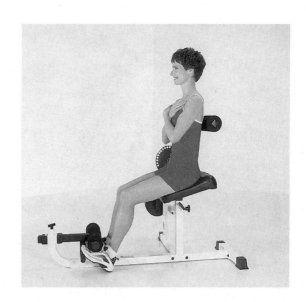

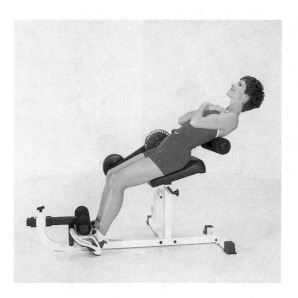

MUSCLES TARGETED **ERECTOR SPINAE**

HOME OR GYM EXERCISE • **Good morning**

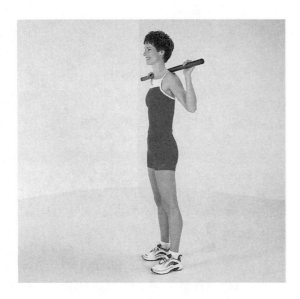

Stand with a barbell resting on your shoulders, your hands holding the bar with an overhand grip, spaced wider than shoulder-width apart. Your knees should be slightly bent.

Slowly bend at the waist until your torso is parallel to the floor, then slowly return to the starting position.

REPETITIONS

Beginner · 12 to 15 repetitions

Experienced · 10 to 12 repetitions at a higher weight

DO IT RIGHT

▶ Keep a firm grip on the bar.

▶ Keep looking up as you bend forward.

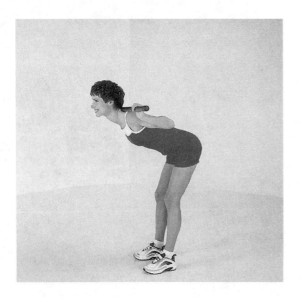

Reshape Your Legs, Hips, and Butt

When *Psychology Today* magazine surveyed readers about how they felt about their bodies, more than 3,400 women wrote back. While most (71 percent) were dissatisfied with the state of their abs, nearly as many (61 percent) were displeased with their hips or upper thighs.

Women are endowed with wider hips than men to accommodate childbearing, and we tend to store fat below the belt to use as fuel for possible pregnancies, whether we have children or not. These factors help contribute to the common "pear-shaped" silhouette that many women would rather see in the produce section than in their dressing room mirror.

Fortunately, this fat doesn't put women at as high a risk for coronary artery disease as fat around their abdomen, says Dr. Weltman. However, this below-the-belt fat "is not very metabolically active," he says, which means it's harder for your body to part with.

When combined with the Fit Not Fat Food Plan in part 3 and some form of aerobic activity from chapter 9, this portion of the 40-Plus Exercise Plan, designed by Dr. Weltman, can work wonders to shape up your lower half.

The following exercises will tone and tighten a soft butt and hips, firm up flabby thighs, and strengthen slack leg muscles. Not only will you feel better when there's a mirror behind you, but also you'll feel stronger when you're marching up the hills and flights of stairs in front of you.

The muscles you'll be working with these exercises include:

▶ The gluteus maximus, in your butt

▶ The adductor and abductor muscles, in your inner and outer thighs

▶ The quadriceps, along the fronts of your thighs

▶ The hamstrings, at the backs of the thighs

▶ The gastrocnemius and soleus muscles, in your calves

Do these exercises two or three times a week, alone or in combination with other workouts in this section.

MUSCLES TARGETED **QUADRICEPS**

HOME EXERCISE • **Seated leg lifts with ankle weights**

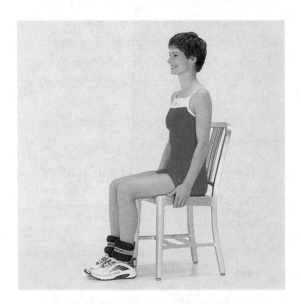

Attach an ankle weight to each leg, and sit on a sturdy chair or bench, your feet flat on the floor in front of you.

Holding the sides of the chair for support if necessary, slowly lift your left foot so your leg is straight in front of you. Pause briefly, then slowly lower your foot. Repeat with the opposite leg.

REPETITIONS

Beginner · 12 to 15 repetitions with each leg

Experienced · 10 to 12 repetitions with each leg at a higher weight

DO IT RIGHT

▶ Don't swing your legs up and down. Use a steady, controlled motion to lift the weight.

MUSCLES TARGETED **QUADRICEPS**

GYM EXERCISE • **Knee extension machine** •

Sit on the padded bench and fasten the seat belt, if available. Choose the desired weight and tuck your shins under the bottom pads that you'll push against to lift the weight. Grasp the handles near the seat.

Press both shins against the pads until your legs are straight in front of you. Pause momentarily and slowly lower the weight to the starting position.

REPETITIONS

Beginner · 12 to 15 repetitions

Experienced · 10 to 12 repetitions at a higher weight

DO IT RIGHT

▶ Use a steady motion, and don't rely on momentum to help.

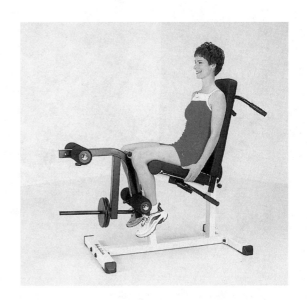

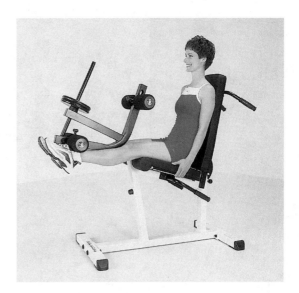

HOME EXERCISE • **Leg curls with ankle weights**

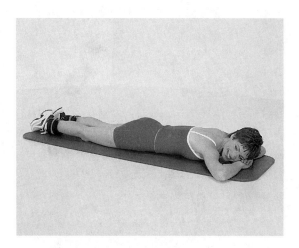

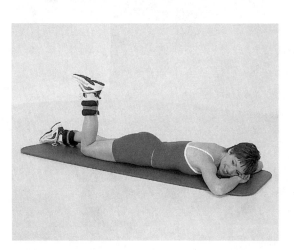

Attach ankle weights to your legs and lie facedown on an exercise mat. You can turn your head to one side, fold your arms, and rest your head on your arms.

Slowly lift your right foot toward your bottom until your leg is at a 90-degree angle. Pause briefly and slowly lower your foot back to the mat. Repeat with your other foot.

REPETITIONS

Beginner · 12 to 15 repetitions with each foot

Experienced · 10 to 12 repetitions with each foot at a higher weight

DO IT RIGHT

▶ Lie flat on your belly with your head resting on your crossed arms. Don't support your upper body on your elbows or arch your back.

▶ Keep your hips planted on the floor throughout the motion.

▶ Lift your foot only until your lower leg is pointed straight up in the air.

MUSCLES TARGETED **HAMSTRINGS**

GYM EXERCISE • **Leg curl machine** •

Set the weight to the desired amount and lie facedown on the padded bench. Tuck the backs of your lower legs under the pads that you'll press against to lift the weights, making contact with them just under your calves.

Press against the pads and pull them in an arc toward your buttocks as far as is comfortable. Pause for a moment, then steadily lower them to the starting position.

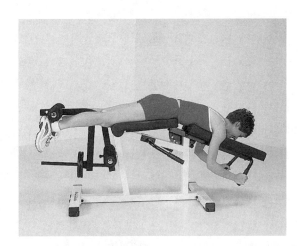

REPETITIONS

Beginner · 12 to 15 repetitions

Experienced · 10 to 12 repetitions at a higher weight

DO IT RIGHT

▶ You'll use less weight for this exercise than for the knee extension machine because the muscles behind your thighs aren't as strong as the ones on the front.

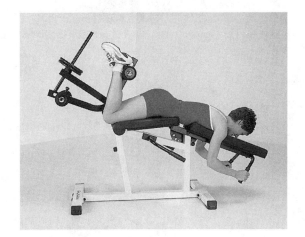

HOME AND GYM EXERCISE · **Calf raises**

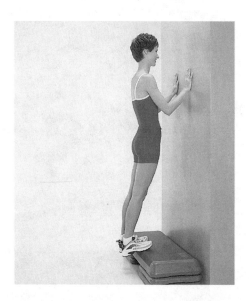

Stand on the edge of a step with your feet about hip-width apart, and ease your heels back over the edge so your weight is on your forefeet and your heels are below the level of the step. Beginners should try this first on a flat floor.

Touching a wall or holding a railing with one hand for balance if necessary, slowly rise on your toes, using your calf muscles to lift you. Pause momentarily, then slowly lower your heels to the starting position.

For an advanced version, hold a dumbbell in the hand that's not holding a wall or handrail for support.

REPETITIONS

Beginner · 12 to 15 without extra weight

Experienced · 10 to 12 with a dumbbell

DO IT RIGHT

▶ Don't lock your knees during the motion.

▶ Don't lean forward.

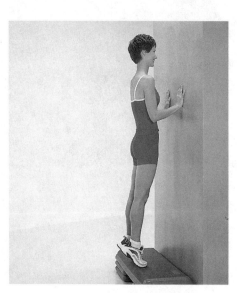

<u>MUSCLES TARGETED</u> **GLUTEUS MAXIMUS** AND **QUADRICEPS**

HOME EXERCISE • **Squats with dumbbells** •

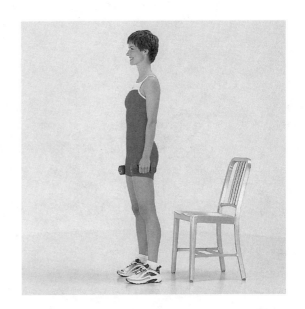

Stand with a chair directly behind you, your feet spaced a bit more than shoulder-width apart. Hold a pair of dumbbells to your sides.

Bend at your hips and knees and lower your bottom until it's almost touching the chair. Your back should be straight and your toes should stay visible past your knees at all times. When you get to the bottom of the motion, slowly stand back up.

REPETITIONS

Beginners • 12 to 15

Experienced • 10 to 12 at a higher weight

DO IT RIGHT

▶ If you have knee pain, lower yourself only partway to the chair.

▶ Don't let your knees go beyond your toes.

▶ You may also want to wear a compression wrap around your knees during this exercise if they hurt.

▶ If you work your way up to using high weights for squat exercises, you might consider using a weightlifting support belt around your waist and using a helper to spot you during the exercise.

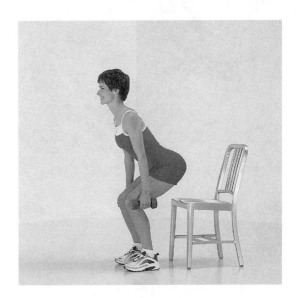

MUSCLES TARGETED **GLUTEUS MAXIMUS** AND **QUADRICEPS**

GYM EXERCISE • **Leg press machine**

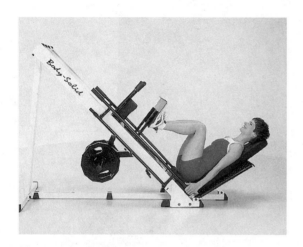

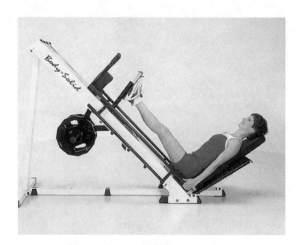

Set the appropriate weight on the machine and adjust the seat so your legs are bent at a 60- to 90-degree angle. Sit back in the seat and place your feet on the platform. If the machine has a mechanism that holds the weight until you're ready, release it and grasp the handles near your hands.

Press the platform with your feet until your legs are straight. Lower it back to the starting point. When you're finished with all your repetitions, set the mechanism that holds the weight back into place if necessary.

REPETITIONS

Beginners · 12 to 15 repetitions

Experienced · 10 to 12 repetitions at a higher weight

MUSCLES TARGETED **ABDUCTOR** AND **ADDUCTOR**

HOME EXERCISE • **Inner- and outer-thigh lifts with ankle weights**

Inner-thigh lift: Lie on your left side with your left leg extended. Your right leg should be bent, with your right foot flat on the floor behind your left knee. Bend your left arm and support your head with your left elbow resting on the ground to support you. Your right hand should be resting on the floor in front of you.

Use the muscles in your left inner thigh to lift your left foot at least 6 inches off the floor. Hold briefly and slowly lower it. Repeat all your repetitions, then switch to the other side.

Outer-thigh lift: Start in the same position as the previous exercise, but stretch both legs out straight. Keeping your top leg straight—the right one—raise it until it forms an 80-degree angle between your legs. The muscles on your outer thigh should be doing the work. Repeat through your repetitions, then switch sides.

REPETITIONS

Beginners · 10 to 12 repetitions

Experienced · 12 to 15 repetitions with a heavier weight

Inner-Thigh Lift

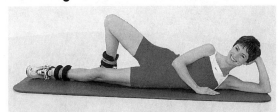

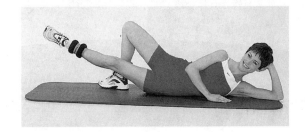

Outer-Thigh Lift

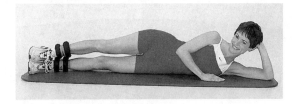

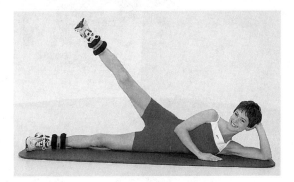

MUSCLES TARGETED **ABDUCTOR** AND **ADDUCTOR**

GYM EXERCISE • **Adduction and abduction cable pull**

Adduction

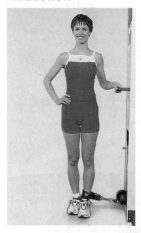 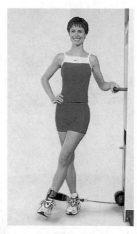

Abduction

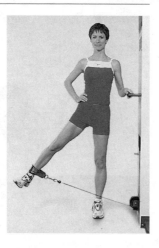

Adduction cable pull: Stand with your left side to the weight stack and select an appropriate weight. Fasten the padded cuff securely around your left ankle, then hold the hand rest with your left hand.

Stand with your feet less than shoulder-width apart, lift your left foot slightly, and sweep it to the right in front of your right foot. Your left foot will end up several inches to the right of your right foot; only move as far as is comfortable. Return to the starting position and repeat. When you're finished, remove the cuff, face the other way, and repeat with the cuff on the right foot.

Abduction cable pull: Stand with your left side to the weight stack and select an appropriate weight. Fasten the padded cuff securely around your right ankle, then hold the hand rest with your left hand.

Standing with your feet less than shoulder-width apart, pull your right foot out to the right side, keeping your leg extended. Pull as far as is comfortable. The cable should be running in front of your left leg. Return to the starting position and repeat. When finished, remove the cuff, face the other way, and repeat with the cuff on the left foot.

REPETITIONS

Beginners · 12 to 15

Experienced · 10 to 12 with a heavier weight

MUSCLE TARGETED **GLUTEUS MAXIMUS**

HOME EXERCISE • **Bent-leg kickbacks** •

Get on your hands and knees on a padded mat or thick carpet. Your back should be parallel with the floor and in a straight line with your head and neck. Place your hands under your shoulders and your knees under your hips, and point your face toward the floor through the entire exercise.

Slowly lift your right foot toward the ceiling as high as possible, which should bring your thigh slightly higher than your torso. At its highest point, your foot should be parallel to the ceiling. Tighten your buttocks to help in the lift.

Pause briefly, then lower your leg. Repeat all your repetitions and switch sides. This exercise also works your hamstrings.

REPETITIONS

Beginners · 12 to 15 repetitions

Experienced · 10 to 12 repetitions with an ankle weight

DO IT RIGHT

▶ Don't look up toward the ceiling or back toward your belly.

▶ Don't arch your back or lock your elbows.

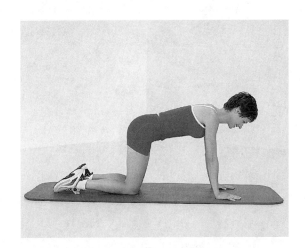

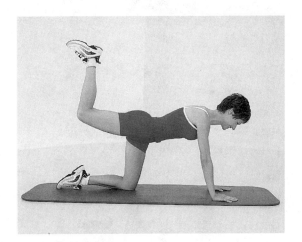

MUSCLE TARGETED **GLUTEUS MAXIMUS**

GYM EXERCISE • **Gluteal extension machine**

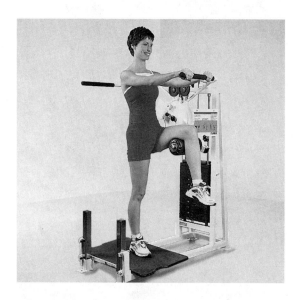

Set the weight to the proper amount, and adjust the padded peg that you'll be pressing against so it's about waist high. Grasp the handle on the machine with both hands and drape your left leg over the padded peg so it fits behind your left knee. Keep your right foot planted firmly on the platform of the machine.

Slowly push your left leg down and back, using the muscles in your buttocks and thigh to press against the pad. Keep pressing until your left leg is straight. Repeat through your repetitions and switch sides.

REPETITIONS

Beginner · 12 to 15 repetitions

Experienced · 10 to 12 repetitions with a higher weight

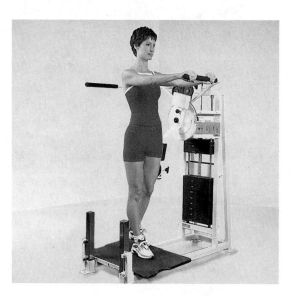

Tone Your Arms, Bustline, Upper Back, and Shoulders ●

Women who haven't worn a halter top since college would love to look good in sleeveless dresses, tank tops, and other torso-flattering styles. Adding a few resistance exercises to your toning program can help you sculpt sleeker back and shoulder muscles, lift and firm the bustline, get rid of bra lines and bulges, and tighten flabby upper arms. When larger-chested women shed fat all over and strengthen the chest muscles under the breasts, they can minimize their breasts. Women more modest in size can make their breasts appear somewhat larger by toning these chest muscles.

Plus, stronger shoulders, arms, and chest muscles will allow you to complete "activities of daily living" more easily, says Dr. Weltman. Whether you're hefting a toddler, dog food, kitty litter, or golf clubs, these muscles will help you do it better.

The muscles you'll be strengthening and toning with the exercises recommended by Dr. Weltman in this section include:

▶ The deltoids, at the outer corners of your shoulders

▶ The biceps, on the fronts of your upper arms

▶ The triceps, underneath your upper arms

▶ The trapezius, atop your shoulders at either side of your neck

▶ The latissimus dorsi, alongside your torso

▶ The pectorals, underneath your breasts

Do these exercises two or three times a week, alone or in combination with other workouts in this section.

MUSCLES TARGETED **PECTORALIS MAJOR** AND **DELTOIDS**

HOME AND GYM EXERCISE • **Chest presses with dumbbells**

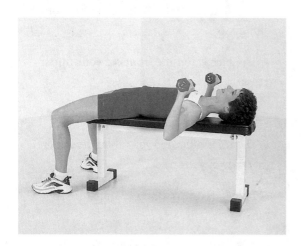

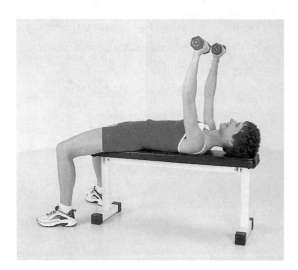

Lying back on a padded bench with your head resting on the bench, hold dumbbells over your chest. If you don't have a bench at home, lie on the floor in the same position. The weights should be pointed end-to-end and your elbows pointed out to the sides and to-ward the floor. Your feet should be flat on the floor to either side of the bench.

Slowly lift the dumbbells straight up as you extend your arms. Pause a moment, then slowly lower them to your chest.

REPETITIONS

Beginner · 12 to 15 repetitions

Experienced · 10 to 12 repetitions at a higher weight

DO IT RIGHT

▶ Avoid bouncing the weights off your chest.

▶ Keep the small of your back pressed down toward the bench.

MUSCLES TARGETED **PECTORALIS MAJOR** AND **FRONT DELTOIDS**

HOME EXERCISE • **Dumbbell flies**

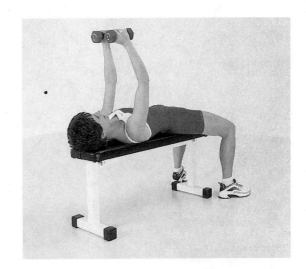

Lie on your back on a padded bench, your head resting on the bench and your feet flat on the floor to either side. If you don't have a bench at home, lie on a mat on the floor in the same position. Hold the dumbbells above your chest, with your arms slightly bent. Grasp the dumbbells so they're touching and their handles are parallel to each other. Your palms should be facing each other.

Keeping your arms slightly bent, slowly lower the weights out to your sides until your arms are at shoulder level, then slowly bring them back to the top. Imagine you're hugging and releasing an invisible barrel lying on the center of your chest.

REPETITIONS

Beginner · 12 to 15

Experienced · 10 to 12 at a higher weight

DO IT RIGHT

▶ Don't use too much weight when you first do this exercise because it can stress your elbows.

▶ Keep your arms slightly bent. Doing this with straightened arms puts you at greater risk of injury.

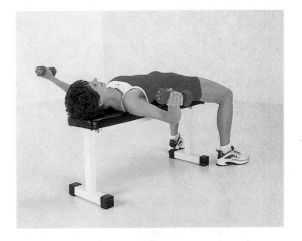

MUSCLES TARGETED **PECTORALIS MAJOR** AND **FRONT DELTOIDS**

GYM EXERCISE • **Fly machine**

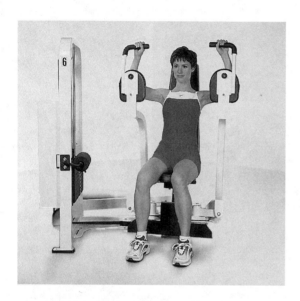

Adjust the seat to the proper height so your upper arms are perpendicular to your chest, and choose the desired weight. Sit down, use the seat belt if one is available, and lean back against the backrest. Place your forearms against the arm pads.

Slowly press against the pads with your forearms as far as you can, pushing them toward each other in front of your chest. Your forearms should remain vertical and parallel with each other through the whole movement. Pause, then slowly bring them back to the beginning position.

REPETITIONS

Beginner · 12 to 15

Experienced · 10 to 12 at a higher weight

DO IT RIGHT

▶ You should feel a little pull in your chest muscles at the starting position.

▶ Don't bend your head forward as you perform this move.

<u>MUSCLES TARGETED</u> **TRAPEZIUS, RHOMBOIDS,** AND **DELTOIDS**

HOME AND GYM EXERCISE • **Shoulder shrugs** •

Hold your dumbbells in front of you with an overhand grasp, letting them hang at arm's length in front of your upper thighs.

Keeping your arms straight, lift the weights by slowly raising your shoulders toward your ears, as if shrugging. Rotate your shoulders backward, then lower them to the starting point.

REPETITIONS

Beginner · 12 to 15 repetitions

Experienced · 10 to 12 repetitions at a higher weight

DO IT RIGHT

▶ Be sure you're using your shoulders to do the work and not your legs.

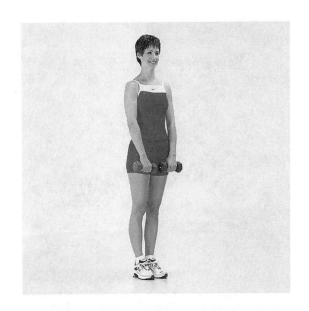

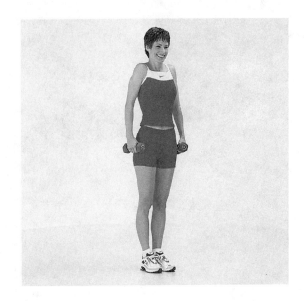

MUSCLES TARGETED **LATISSIMUS DORSI**

HOME EXERCISE • **Dumbbell pullovers**

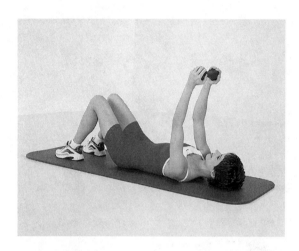

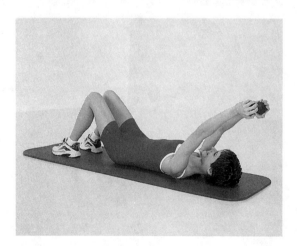

Lie on your back on an exercise mat, your legs bent and your feet flat on the mat about hip-width apart. Pick up a dumbbell, each hand clutching one knobby end. Hold the weight above your chest with both hands, your arms slightly bent.

Now slowly lower the weight in an arc behind your head, keeping your arms slightly bent. When the weight goes more than halfway to the floor, pause, then slowly bring the weight in an arc back to the starting point. This also works your chest muscles.

REPETITIONS

Beginner · 12 to 15

Experienced · 10 to 12 at a higher weight

DO IT RIGHT

▶ When your arms are out, don't lock your elbows.

▶ Press your lower back into the floor.

▶ Keep your feet hip-width apart.

MUSCLES TARGETED **LATISSIMUS DORSI**

GYM EXERCISE • **Lat pulldowns** •

If there is a brace, adjust the seat so your knees fit securely under it. Set the weight appropriately. Reach up and grasp the bar with an overhand grip, your hands wider than shoulder width.

Slowly pull the bar down to your upper chest, using the muscles in your upper back to do the pulling, instead of your arms. Pause at your chest, then slowly let the bar back up. This also works the biceps muscles.

REPETITIONS

Beginner · 12 to 15

Experienced · 10 to 12 at a higher weight

DO IT RIGHT

▶ Pull the bar to your upper chest, not the back of your neck. You're more likely to injure your neck if you draw the bar down behind your head.

▶ Stay in control of the bar—use your muscles, not momentum, to pull.

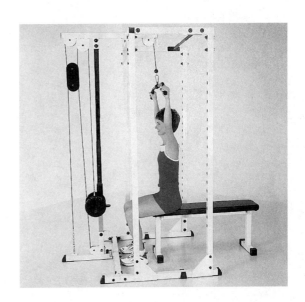

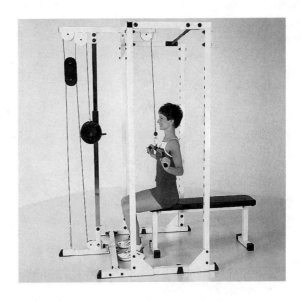

HOME AND GYM EXERCISE　•　**Biceps curls with dumbbells**

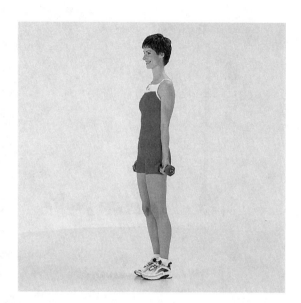

While standing, hold a dumbbell in each hand at thigh level, your palms facing outward and your feet shoulder-width apart. Keeping your elbows close to your body, slowly raise the weights toward your shoulders. Pause at the top, then slowly lower them to the starting point.

REPETITIONS

Beginner · 12 to 15

Experienced · 10 to 12 at a higher weight

DO IT RIGHT

▶ Stay in control of the weights, instead of letting momentum assist.

▶ Avoid leaning back to help you finish the last repetitions—that lets you use other muscles, instead of your biceps. If you have to do this to finish, you need to lower the weight or the number of reps.

MUSCLES TARGETED **TRICEPS**

HOME EXERCISE • **Triceps kickbacks with dumbbell** •

Place your right knee on the edge of a chair, then lean across the seat and plant your right palm on the other edge. Keep your left foot on the floor next to the chair. Keeping your back flat, look down so your neck is in line with your back.

Grasp a dumbbell with your left hand and pull it up to the side of your abdomen, with your left elbow pointed at the ceiling. The handle of the weight will be parallel to the floor.

Keeping your elbow pressed to your side, slowly lift the weight up and back until your arm is straight and at shoulder height. The weight will end up at the side of your left buttock, and your palm will face your body. Pause, then slowly return the weight to the starting place. After all your repetitions on that side, switch sides; now your left knee and palm will be on the bench and your right foot on the floor and your right hand holding the weight.

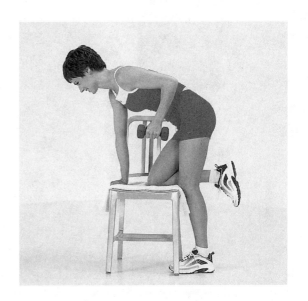

REPETITIONS

Beginner · 12 to 15

Experienced · 10 to 12 at a higher weight

DO IT RIGHT

▶ Don't lock the arm that's holding you up off the chair.

▶ Keep your lifting arm close to your body.

▶ Lift your forearm to shoulder height.

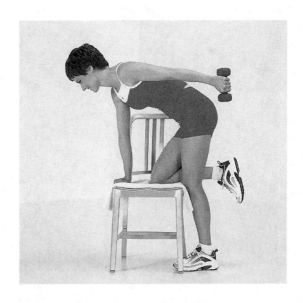

GYM EXERCISE • **Triceps pushdowns**

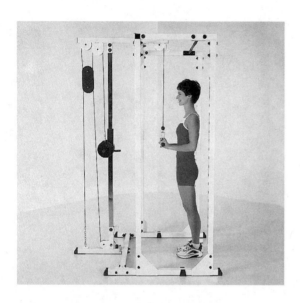

Stand facing a cable pulldown device. Select the appropriate weight, and attach the proper handle to the end of the cable. You can use a short, padded handle to grasp, but another option may be a short, thick rope.

Hold the handle with both hands in an overhand grip, or grip the ends of the rope with both hands. Pull it down to chest level, bringing your elbows down to your sides.

Keeping your elbows in place, slowly force the handle down to the tops of your thighs. Pause briefly, then allow the handle to rise to chest level. Repeat.

REPETITIONS

Beginner · 12 to 15

Experienced · 10 to 12 at a higher weight

DO IT RIGHT

▶ Don't lean forward and force the handle down with your body weight—you'll deprive your triceps of a workout.

▶ Keep your elbows stationary at your sides throughout the exercise.

MUSCLES TARGETED **DELTOIDS, TRICEPS,** AND **TRAPEZIUS**

HOME EXERCISE • **Overhead presses with dumbbells**

Hold the dumbbells, ends facing each other, in an over-hand grip in each hand. Sit up straight in a chair with your feet flat on the floor and pointed forward. Lift the dumbbells in front of your shoulders.

Slowly lift the weights directly overhead until your arms are almost straight. Pause briefly, then bring them back to the starting point.

REPETITIONS

Beginner · 12 to 15

Experienced · 10 to 12 at a higher weight

DO IT RIGHT

▶ Keep your back straight, not arched.

▶ Don't arch your neck; look forward throughout the motion.

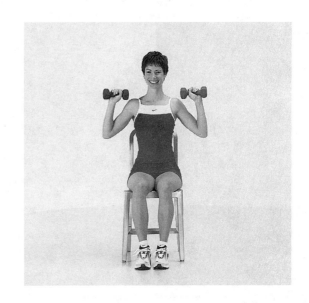

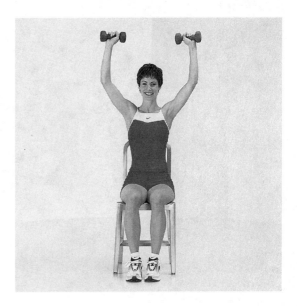

MUSCLES TARGETED **DELTOIDS, TRICEPS,** AND **TRAPEZIUS**

GYM EXERCISE • **Overhead press machine**

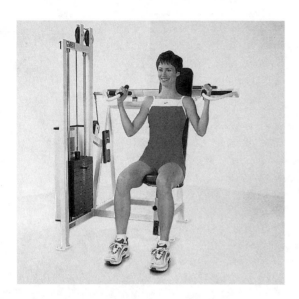

Adjust the seat so the handles are just above your shoulders, and choose the weight you want. Take a seat and put on the seat belt if one is available. Grasp the handles with your palms facing inward and slowly press the weight upward until your arms are extended, your elbows slightly bent. Pause briefly at the top, then slowly lower the handles to the starting point.

REPETITIONS

Beginner · 12 to 15

Experienced · 10 to 12 at a higher weight

DO IT RIGHT

▶ Keep your back straight, not arched.

▶ Don't arch your neck during the exercise; keep eyes facing forward.

A Head-to-Toe Shape-Up Plan

If you're more concerned with overall slimming and toning than with focusing on one particular figure problem, this workout is for you. Composed of selected exercises from the three previous sections, the head-to-toe routine works opposing muscle groups—like the biceps and triceps in your arms, the quadriceps and hamstrings in your legs, and so on. As a result, you build muscle and reduce body fat while firming up your abdomen, toning your butt, strengthening your back, and developing stronger arms, says Dr. Weltman.

When you strengthen your entire body from top to bottom, you prepare all your parts—arms, shoulders, back, legs—for any challenge, from gardening and swimming to hiking, biking, and skiing. At the same time, you'll increase your bone mass and strengthen your ligaments and tendons, Dr. Weltman says.

And strength training seems to be the *only* effective self-care technique you can use to help keep your skin toned and taut as you lose weight. Ideally, your muscles hold up and give shape to your skin, with an even layer of fat in between. If you lose too much muscle along with the fat during your weight loss, your skin can become loose and uneven. Keep strength training with light weights and high repetitions as you lose weight, and with enough time your skin should become tauter and shapelier.

Do your head-to-toe workout two or three times a week, recommends Dr. Weltman. As with the workouts in the previous chapters, one set of repetitions will suffice—welcome news for time-pressed women who want to stay in shape.

Start with a weight that you can lift 12 to 15 times, but no more. Once you're able to start lifting it more than 15 times, move up to a heavier weight.

Feel free to do these exercises in whichever order you choose, Dr. Weltman says. However, you may find it easiest to progress through exercises that target different parts—say, arms, shoulders, back, abs, legs—so each part is allowed to rest before it has to perform again.

MUSCLES TARGETED **PECTORALIS MAJOR** AND **DELTOIDS**

HOME OR GYM EXERCISE • **Chest presses with dumbbells**

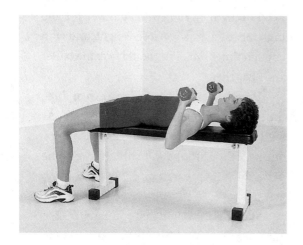

Lying back on a padded bench with your head resting on the bench, hold dumbbells over your chest. If you don't have a bench at home, lie on the floor in the same position. The weights should be pointed end-to-end and your elbows pointed out to the sides and toward the floor. Your feet should be flat on the floor to either side of the bench.

Slowly lift the dumbbells straight up as you extend your arms. Pause a moment, then slowly lower them to your chest.

REPETITIONS

Beginner · 12 to 15 repetitions

Experienced · 10 to 12 repetitions at a higher weight

DO IT RIGHT

▶ Avoid bouncing the weights off your chest.

▶ Keep the small of your back pressed down toward the bench.

MUSCLES TARGETED **DELTOIDS, TRICEPS,** AND **TRAPEZIUS**

HOME EXERCISE · **Overhead presses with dumbbells**

Hold the dumbbells, ends facing each other, in an overhand grip in each hand. Sit up straight in a chair with your feet flat on the floor and pointed forward. Lift the dumbbells in front of your shoulders.

Slowly lift the weights directly overhead until your arms are almost straight. Pause briefly, then bring them back to the starting point.

REPETITIONS

Beginner · 12 to 15

Experienced · 10 to 12 at a higher weight

DO IT RIGHT

▶ Keep your back straight, not arched.

▶ Don't arch your neck; look forward throughout the motion.

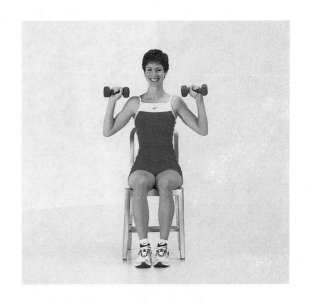

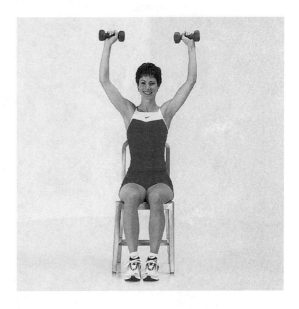

MUSCLES TARGETED **PECTORALIS MAJOR** AND **FRONT DELTOIDS**

GYM EXERCISE • **Fly machine**

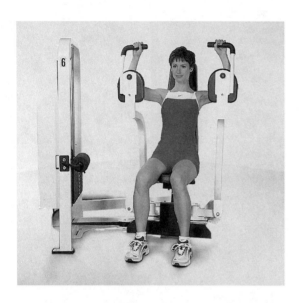

Adjust the seat to the proper height so your upper arms are perpendicular to your chest, and choose the desired weight. Sit down, use the seat belt if available, and lean back against the backrest. Place your forearms against the arm pads.

Slowly press against the pads with your forearms as far as you can, pushing them toward each other in front of your chest. Your forearms should remain vertical and parallel with each other through the whole movement. Pause, then slowly bring them back to the beginning position.

REPETITIONS

Beginner · 12 to 15

Experienced · 10 to 12 at a higher weight

DO IT RIGHT

▶ You should feel a little pull in your chest muscles at the starting position.

▶ Don't bend your head forward as you perform this move.

MUSCLES TARGETED **BICEPS**

HOME OR GYM EXERCISE • **Biceps curls with dumbbells**

While standing, hold a dumbbell in each hand at thigh level, your palms facing outward and your feet shoulder-width apart. Keeping your elbows close to your body, slowly raise the weights toward your shoulders. Pause at the top, then slowly lower them to the starting point.

REPETITIONS

Beginner · 12 to 15

Experienced · 10 to 12 at a higher weight

DO IT RIGHT

▶ Stay in control of the weights, instead of letting momentum assist you.

▶ Avoid leaning back to help you finish the last repetitions—that lets you use other muscles, instead of your biceps. If you have to do this to finish, you need to lower the weight or the number of reps.

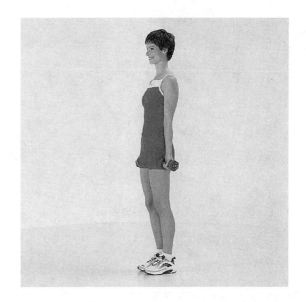

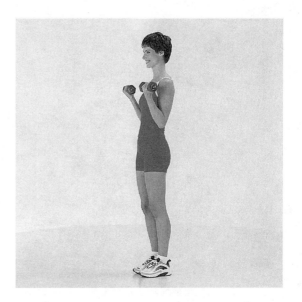

HOME EXERCISE • **Triceps kickbacks with dumbbell**

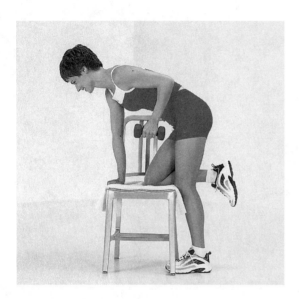

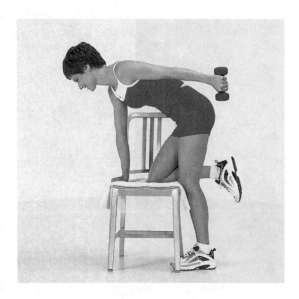

Place your right knee on the edge of a chair, then lean across the seat and plant your right palm on the other edge. Keep your left foot on the floor next to the chair. Keeping your back flat, look down so your neck is in line with your back.

Grasp a dumbbell with your left hand and pull it up to the side of your abdomen, with your left elbow pointed at the ceiling. The handle of the weight will be parallel to the floor.

Keeping your elbow pressed to your side, slowly lift the weight up and back until your arm is straight and at shoulder height. The weight will end up at the side of your left buttock, and your palm will face your body. Pause, then slowly return the weight to the starting place. After all your repetitions on that side, switch sides; now your left knee and palm will be on the bench and your right foot on the floor and your right hand holding the weight.

REPETITIONS

Beginner · 12 to 15

Experienced · 10 to 12 at a higher weight

DO IT RIGHT

▶ Don't lock the arm that's holding you up off the chair.

▶ Keep your lifting arm close to your body.

▶ Lift your forearm to shoulder height.

MUSCLES TARGETED **LATISSIMUS DORSI**

HOME EXERCISE • **Dumbbell pullovers**

Lie on your back on an exercise mat, your legs bent and your feet flat on the mat about hip-width apart. Pick up a dumbbell, each hand clutching one knobby end. Hold the weight above your chest with both hands, your arms slightly bent.

Now slowly lower the weight in an arc behind your head, keeping your arms slightly bent. When the weight goes more than halfway to the floor, pause, then slowly bring the weight in an arc back to the starting point.

REPETITIONS

Beginner · 12 to 15

Experienced · 10 to 12 at a higher weight

DO IT RIGHT

▶ When your arms are out, don't lock your elbows.

▶ Press your lower back into the floor.

▶ Keep your feet hip-width apart.

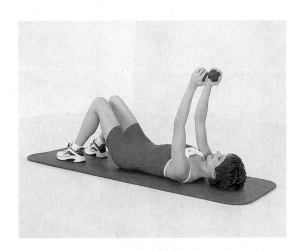

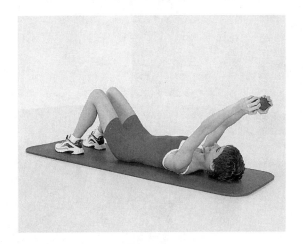

MUSCLES TARGETED **TRAPEZIUS, RHOMBOIDS,** AND **DELTOIDS**

HOME OR GYM EXERCISE • **Shoulder shrugs**

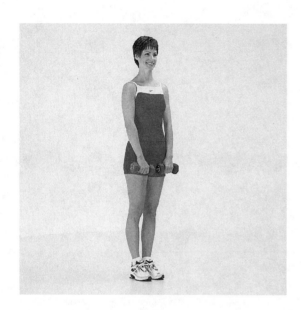

Hold your dumbbells in front of you with an overhand grasp, letting them hang at arm's length in front of your upper thighs.

Keeping your arms straight, lift the weights by slowly raising your shoulders toward your ears, as if shrugging. Rotate your shoulders backward, then lower them to the starting point.

REPETITIONS

Beginner · 12 to 15 repetitions

Experienced · 10 to 12 repetitions at a higher weight

DO IT RIGHT

▶ Be sure you're using your shoulders to do the work and not your legs.

MUSCLES TARGETED **ERECTOR SPINAE**

GYM EXERCISE • **Back machine** •

Adjust the seat or foot platform so it's in the appropriate position for you, and set the weight to the desired amount. Sit on the seat and fasten yourself in with the seat belt, if it's provided.

Cross your arms in front of your chest. Lean back against the pads behind your back. Without arching your back, slowly press against the pads and push them down. Pause briefly at the bottom, then slowly lean forward to the starting point.

REPETITIONS

Beginner · 12 to 15

Experienced · 10 to 12 at a higher weight

DO IT RIGHT

▶ Move slowly, and don't bob up and down.

▶ Don't arch your back or neck during the movement.

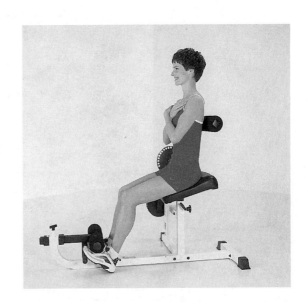

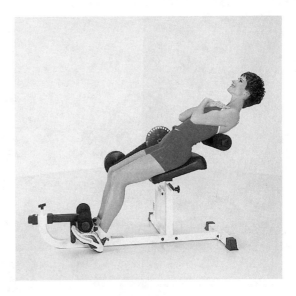

MUSCLE TARGETED **RECTUS ABDOMINIS**

GYM EXERCISE • **Ab machine**

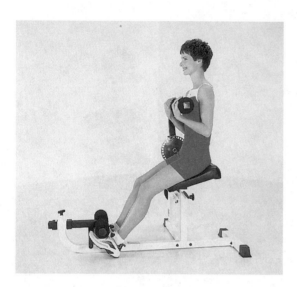

Adjust the seat so it's the appropriate height, and choose the desired weight. You should be sitting straight up.

Place your chest against the padded bar. Lightly wrap your hands around the bar. Slowly lean forward, using your abdominal muscles to push yourself down and forward as far as you can comfortably go. Pause a moment, then slowly lean back to the beginning point.

REPETITIONS

Beginner · 12 to 15 repetitions at a weight you can do comfortably only that many times

Experienced · 10 to 12 repetitions at a higher weight

DO IT RIGHT

▶ Don't bend your head forward as you push your body down

▶ Don't use your hands to pull the bar forward.

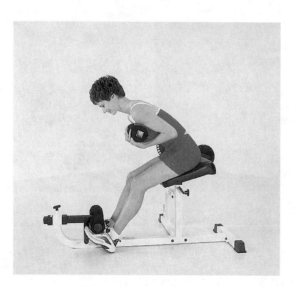

MUSCLES TARGETED **QUADRICEPS**

HOME EXERCISE • **Seated leg lifts with ankle weights**

Attach an ankle weight to each leg, and sit on a sturdy chair or bench, your feet flat on the floor in front of you.

Holding the sides of the chair for support if necessary, slowly lift your left foot so your leg is straight in front of you. Pause briefly, then slowly lower your foot. Repeat with the opposite leg.

REPETITIONS

Beginner · 12 to 15 repetitions with each leg

Experienced · 10 to 12 repetitions with each leg at a higher weight

DO IT RIGHT

▶ Don't swing your legs up and down. Use a steady, controlled motion to lift the weight.

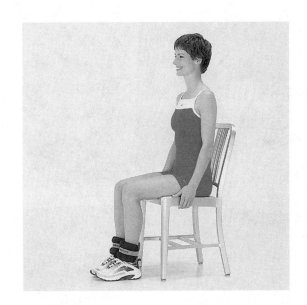

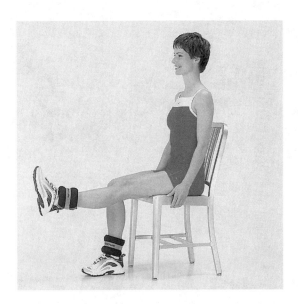

HOME EXERCISE • **Leg curls with ankle weights**

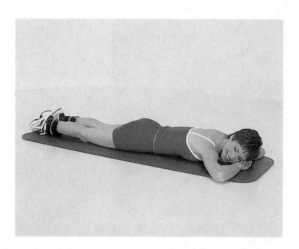

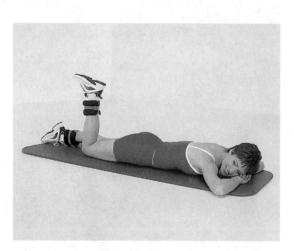

Attach ankle weights to your legs and lie facedown on an exercise mat. You can turn your head to one side, fold your arms, and rest your head on your arms.

Slowly lift your right foot toward your bottom until your leg is at a 90-degree angle. Pause briefly and slowly lower your foot back to the mat. Repeat with your other foot.

REPETITIONS

Beginner · 12 to 15 repetitions with each foot

Experienced · 10 to 12 repetitions with each foot at a higher weight

DO IT RIGHT

▶ Lie flat on your belly with your head resting on your crossed arms. Don't support your upper body on your elbows or arch your back.

▶ Keep your hips planted on the floor throughout the motion.

▶ Lift your foot only until your lower leg is pointed straight up in the air.

<u>MUSCLES TARGETED</u> **GLUTEUS MAXIMUS** AND **QUADRICEPS**

HOME EXERCISE • **Squats with dumbbells** •

Stand with a chair directly behind you, your feet spaced a bit more than shoulder-width apart. Hold a pair of dumbbells to your sides.

Bend at your hips and knees and lower your bottom until it's almost touching the chair. Your back should be straight and your toes should stay visible past your knees at all times. When you get to the bottom of the motion, slowly stand back up.

REPETITIONS

Beginners · 12 to 15
Experienced · 10 to 12 at a higher weight

DO IT RIGHT

▶ If you have knee pain, lower yourself only partway to the chair.

▶ Don't let your knees go beyond your toes.

▶ You may also want to wear a compression wrap around your knees during this exercise if they hurt.

▶ Also, if you work your way up to using high weights for squat exercises, you might consider using a weightlifting support belt around your waist and using a helper to spot you during the exercise.

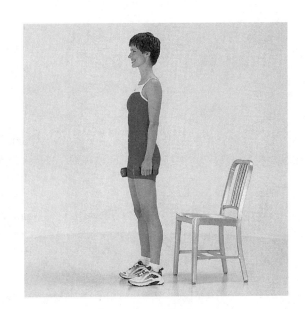

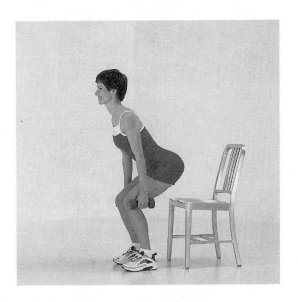

MUSCLES TARGETED **GASTROCNEMIUS** AND **SOLEUS**

HOME OR GYM EXERCISE · **Calf raises**

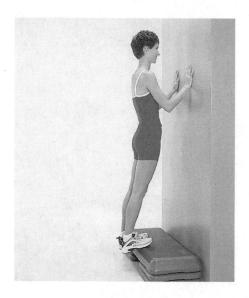

Stand on the edge of a step with your feet about hip-width apart, and ease your heels back over the edge so your weight is on your forefeet and your heels are below the level of the step. Beginners should try this first on a flat floor.

Touching a wall or holding a railing with one hand for balance if necessary, slowly rise on your toes, using your calf muscles to lift you. Pause momentarily, then slowly lower your heels to the starting position.

For an advanced version, hold a dumbbell in the hand that's not holding a wall or handrail for support.

REPETITIONS

Beginner · 12 to 15 without extra weight
Experienced · 10 to 12 with a dumbbell

DO IT RIGHT

▸ Don't lock your knees during the motion.
▸ Don't lean forward.

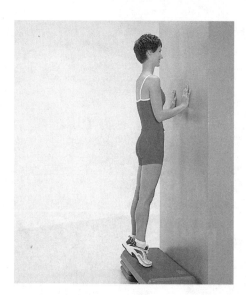

<u>MUSCLE TARGETED</u> **GLUTEUS MAXIMUS**

HOME EXERCISE · **Bent-leg kickbacks** ·

Get on your hands and knees on a padded mat or thick carpet. Your back should be parallel with the floor and in a straight line with your head and neck. Place your hands under your shoulders and your knees under your hips, and point your face toward the floor through the entire exercise.

Slowly lift your right foot toward the ceiling as high as possible, which should bring your thigh slightly higher than your torso. At its highest point, your foot should be parallel to the ceiling. Tighten your buttocks to help in the lift.

Pause briefly, then lower your leg. Repeat all your repetitions and switch sides.

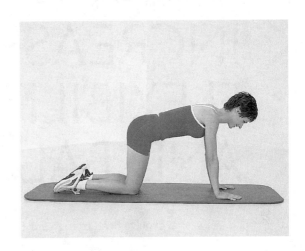

REPETITIONS

Beginners · 12 to 15 repetitions

Experienced · 10 to 12 repetitions with an ankle weight

DO IT RIGHT

▶ Don't look up toward the ceiling or back toward your belly.

▶ Don't arch your back or lock your elbows.

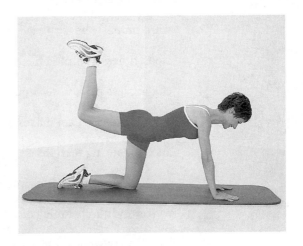

FIT NOT FAT BASICS:
INCREASE FLEXIBILITY AND BALANCE

If you've been trying your hardest to lose weight, you may be tempted to skip stretching and balance exercises in favor of those that offer "better" results. But you'd probably be surprised to know that flexibility and grace are two very precious fitness commodities that offer immediate and long-term benefits, including less pain, fewer injuries, and more self-confidence. That's why the Fit Not Fat Exercise Plan makes a point of including three to six flexibility- and balance-enhancing sessions every week.

While you are setting your Master Plan goals, pair one flexibility session with every muscle-toning or calorie-burning session. Delight in the sensation of lengthening your muscles and relieving tension—think of it as a free massage you give to yourself.

To fill out the rest of your Fit Not Fat Basics goal, pick one balance exercise to try, gradually increasing to two or more each week. You may find them surprisingly challenging at first, but don't give up—that increased sense of coordination and grace will translate into everything you do, whether running on the treadmill or just walking down the street, flaunting your new, fit body!

Limber Up

You may have taken your flexibility for granted when you were in your teens and twenties. But as you get older, you might find it difficult to hook your bra, bend over to tie your shoelaces (or your kids' shoelaces), or turn your head when you back your car out of a parking spot. That's because you lose flexibility with age due to a decrease in tendon strength and an increase in tendon rigidity, making your muscles and joints difficult to move.

Stretching slowly and deliberately at least 3 days a week enhances your range of motion and improves your flexibility. Especially after doing weight training and aerobic exercise, stretching is essential to keep muscles limber and to prevent cramping.

"Increasing your flexibility will enhance your life and allow you to continue performing activities that may get harder as you get older," says Kathleen Cercone, P.T., professor of exercise science and physical therapy at Housatonic Community College in Bridgeport, Connecticut. "Putting socks on, a simple activity of daily living, can become a challenge as flexibility decreases. By staying flexible, you can help maintain your own way of life longer."

An Essential Part of Fitness over 40

When incorporated with weight lifting, stretching improves the benefits women over 40 gain from weight training. In a study by Wayne Westcott, Ph.D., fitness research director at the South Shore YMCA in Quincy, Massachusetts, a group of exercise enthusiasts (age 50 and over) stretched after each muscle group was worked in a weight-lifting routine. After 10 weeks of lifting weights and stretching in between (holding each stretch for 20 seconds), the group had improved their strength by 20 percent more than a similar group who had only lifted weights.

"If you condition a muscle by stretching, you get some strength benefit, and vice versa," Dr. Westcott says. "Most people save stretching until the end of their workouts—and find they don't have time left to do it. But with this combination, you use your time more productively."

Stretching also:

▶ Improves circulation to your arms and legs

▶ Improves muscle control

▶ Increases stride length

▶ Improves sports performance

▶ Maximizes the benefits of strength training

▶ Improves balance and coordination

▶ Helps muscles recover from exercise

▶ Increases range of motion

▶ Decreases risk of injury

▶ Decreases amount of time needed to recover from injuries

▶ Relieves and prevents pain

▶ Improves posture

▶ Improves self-esteem and self-confidence

▶ Relaxes and invigorates your body

▶ Improves overall mood

▶ Provides an opportunity to take time out for yourself

Add up the benefits, and it's easy to see why experts say stretching rounds out a complete exercise program.

"No matter what your age, you can improve your flexibility," says Cercone. In fact, the older you get, the more you need to stretch.

FIT | FLASH

Stretch Your Muscles, Build Self-Esteem

Stretching not only increases flexibility and range of motion; it also improves your self-esteem.

Researchers at the University of Illinois–Urbana invited 153 nonexercising men and women to participate in a 6-month exercise study. Some were assigned to aerobic walking, and the others were assigned to a toning/stretching routine. Both groups worked out three times per week, in 40-minute increments.

After 6 months, researchers found that the toning/stretching group got the same self-esteem benefits as the aerobic walking group.

"Regular, light to modest activity can result in improvements in esteem," says lead study author Edward McAuley, Ph.D., professor of kinesiology and psychology at the university.

BESTBET

Morning Stretches

Simple stretches in the morning can go a long way toward getting your muscles ready for the day, getting your blood circulating, and giving you some much-needed time to focus peacefully on your body and yourself. That leaves you invigorated. You can do these three stretches while you're comfortably resting in bed, and they require no warmup.

MORNING STRETCH 1

While lying on your back, reach your arms over your head and straighten your legs, making yourself longer. Imagine you're being pulled in opposite directions; reach out your arms as far as you can, and push your legs as far as they'll go. If you're prone to calf cramps, keep your feet flexed. Hold this stretch for three deep breaths and release, letting your body relax into the bed.

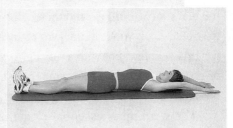

MORNING STRETCH 2

Sit on the edge of your bed and slump your body over your legs. You should look like a rag doll bent at the waist. Starting from your lower back, slowly roll to a sitting position. To finish, slowly roll your shoulders back to correct posture—this should take

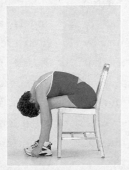
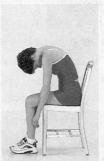
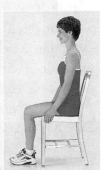

approximately 6 to 8 seconds—and look straight ahead. Just as slowly—again, taking 6 to 8 seconds—roll back down to the rag doll position, first tucking your head in to your chest, then rolling your shoulders forward, and finally curling down toward your knees.

MORNING STRETCH 3

In the rag doll position, wrap your arms under your knees and push your back out to stretch out your upper, middle, and lower spine. Hold for three deep breaths and release.

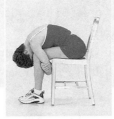
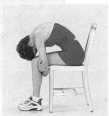

Warm Up First

To increase your flexibility and range of motion, it's important to warm up for at least 5 minutes before stretching. The warmup should be a lighter version of the workout to come. For instance, if you're about to set off on a power walk, take an easy walk around the block for 5 minutes, and then come back to stretch. Or, if you're at the gym ready to lift weights, do a few reps with a very light weight or no weight at all. And remember to stretch between sets to improve strength gains.

The warmup is essential to get blood circulating throughout your body, giving oxygen and energy to muscles tight from inactivity. It also prepares your body for the workout ahead. Plus, warming up before stretching decreases your risk of injury by preventing pulls or strains of muscles that are overworked, tight, or out of shape. In a study of U.S. male military recruits during basic training, soldiers who stretched three times a day, in addition to their normal basic training program, had half the injuries of those who didn't take time to stretch. According to Cercone, the same results apply to women. In addition, you should follow your workout with a brief stretching routine in order to maximize the flexibility you've gained.

"Think of cold taffy; if you tried to stretch it, it would break in half," says Cercone. "But if you warm up taffy first and then pull it, it stretches."

After warming up, stretch gradually and slowly. Avoid bouncing your way through a stretch, advises Cercone. Jerky movements—like bouncing—make your muscles contract and become rigid, counteracting the goal of stretching, which is to make your muscles pliable for easy movement. After stretching, your body should feel relaxed and revived, not sore and tense, which can often happen after bouncy stretching. So don't bounce!

Perform the following head-to-toe stretches in the order given. That way, you'll work the larger muscles, like your back and quads, before working the smaller muscles underneath, like the hip flexors. Hold each stretch for 20 to 30 seconds, imagining your muscles getting longer and looser. Exhale as you stretch; do not hold your breath.

You know you're getting a good stretch when you feel your muscles pull. This might be uncomfortable, but it shouldn't be painful, according to Cercone. Shooting pains or tenderness in one specific area is a sign of injury, and you should contact your physician.

Don't rush through your stretching routine. Never force a stretch. If you have difficulty completing some of the stretches, work slowly. Don't do the advanced stretches until you can do the regular stretches comfortably. In time you'll gain flexibility, so be patient.

MUSCLES TARGETED
ABDOMINALS, DELTOIDS, TRICEPS, TRAPEZIUS, LATISSIMUS DORSI, AND ERECTOR SPINAE

Whole-body stretch

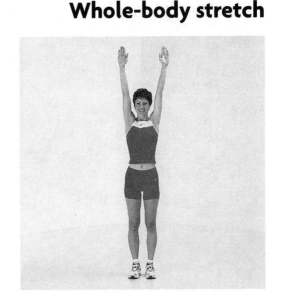

Stand with feet shoulder-width apart and raise your arms above your head to reach for the sky. Feel the stretch from your feet to your fingertips. Imagine yourself getting taller. Slowly lower your arms to your sides. Repeat three times.

MUSCLES TARGETED **TRAPEZIUS**

Neck stretch

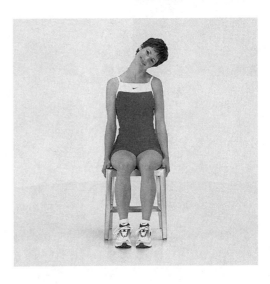

Sit straight back in a firm chair (or a bench, if you're outdoors). Hold on to the seat for support if you need to. Drop your chin to your chest. Roll your head to the left side, trying to touch your ear to your shoulder. Return your chin to your chest. Roll your neck to the right side, again trying to touch this ear to your shoulder. Return your chin to your chest. Imagine your shoulders sinking into the ground and your head touching the floor.

Note: Never roll your head in a complete circle; doing so can injure the occipital joint at the base of your head and neck.

MUSCLES TARGETED **REAR DELTOIDS** AND **TRICEPS**

Shoulder stretch 1

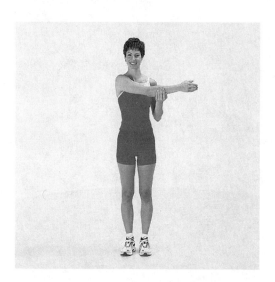

Straighten your right arm in front of you. With your left hand, grab either below or above your elbow (not right on the joint). Pull your right arm across your chest. Repeat on the left side.

MUSCLES TARGETED **DELTOIDS, TRICEPS,** AND **LATISSIMUS DORSI**
Shoulder stretch 2

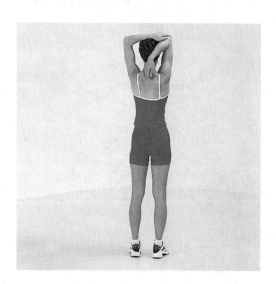

Reach your right arm over your head and bend it at the elbow so the palm of your hand touches the back of your head. Take your left hand and grab your right elbow. Pull your elbow toward the left side of your head, making your right hand reach for the middle of your back. Repeat on your left side.

MUSCLES TARGETED
DELTOIDS, LATISSIMUS DORSI, TRICEPS, ABDOMINALS, TRAPEZIUS, AND **ERECTOR SPINAE**

Short shirt pull

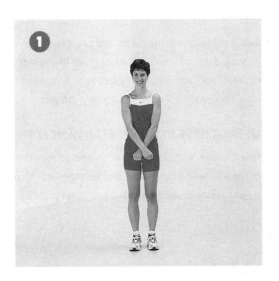

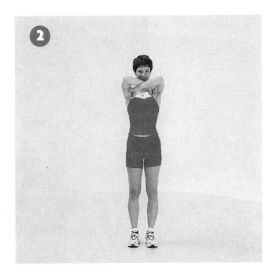

Cross your arms at the wrists as if to pull a shirt off over your head (1). Inhaling, tilt your face upward, and pull your crossed arms up, (2) raising them and uncrossing them until they are fully stretched overhead. Without arching your back, lengthen your torso as you reach toward the sky (3). As you exhale, return your head to level and lower your arms, dropping your shoulders like a shirt resting on a hanger (not shown).

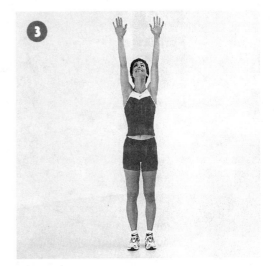

Upper-chest stretch 1

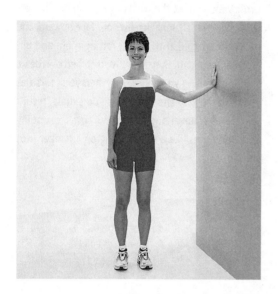

Reach out with your left arm and press the palm of your hand against a wall, a door, or a tree (if you're outdoors). Turn your torso away from the arm, keeping your back straight. Repeat using your right arm.

UPPER-CHEST STRETCH 2 (ADVANCED)

Face a corner of the room. Put both arms on either side of the wall, with elbows bent, and lean forward. (Don't stand so close to the corner that you bump your head.)

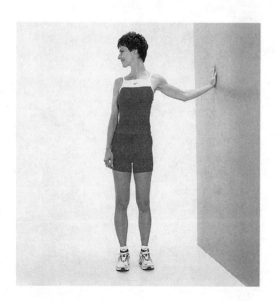

MUSCLE TARGETED **ERECTOR SPINAE, LUMBAR,** AND **GLUTEUS**

Lower-back stretch

Lie on your back. Bring both knees in toward your chest. Clasp your hands underneath your right knee (not on top) and hold for a great lower-back stretch. Repeat with your left leg.

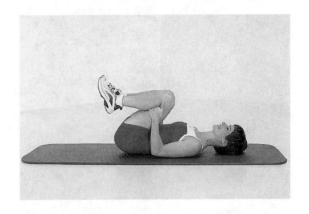

MUSCLES TARGETED **QUADRICEPS** AND **HIP FLEXORS**

Quadriceps stretch

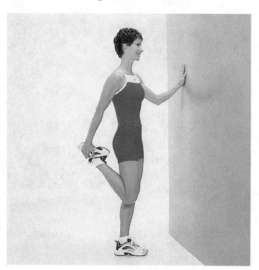

Stand up straight, holding a wall (or, if you're outdoors, a tree) for support. Bend your right knee behind you and grasp your foot with your right hand, pulling the heel toward your butt. To avoid arching your back, keep your pelvis level. Repeat on your left leg.

MUSCLES TARGETED **HAMSTRINGS** AND **GLUTEUS**

Hamstring stretch 1

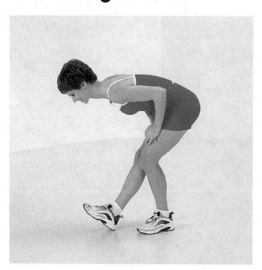

Standing, place your right heel about 6 to 12 inches in front of you, your toes pointing up. Put your hands on your left thigh for support. Bending your left knee, lean forward from your hips. Shift your weight back and stick your butt out until you feel a stretch in the back of your right leg. (It'll look as if you're half sitting.) Keep your back straight. Do two or three stretches with each leg.

MUSCLES TARGETED **HAMSTRINGS**

Hamstring stretch 2

Lie on your back with your left foot flat on the floor and your right leg extended. Slowly raise your right leg as far as is comfortable. You can use your hands, a towel, or a rope to hold your leg in position. (Or you can rest your leg against the corner of a wall.) Keep your back flat on the floor. You should feel the stretch in the back of your right leg. Repeat using your left leg.

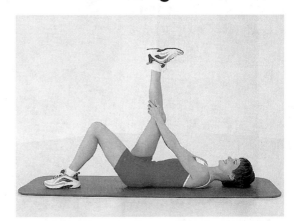

COOL TOOL

Stretching or Yoga Mat

Stretching mats look like standard gymnastics or wrestling mats. If you're stretching on a hard surface, your back or other bony surfaces may become sore. A stretching or yoga mat can provide a little extra cushion.

WHAT THE EXPERT SAYS: A stretching mat, with extra foam padding, can be great for flexibility work on the floor, says Kathleen Cercone, P.T., professor of exercise science and physical therapy at Housatonic Community College in Bridgeport, Connecticut. And a yoga mat, with its nonslip rubbery surface, is perfect for those stretches or yoga positions where you might slide or slip.

PURCHASING TIPS: Stretching and yoga mats can be found at any sporting goods store and most discount stores. Look for mats with extra cushioning and a nonslip surface. They cost anywhere from $15 to $25.

Hamstring stretch 3 (with resistance band)

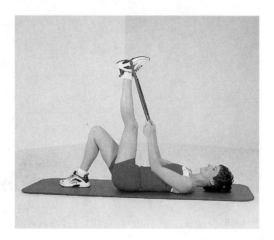

If your muscles are too tight for you to hold your leg with your hands, use a resistance band to stretch your hamstrings. Repeat several times with each leg.

MUSCLES TARGETED **GASTROCNEMIUS** AND **SOLEUS**

Calf stretch 1 (advanced)

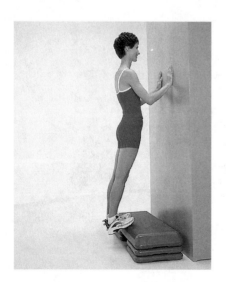

Place a small, sturdy footstool near a wall, or stand on the bottom step of a flight of stairs. (Or purchase a stretch step, available at discount and sporting goods stores.) If you're outdoors, find a step or a curb near a pole, tree, or something sturdy to hold on to for support. Grasp the wall or pole to maintain balance. Place your toes on the edge of the step. Keeping your legs straight (don't lock your knees), lower your heels slowly and feel the stretch in your calf. An alternative is to stretch one calf at a time, using your other leg to maintain balance; repeat on the other leg.

MUSCLES TARGETED **GASTROCNEMIUS** AND **SOLEUS**

Achilles tendon stretch

Stand an arm's length from a wall or tree (if you're outdoors). Lean in to the surface, bracing yourself with your arms. Place your left leg forward, with your knee bent. Keep your right leg back, the knee straight and your heel down. Stretch out the back leg. Repeat with the other leg.

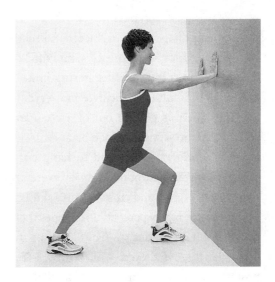

Improve Your Balance

You probably don't give your sense of balance much thought, but being able to maintain your balance in a variety of situations is a very real marker of personal fitness. For women especially, poor balance combined with brittle bones, weak muscles, and inflexible joints can result in a life-altering injury, making it difficult to participate in everyday activities such as getting out of a chair or walking. At the very least, good balance gives you the confidence you need to hang curtains, paint your bedroom, or enjoy exercise like hiking, biking, and cross-country skiing.

Yet small, barely perceptible changes that occur as you hit the age of 40 or older can affect balance, says Steven Wolf, Ph.D., P.T., professor in the department of rehabilitation medicine at the Emory University School of Medicine in Atlanta, who studies the change in balance in older adults. As you age, tiny wavelike hairs in your inner ear that play a role in equilibrium lose sensitivity, decreasing your ability to detect changes in balance. Nerve cells become less sensitive, and the reaction time and flexibility of your muscles decrease.

Not Just for Gymnasts

You can maintain good balance indefinitely. Research suggests that over time, exercise, particularly resistance-training routines like those in chapter 10, can help maintain your sense of balance at midlife or older.

To focus specifically on improving your balance, add the following exercises into your regular fitness routine at least 3 days a week. For exercises that require holding on to a table or chair, try using only one hand as your steadiness increases. Progress to using only one finger, then without holding on at all, and finally with your eyes closed, suggests Dr. Wolf.

BESTBET

A Simple Way to Test Your Balance

How steady are you on your feet? Try any or all of these simple tests.

▶ Walk backward, first with your eyes open and then with your eyes closed. You should be able to walk at least 10 feet without stumbling.

▶ Walk heel-to-toe: Position your heel just in front of the toes of your opposite foot each time you take a step. Your heels and toes should touch or almost touch. How long you can do this test will vary, but you should be able to do at least a few steps.

▶ Stand on one foot for 10 seconds. Alternate feet. You should be able to do this at least 10 times.

▶ Stand up and sit down without using your hands. You should be able to do this at least five times.

Rock and roll

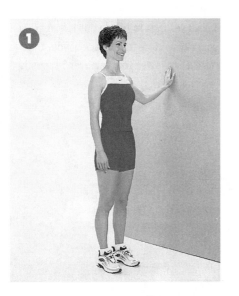

Stand next to a wall for support, facing sideways, your feet about hip-width apart (1). Without bending your knees, slowly shift your weight to your toes, leaning slightly forward as far as you can without tipping or letting your heels come off the floor (2). Then shift your weight back to your heels, tilting backward without lifting your toes (3). Next, still keeping your feet flat on the floor, sway to the left and then to the right as far as possible (not shown). For more of a challenge, bring your feet closer together, and then try it with your eyes closed.

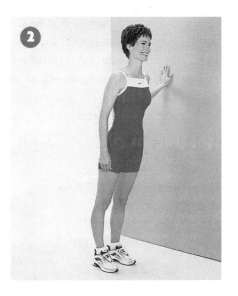

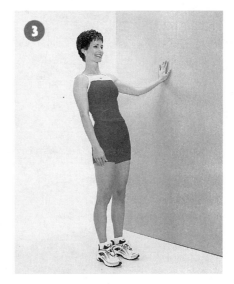

Kick your butt

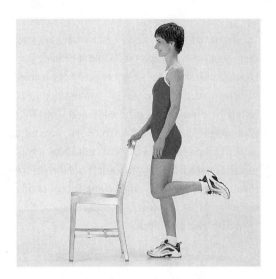

Stand straight, holding a table or chair for balance. Take 3 seconds to bend your left knee, trying to get your calf as close to the back of your thigh as possible. Hold, then lower your leg over 3 seconds. Repeat on your right leg.

The march

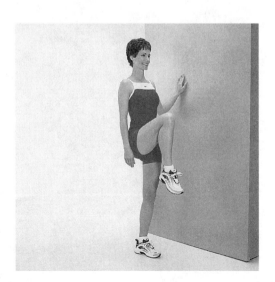

Stand next to a wall for support and face sideways. Slowly raise your right knee over 3 seconds, bringing it as close to your chest as possible. Don't bend at the waist or hips. Hold for a second or two, then lower your leg over 3 seconds. Repeat on your left leg.

Scissor kick

Stand straight, holding a table or chair for support. Slowly lift your left leg 6 to 12 inches to the side; do not bend your knee or upper body. Hold. Slowly lower, and repeat on your right side. Once you've mastered this, hold the table with one hand, then one finger, then no hands, then eyes closed, to further improve your balance.

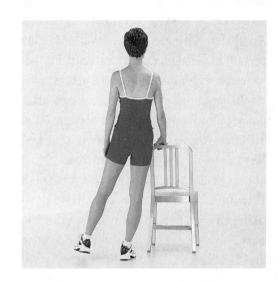

FITNESS MYSTERIES

How do tightrope walkers maintain their balance on such shaky footing?

The key to maintaining balance and poise on a ⅝-inch cable 40 feet above the circus ring is posture, says Lisa Wallenda, an eighth-generation member of the Flying Wallendas, a family of high-wire walkers performing for more than 25 years with Ringling Brothers and Barnum and Bailey Circus. Good posture comes naturally if you tighten your abs and visualize pulling your belly button in toward your spine. And you can do that while walking on solid ground!

Tightrope walkers must keep their upper bodies perfectly still (from hip to head). Having strong abdominal and back muscles is vital to keeping your body taut and stable, Wallenda says. Without this, tricks where performers balance on each other's head or form pyramids would be impossible.

To stay in shape between performances, Wallenda says, her family incorporated lots of little activities into the day that would help them maintain their strength and flexibility on the road. Sitting on a chair or couch while watching TV was forbidden; instead, they had to sit on the floor and stretch or do crunches—an activity she has carried over to this day.

Go Steady with Tai Chi

If you're interested in a formal balance-training activity that incorporates strength training and flexibility work, and offers a moderate cardiovascular workout, try tai chi. An ancient Chinese practice that originally served as a starting point for studying advanced-level training for martial arts experts, tai chi has grown into its own respected place among fitness gurus and practitioners. Tricia Yu, director of the Tai Chi Center in Madison, Wisconsin, a certified tai chi instructor, and author of *Tai Chi Fundamentals for Health Professionals and Instructors*, has been practicing tai chi 15 to 20 minutes daily for the past 30 years and credits it for her balance and flexibility.

"Tai chi teaches us to maintain balance in all physical activities, such as standing, lifting, pushing, pulling, walking, and running. It trains you to bring your mind and body together so you're aware of your posture, your body, and your movement," says Yu. These benefits don't only help women in their forties. In several studies conducted by Dr. Wolf, tai chi reduced the onset of falls by almost 50 percent in adults over age 70, reduced their fear of falling, and increased their confidence in doing activities they enjoy. Other studies linked the practice of tai chi with improved emotional health, increased immune system function, and decreased blood pressure.

Easy, rhythmic movements are slowly and gradually worked into the tai chi routine. By concentrating on the movements, their sequence, and how your body is moving, you become better able to compensate for a declining ability to multitask as you get older. This compromised ability to perform multiple tasks at one time probably contributes to balance problems later in life. "It's the old 'can't walk and chew gum' phenomenon," says Dr. Wolf.

"With tai chi, every movement is deliberate, and it trains you to think about what you're doing," he says. Doing so will make you less likely to stumble or fall and will decrease your risk of sustaining a life-altering injury.

For more on how to locate and enroll in tai chi classes, along with tips on how to get the most out of a tai chi workout, see page 162 in chapter 9.

CHAPTER 12

CUSTOMIZING YOUR WORKOUT:

FITNESS PRESCRIPTIONS FOR BUM BACKS, HIPS, KNEES, AND MORE

Exercisers and would-be exercisers need their own serenity prayer: *Grant me the courage to work through mild discomfort so in the long run I have less pain; the serenity to baby my joints and muscles when they really need it; and the wisdom to know the difference.*

Any active woman occasionally experiences backaches, shoulder strain, knee pain, or other bone, muscle, or joint discomfort. Some women earnestly want to exercise but are hampered by chronic pain.

If discomfort is moderate to severe or lasts longer than 3 to 4 days; if you have any redness, bruising, or swelling; or if the pain is too intense to work through, you need to see a doctor. If you have shooting pain or numbness radiating down your arms or legs, stop exercising at once and consult your doctor. You may be referred to an orthopedist or physiatrist, to prevent nerve damage.

Mild discomfort is usually nothing to worry about, though. Most likely you need to warm up or cool down more effectively. (See chapter 11 for how to do so.) Or it may be time to replace your workout shoes. (See "Exercise in Comfort with the Right Shoes" on page 257.)

After the age of 40, men and women alike have less elastin, a specialized protein that keeps skin, muscles, tendons, ligaments, and other connective tissue flexible. As a result, your muscles feel more irritated when stretched, and you are sorer after a hike on the trails, a tennis match, or a day at the pool than you were when you were 25.

If you feel achy after exertion, fight the urge to lunge for the couch, says Dan Hamner, M.D., a physiatrist and sports medicine specialist in New York City.

Inactivity can worsen mild joint and muscle pain because it prevents blood from flowing to that area. Plus, if you stop working out and begin *filling* out, added weight will cause more stress to your musculoskeletal system.

Cut back on the intensity of your workouts, but not the frequency, says Willibald Nagler, M.D., professor of rehabilitation medicine at New York Weill Cornell Medical Center in New York City. If anything, you want to exercise *more* regularly, in order to condition all your muscle groups and keep them from getting even stiffer.

"Your muscles and joints are better off with a little conditioning every day rather

BESTBET

Lighten Up Your Backpack, Purse, or Workout Bag

The first way to take daily stress off your shoulders, knees, back, hips, and feet is to clean out your backpack or purse weekly," says Mary Margaret Sloan, president of the American Hiking Society in Silver Spring, Maryland. A savvy packer who's scaled Mount Kilimanjaro, Sloan once discovered that she'd been walking around for a week with a pair of lost sandals at the bottom of her backpack.

Other back-friendly tips:

▶ Choose nylon over leather or heavy cotton.
▶ If you must carry aspirin, hair products, or hand cream, buy travel-size containers.
▶ Choose double-strap backpacks, which keep weight closer to your center of gravity, or choose a flat purse with a long enough strap to wear across your shoulder.

<u>COOL</u>
TOOL

Abdominal Exercise Devices

Sporting goods stores and TV ads offer a variety of devices, including the Torso Track, Ab Roller, and Ab Rocker, designed to flatten your abs by targeting your midsection and working your abdominal muscles.

WHAT EXPERTS SAY: Contraptions designed to exercise your abdominal muscles don't work any better than traditional crunches. Using special equipment to measure the muscle activity, researchers in the Biomechanics Lab at San Diego State University tested several abdominal devices and exercises in a group of 30 men and women age 20 to 45. The Ab Rocker device generated 79 percent *less* activity than a traditional crunch. The Torso Track was a bit better than a crunch, but caused lower-back discomfort in many of the study participants.

The most effective home equipment they tested was the exercise ball, which generated 39 percent more activity in the participants' rectus abdominis muscles than a traditional crunch.

TO WORK YOUR ABS WITH AN EXERCISE BALL: Sit on the ball with your feet flat on the floor, then let the ball roll back slowly until you're lying on it with your thighs and torso parallel to the floor. Cross your arms over your chest and slightly tuck in your chin. Raise your torso to 45 degrees at the most, using your abdominal muscles to lift you. Exhale as you contract your muscles and inhale as you lower yourself back down.

than heroic efforts once a week," says Dr. Nagler. Daily stretching, for instance, renders muscles more flexible, in effect giving them the same properties they had in younger years, when elastin was more plentiful.

Yet even with serious injuries or physical problems such as a herniated disc or torn ligament, the goal is to return you to a fitness routine after getting the proper treatment from your doctor, Dr. Hamner explains. If you've been sidelined by a serious injury, don't be surprised if your doctor prescribes a well-designed exercise program in addition to ice, heat, and medications.

If you're certain that regular exercise will help, not hinder, your achy body, these doctor-designed workouts can help you stay fit not fat at 40-plus. Use these exercises for mild discomfort or if approved by your doctor for more serious problems.

Back-Friendly Fitness ●

Based on his experience, almost 9 out of 10 women who complain about having a "bad back" are experiencing discomfort because of a basic musculoskeletal problem, says Dr. Hamner. Some are simply more prone to muscle spasm. For most, the lumbar muscles supporting the lower back are too tight or too weak, or there is an imbalance and one muscle, like the hip flexor, overcompensates for a weaker one, like the hip extensor, explains Dr. Hamner.

You may also be feeling an imbalance in more than just the muscles of your back. When muscles in the shoulders and neck are too tight, back muscles are forced to overcompensate. And since tight hamstrings, at the backs of the thighs, pull on your pelvis and tight hip muscles like the piriformis prevent you from rotating properly, you'll also want to keep your lower body limber. Along with strengthening and stretching the back muscles themselves, you need to condition the abdominal muscles, to help support your spine.

If you have the classic "bad back," which is usually caused by either tight or weak muscles, check with your doctor to see if you'll benefit from these moves. Your doctor will probably need to rule out a disk problem or another abnormality that needs special therapy before you begin.

Note: All exercises should be done on an exercise mat or soft carpeting.

FITNESS PRESCRIPTIONS FOR THE **BACK**

The bicycle

Lie on your back, and raise your legs straight in the air. Tuck in your pelvis, and put your hands on your abdomen. "Bicycle pedal" your legs, being sure not to arch your back. Start with 30 seconds, and work up to 1 minute over time.

What makes it back-friendly: Fosters strong thigh muscles while loosening up the back muscles.

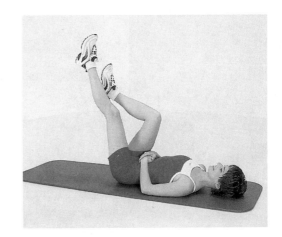

The bridge

Lie on your back with your knees bent and arms stretched out at your sides. Slowly squeeze your buttocks together while raising your hips and lower back as far as you can while still maintaining floor contact with your upper back, neck, and shoulders. Try to form a straight line between your knees and shoulders. Hold for 2 to 3 seconds, then gently lower yourself to the floor. Repeat 10 times.

What makes it back-friendly: Releases tension in the lower back and hips and strengthens muscles in the upper and lower body that foster good posture.

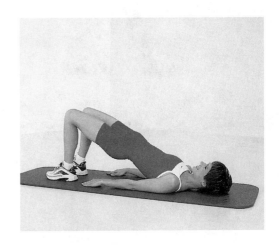

Cow and cat

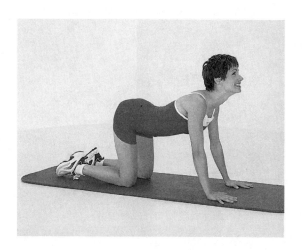

Start on your hands and knees, with your weight evenly distributed among all four limbs—think of your body as resting in "neutral," not forward, not back. Place your hands under your shoulders, and your knees under your hips. Inhale and arch your spine as you look up. This is the cow pose. Then exhale while rounding your back, tucking your tailbone under and dropping your chin toward your chest. This is a cat pose. Repeat several times, alternating between the two poses.

What makes it back-friendly: Loosens entire spine while strengthening back and abdominal muscles.

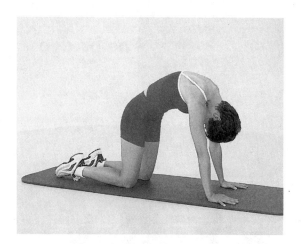

Other Back-Friendly Exercises

**BACK
MACHINE**
(page 183)

**NECK
STRETCH**
(page 229)

FITNESS PRESCRIPTIONS FOR THE **BACK**

Baby pose

Sit on your heels, with your knees apart and your ankles together. Slowly lean forward over your legs until your forehead touches the floor (or as close to it as you can comfortably get). Rest your arms overhead on the floor and breathe deeply, expanding your lower back as you breathe.

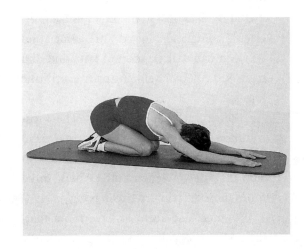

What to Avoid

If you have a bad back, you should avoid exercises with a lot of twisting, and anything that sends shooting pain through your back. And while it is important to strengthen the abdominal muscles to support good posture, never do full situps—come up only halfway. The following exercises put a lot of strain on backs that are achy or injured, so they are *not* recommended unless you do them under the supervision of a physical therapist or have recovered from your bad back:

▶ Crossover crunches (page 178)

▶ Rotary torso machine (page 179)

▶ Good morning (page 184)

▶ Overhead presses with dumbbells (page 207)

▶ Overhead press machine (page 208)

Knee-Saving Exercises

The knee is a sensitive joint, and at one time it was feared that vigorous exercise would in time wear out the knee, eventually leading to osteoarthritis. Not so. Actual research—including data on 150 lifetime female exercisers in England—found little association between habitual exercise of any kind and increased risk of developing painful arthritic knees.

Still, things can go wrong. The most common forms of sudden injury are tears to the anterior cruciate ligament (ACL), deep inside the knee. Women suffer about three times more ACL injuries than men.

Women also seem to have more than their share of painful kneecap problems, such as bursitis and tendinitis (two types of inflammation) and iliotibial band syndrome (tight tendons that rub the bones and cause irritation) and chondromalacia (softening of cartilage).

But bad knees don't have to stand in the way of your fitness program. Muscle-strengthening exercises can help prevent most kneecap problems.

"The secret to keeping a knee healthy throughout your life is to condition the long muscles and tendons connected to it," says Dr. Hamner. Your hamstring muscle runs up and down the entire back of your leg, not only supporting the ligaments and tendons surrounding the knee but also stabilizing your ankle. In front, your mighty quadriceps supports your kneecap by connecting it to the entire front of your thigh and the tendons across your hip.

A torn ACL usually calls for surgery. But the more supported your knee is by the connecting muscles and tendons, the better you avoid or recover from injury. And since we lose protective cartilage around our kneecaps as we age, it's all the more important to strengthen our legs to reduce stress to the knees. Maintaining strength and flexibility of your entire leg can also lessen the discomfort of any knee overuse condition, such as bursitis, tendinitis, or arthritis.

If you have had a previous knee injury, you are at greater risk for developing osteoarthritis in your knee. Under your doctor's direction, a physical therapist or certified fitness instructor can give you a specialized routine.

Otherwise, Dr. Hamner recommends these knee-safe moves to prevent injury or for rehabilitation. (Before beginning exercises for rehabilitation, check with your doctor).

FITNESS PRESCRIPTIONS FOR **KNEES**

Wall squat

Start with your feet shoulder-width apart approximately 18 inches from a wall. Keeping your head and back against the wall, slide down until your knees are at about a 45-degree angle. Hold this position for 60 seconds. Repeat three times. As your knees recover, you can push in to the wall with your back to slide between standing and squatting positions up to 15 times, but never squat so deeply that your hips drop below the level of your knees.

What makes it a knee saver: Conditions quadriceps and hamstrings to stabilize the knee. The wall prevents the tendency to use your back or overflex your knees during squats.

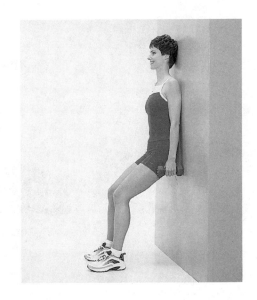

Rotated leg raise

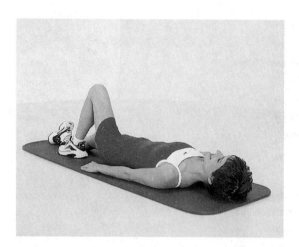

Lie on your back with both knees bent. Straighten your right leg, turning the toes up and out. Keeping your toes turned out, raise your right leg to the level of your bent knee, slowly lower to an inch off the ground, and raise it again. Repeat 15 times, then switch sides. You may add the heaviest ankle weight you can lift without jerking or straining during the 15 reps.

What makes it a knee saver: These moves strengthen the medial quadriceps to prevent knee pain.

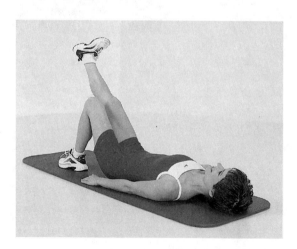

FITNESS PRESCRIPTIONS FOR **KNEES**

Straight and rotated knee extensions

Start with your back against a wall, with your right leg bent and foot flat on the floor. Extend your left leg straight out in front of you, about 8 inches above the ground. Bring your left leg in and extend it back out to a straight leg with your toes up. Do two sets of 15 repetitions. Do a third set of 15 repetitions, but with your leg and ankle turned out. Repeat on the other side.

What makes it a knee saver: The first two sets concentrate on building strength in all four quad muscles. The third set gives special attention to your inner quads, which tend to be weaker than the rest.

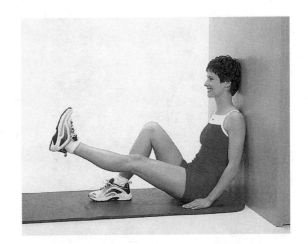

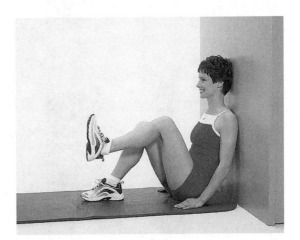

Calf stretch 2

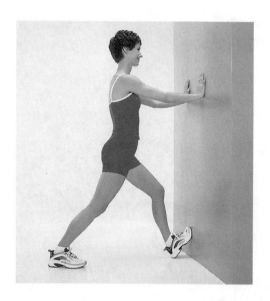

While standing, place your left foot at a 45-degree angle against a wall so that your heel is on the floor and the ball of your foot is on the wall. Bend your knees slightly. As you lean your hips in to the wall, allow your right heel to come off the floor until you feel a stretch in your left calf. Repeat several times with each leg.

What makes it a knee saver: Keeps the gastrocnemius muscle of your calf limber. This muscle connects with the hamstring to stabilize your knee and ankle.

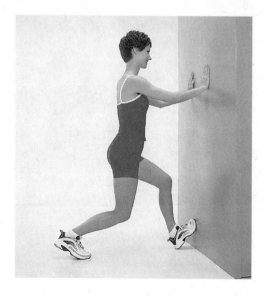

FITNESS PRESCRIPTIONS FOR **KNEES**

Soleus stretch

Stand an arm's length from a wall or tree. Lean in toward the surface, bracing yourself with your arms. Place one leg forward with your knee bent, and keep the other leg back, knee straight, but not locked, and heel down. Shift your weight onto your front leg. Bring the back leg in so your back ankle wraps around your front ankle, and lean in closer and lower until you feel a stretch in your lower calf. Hold for 15 seconds, then repeat on the other side.

What makes it a knee saver: Targets flexibility deep in the lower calf, which is necessary for ankle stability. Stable ankles prevent injury to your knee and foot.

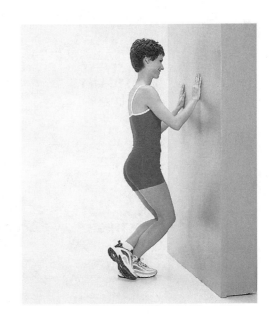

Other Helpful Knee Savers

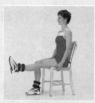

**SEATED
LEG LIFTS**
(page 186)

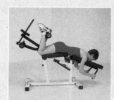

**LEG CURL
MACHINE**
(page 189)

**CALF
RAISES**
(page 190)

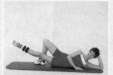

**INNER-THIGH
LIFTS**
(page 193)

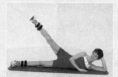

**OUTER-THIGH
LIFTS**
(page 193)

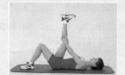

**HAMSTRING
STRETCH 2**
(page 235)

What to Avoid

If you have knee problems, including discomfort, avoid sports that involve sudden twisting motions of the knee. When you jump, land with your knees bent. Don't do any exercise where you'd have to lunge into your knees past your toes, and avoid exercise routines where you'd have to do a lot of jumping. Certain exercises are best avoided by women with knees that tend to give out because it's too easy to overextend your knees or overcompensate for weak knees with your back. These include:

▶ Squats with dumbbells (page 191)

▶ Leg press machine (page 192)

▶ Full-arc knee extensions
(not pictured)

▶ Hurdler's stretches (not pictured)

▶ Stepups (not pictured)

Exercise in Comfort with the Right Shoes

By their 40th birthdays, most women have taken 120 million steps, each one sending two to three times their body weight into the muscles and bones of their feet. The cumulative effects can actually alter foot structure—and comfort, says Cherise Dyal, M.D., chair of the American Orthopaedic Foot and Ankle Society (AOFAS) public education committee and in private practice in Wayne, New Jersey. The arch slightly falls, the foot becomes wider and longer, and the padding on the bottom of the heel thins. Also, the ligaments of your foot stretch out and lose some of their supportive quality, she explains.

Combine the aging process with the wrong workout shoes, and women in their forties, fifties, and sixties encounter bunions, "hammer" or "claw" toes, corns, and even arthritis. You may also find that you lose your balance more easily, or you develop the stabbing heel pain known as plantar fasciitis.

Stretching daily can help to avoid or alleviate problems. So can selecting the right—and right-fitting—shoes. Here's what the experts recommend.

▶ If you do a particular sport or workout more than three times a week, get a sport-specific shoe. Walking shoes, for example, have a slightly rounded sole that smoothly shifts the weight from heel to toes. Running shoes are designed for intense shock absorption.

▶ For hiking, look for high-top style hiking boots that are lightweight, like a running shoe, but with better traction so that your soles stay put on wet rocks and muddy slopes. The more the shoe feels like it contours to your foot and calf, the better you will avoid heel pain.

▶ If you already have chronic foot or ankle problems, an orthopedic surgeon can modify your exercise shoe with custom supports and inserts.

▶ No matter what shoe you get, be certain you have the right fit by allowing for adequate space in the front and the sides. The big toes on both feet should have $\frac{3}{8}$ to $\frac{1}{2}$ inch to the tip of the shoe to move around. You shouldn't feel tightness anywhere, but you also don't want your heel to slip around.

▶ Try on shoes at the end of the day, when your feet are fully spread, and wear socks you usually wear for exercise. Go by measurement and fit, not size, which varies with shoe type and brand.

▶ Even if your exercise shoes don't appear worn down on the outside, replace them after 300 to 500 hours of running or 300 hours of aerobic activity. Maximum cushioning and heel control are necessary to prevent shin splints, tendinitis, heel pain, stress fractures, and other injuries.

Hip-Helping Workouts

Hip pain is commonly caused by strained or pulled muscles anywhere from the lower back to the buttocks and upper legs. As we age, many of us also endure the ache of osteoarthritis in our hips, the wearing down of the cartilage cushion between the ball and socket of the joint.

"A woman with mild to moderate arthritis can benefit tremendously from keeping up with her normal exercise program while taking glucosamine and chondroitin supplements," says Dr. Hamner. Note that if you are taking chondroitin alone or with glucosamine, it may increase the effects of blood-thinning drugs and herbs. "A woman with advanced arthritis will need to work with a therapist or doctor to modify her activities," he says.

See a doctor to evaluate any hip pain and to see what exercises might be right for you. If hip pain radiates down the front of your leg or into your groin or the pain keeps you from bearing weight, the following exercises won't be for you. For mild pain or discomfort, focus on improving flexibility and strength in the entire greater hip area. One safe and comfortable way to achieve this goal is swimming. The following moves will also help put the tilt back in your pelvis.

COOL TOOL

Nordic Walker or Leki Trekking Poles

Specially designed for traversing trails and other walking surfaces, walking poles look like ski poles with rubber tips, instead of pointed ends, and rubber rings. And they're lightweight.

WHAT THE EXPERT SAYS: Walking poles "unweight" your lower body and lighten the load on your legs (sort of like walking with a cane), making the poles a useful tool for women with arthritis or orthopedic problems. But walking poles can add to your workout while taking stress off your knees, back, and hips. John Porcari, Ph.D., professor of exercise and sports science at the University of Wisconsin–La Crosse, studied the use of walking poles during exercise and found that using walking poles can help you burn up to 25 percent more calories, boost your upper-body endurance by 40 percent, increase your heart rate, and decrease strain on your legs.

"It's not the weight of the poles that's giving all these benefits; it's how you use them," he says. "To benefit fully, swing your arms, plant the poles, and pull yourself along as you walk."

PURCHASING TIPS: You can choose between two types of walking poles. One type comes at a set length and tends to be more rigid and stable. The other type is adjustable but has a greater tendency to rattle and vibrate as you walk. Try the poles out in the store to determine which type you like better. Look for poles at your local sporting goods store, and expect to pay between $70 and $150.

FITNESS PRESCRIPTIONS FOR **HIPS**

Gentle twist

Lie on your back with your legs straight. Bend your left leg, then drop it over your right leg so your left foot is up near your right knee and your left knee points to the right. Using your right hand, gently press your left leg toward the floor. Trying to keep both shoulders on the ground, turn your head to the left so your spine feels like it is rotating and you feel a deep release in your hip and buttocks. Hold for 30 seconds. Repeat three times on each side.

How it helps the hips: A classic hip stretch known to runners, swimmers, dancers, and yoga students worldwide, this stretches all the gluteus muscles as well as the whole back.

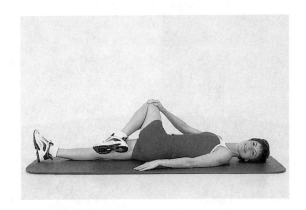

Hip stretch

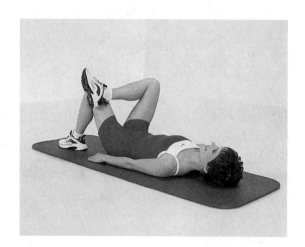

Starting on your back with both knees bent, cross your right foot over your left knee. Clasp both hands behind your left knee and bring it toward your chest until you feel a deep stretch in your right buttock area. For a deeper stretch, push your raised knee away from you with your right elbow. Breathe slow and deep while you hold the stretch for 30 seconds. Do the stretch four times on each side.

How this helps the hips: Tight gluteal muscles contribute to a feeling of stiffness in the hip; this exercise releases the buttocks and surrounding area.

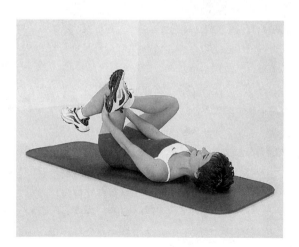

FITNESS PRESCRIPTIONS FOR **HIPS**

The sphinx

From a belly-down position on bent elbows, push your arms to the ground and lift your upper body off the floor while your hips remain grounded. Hold this position for 60 seconds, trying to widen the space between your shoulders and relax your back. Repeat three times.

How it helps the hips: A basic yoga pose, this stretches and relaxes the back, abdomen, and hips when they are sore or tight.

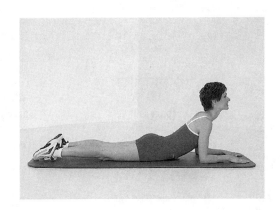

The cobra

From a belly-down position with palms beside your rib cage, engage your arms to lift your upper body. Straighten your arms as much as possible while keeping your lower back relaxed and buttocks firm. Look up; hold for 3 seconds. Gently lower yourself to the ground, then push back into cobra. Repeat 15 more times.

How it helps the hips: Also a yoga pose, this is a more advanced version of the sphinx that greatly stretches hips while also strengthening the hip-supporting muscles of the abs and lower back.

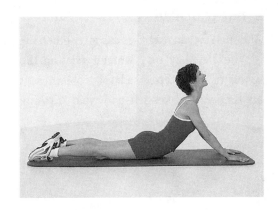

Other Helpful Exercises for the Hips

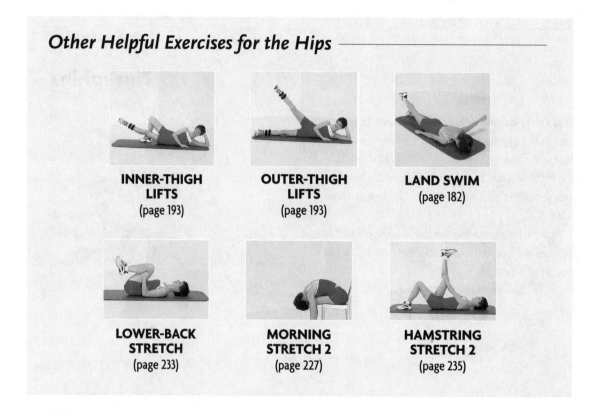

**INNER-THIGH
LIFTS**
(page 193)

**OUTER-THIGH
LIFTS**
(page 193)

LAND SWIM
(page 182)

**LOWER-BACK
STRETCH**
(page 233)

**MORNING
STRETCH 2**
(page 227)

**HAMSTRING
STRETCH 2**
(page 235)

What to Avoid

Although certain exercises can strengthen the hip flexors, they may worsen existing hip problems or exacerbate a back problem, says Dr. Nagler. It makes sense to avoid anything that hurts your hips, but if you have a hip problem, he cautions against quadriceps stretches (see the photo on page 234), whether performed standing or lying on the side.

Shoulder-Savvy Moves

Athletes commonly develop aching shoulders from not stretching them enough before and after a workout. But even nonathletes fall prey to tight shoulders when they walk and sit with poor, head-forward and rounded-shoulder posture. Every woman should stretch her upper body daily, especially in midlife, when she's more prone to the added shoulder discomfort of tendinitis, says Dr. Hamner. The best time to do this is while you're taking a warm shower or right afterward, he says.

In addition, maintaining upper-body strength—particularly in the commonly neglected back of the torso—will foster better posture and make it easier to execute daily activities, whether your goal is to trim the hedges or spike a mean volleyball.

If you've had a rotator cuff injury, check with your doctor before doing the following shoulder-savvy moves.

FITNESS PRESCRIPTIONS FOR **SHOULDERS**

The pullup

Using a chinup bar or a gym set bar, with your palms facing away from you, boost yourself into chinup position and hold for as long as you can. *(Alternative)* On a Gravitron-style machine: Adjust the device to absorb approximately half your weight so that you can do six to eight pullups at a time. Gripping the bar with your palms facing away from you, do three sets of eight.

How it helps the shoulders: Because the pullup strengthens the entire upper body, it's probably the best exercise you can do to condition the shoulders.

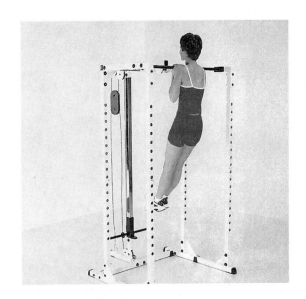

Dips

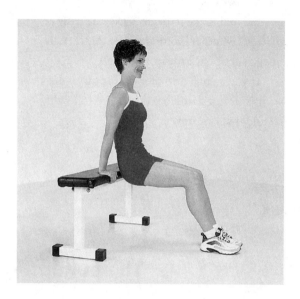

Sitting on the edge of a workout bench (or a stable, knee-level piece of furniture such as a chair or the arm of a couch) with palms down at your sides, place your weight on your palms, and walk your feet out approximately 24 inches. Straighten your arms as you lift your hips off the bench. Bending your elbows directly behind you, lower your hips 12 to 18 inches (be careful not to go any lower). Keeping your arm muscles fully engaged, push yourself back up. Repeat 8 to 10 times. Do three sets.

How it helps the shoulders: Dips give your upper body a good stretch and strengthen the lateral, deltoid, and triceps muscles while also working your abdominal muscles.

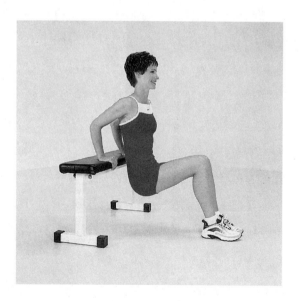

FITNESS PRESCRIPTIONS FOR **SHOULDERS**

Internal and external rotator raise

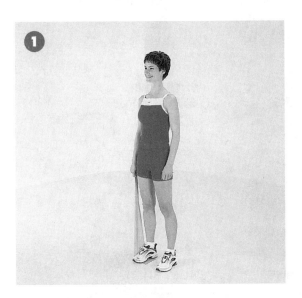

Stand on one end of a 5-foot-long resistance band and take approximately a foot's worth of the other end into your right fist, holding it palm-down at your hip (1). Straighten your arm, and gradually raise it straight in front of your body until you get as close to over your head as possible (2). Lower it and raise it five more times, each time moving it farther out to the side of your body with straight arms until your arm is perpendicular to your hip (3). (You may need to turn your palm partially up the farther out you go.) Repeat the five raises on your left side, and do at least three sets a day.

How it helps the shoulders: Helps restore the full range of motion to stiff shoulders.

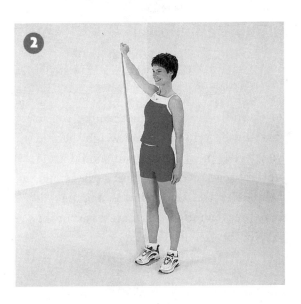

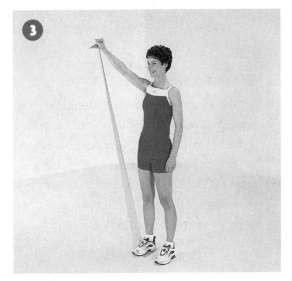

Other Helpful Shoulder Exercises

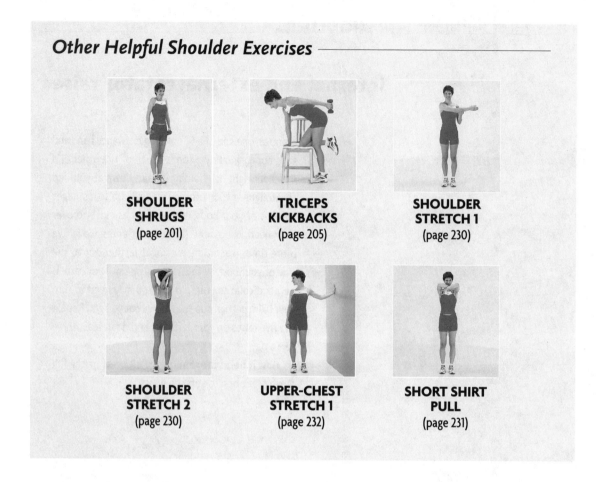

SHOULDER SHRUGS
(page 201)

TRICEPS KICKBACKS
(page 205)

SHOULDER STRETCH 1
(page 230)

SHOULDER STRETCH 2
(page 230)

UPPER-CHEST STRETCH 1
(page 232)

SHORT SHIRT PULL
(page 231)

What to Avoid

Lifting weight can tone and strengthen your arms, but poor form will do your shoulders more harm than good. As you age, it's easier to dislocate your shoulder or develop a rotator cuff injury. When doing a chest press with dumbbells (see the photo on page 198), don't let your elbows drop below the bench level, and avoid moves that require you to take a wide grip or to pull weight behind your head. In particular, you should avoid upright rows, overhead triceps extensions, behind-the-neck lat pulldowns, and the military press, none of which are a part of the Fit Not Fat Exercise Plan.

CHAPTER 13

CUSTOMIZING YOUR WORKOUT:

FITNESS PRESCRIPTIONS FOR ASTHMA, DIABETES, HIGH BLOOD PRESSURE, AND MORE

Typically, women over 40 know they should exercise, want to exercise, and even like to exercise. But any one of a number of health conditions—such as arthritis, a bad back, fibromyalgia, or obesity—may make it difficult for them to become active or stick with a program once they start. Others have specific health conditions for which exercise can help.

While part 4, The 40-Plus Exercise Plan, gives general guidelines for staying fit not fat at 40-plus, this chapter of the Fit Not Fat Program modifies that plan to enable you to overcome personal obstacles, achieve personal goals, and customize your workouts for success despite health conditions that can arise at midlife. And being active can actually help prevent or ease several conditions, such as diabetes, high cholesterol and osteoporosis.

"There are few physical obstacles that should hold people back from exercising," says R. Norman Harden, M.D., director of the Center for Pain Studies at the Rehabilitation Institute of Chicago. The key lies in knowing how to modify your exercise program to fit your needs. Following are expert tips to help you deal with any of the 23 health conditions that commonly affect women over 40. (For more information about specific types of exercises recommended, see chapters 9, 10, and 11.)

Advancing Age

Searching for the Fountain of Youth? You need look no further than your own two feet, because physical activity is the secret to aging gracefully. "Activity will improve and maintain your functioning in life," says Jessie Jones, Ph.D., codirector of the Center for Successful Aging at California State University at Fullerton. "It will maintain your ability to stay independent as you age."

Being active on a regular basis can keep you going strong for about 15 years longer than women your age who are physically inactive, Dr. Jones adds. That means you'll be able to play with your grandchildren, walk the dog, take active vacations, tackle house and yard work, and take care of your personal needs, even into your ripe old age.

And it's never too late to start. You can begin exercising at age 70, 80, or beyond, and still reap tremendous benefits.

Besides allowing you to participate more fully in life, activity helps you improve your posture, look younger, maintain your body weight, reduce the risk of conditions such as osteoporosis, improve your memory, and boost your mood. It can also aid recovery from various health conditions.

Dr. Jones has worked with women who have had paralyzing strokes and then exercised their way back to walking. She's also known older women who have been able to leave nursing homes and live in their own homes, thanks to exercise.

But where do you start, especially if you're not accustomed to activity? First, figure out how much time you spend sitting or lying down each day—you may be surprised at how inactive you are. Then find ways to be less idle. "Move a little more, and do it more often," Dr. Jones says. Stretch while you're watching television, for example. If you can, adopt a dog so you have a reason to walk. Stroll down the street to the grocery store. Take up gardening. Join a fitness class for older adults. Go dancing.

Senior Aerobics Classes

No matter what your age, fitness can and should be a way of life. Health clubs have been increasingly offering more classes specifically designed for men and women over age 60, says Josie Gardiner, Reebok Master Trainer.

You'll probably find a wide assortment of classes such as yoga, tai chi, aerobics, and strength and flexibility training for seniors. These classes might take place on land or in the water. They focus on activities that will help you age gracefully and perform the activities of daily living while improving the quality of your life. The moves are uncomplicated and gentle. You'll also hear music more likely to suit your tastes, such as swing, light country, or the best of the 1950s.

Taking an aerobic class at a health club offers numerous benefits. Instructors are trained to work with older adults. Plus, senior classes are offered when clubs are the quietest— usually late morning through early afternoon—which means you'll avoid the rush of the prime-time crowd. You'll also find a community of friends who can offer support, encouragement, and friendly faces. Perhaps you'll meet for coffee or lunch after class.

If you don't know where to take a class, ask friends for recommendations. And if you're nervous about participating, ask if you can watch a class or two. A good instructor will make repeated eye contact with students, suggest ways to modify moves to individual needs, give clear, precise instructions, and offer positive reinforcement.

Once you join the class, let the instructor know about any health conditions you have. And don't worry about being able to make it through the whole class. If an hour seems intimidating, sign up for a 30-minute class. Or just do as much as you can at first, even if it's just the warmup or 20 minutes of the class. The most important part is to have fun. As Gardiner says, "Enjoy the commitment you've made to your health."

If you're interested in a formal exercise program, first check with your doctor about any health conditions that may interfere with your exercise plan. Then talk to a qualified fitness professional who has experience working with older adults.

Your Fitness Prescription

You'll need to include cardiovascular activity—such as walking, swimming, or water aerobics—plus exercises that build strength and flexibility and help improve your posture.

Aim for 30. Half an hour of cardiovascular activity daily, either all in one session or in increments of 10 minutes throughout the day, is a great goal.

Hoist the weights. Once or twice a week, strengthen your muscles and help boost bone density by lifting weights or using an exercise machine—if your doctor has given you clearance. Start with light weights, or low resistance on a machine, and do one set of 15 repetitions. As you become fitter, increase the weight or resistance and do just 12 repetitions.

Stretch daily. Also, work on improving your posture since poor posture can affect the joints and muscles. Dr. Jones recommends the structured exercise regimen of Pilates, a series of continuously linked yoga-like movements, which can not only enhance your posture but also build strength. Being strong and agile can help prevent falls.

Listen to your body. Exercise at moderate intensity; the workout should feel *somewhat* hard. Should you begin to feel pain, it's a sign that you may be overdoing it, so decrease the intensity. If the pain persists, stop exercising and talk to a qualified fitness professional about modifying your activities. Also, if your joints are inflamed or red, don't do exercises that bend or stress them.

Try chair aerobics. If you have difficulty standing, this low-level fitness exercise can help you do strengthening exercises while seated. Basically, any type of movement can be beneficial—for example, arm raises, arm circles, leg raises, and knee bends. Because sitting can worsen certain problems, however, Dr. Jones recommends that you try to do some activities while standing. You can use a walker or a cane or hold on to a handrail or a wall for support.

Wear well-fitting, good-quality shoes appropriate for the activity. Shoes that offer poor support and inadequate cushioning may cause or aggravate joint problems.

Drink water regularly. As you age, you lose your ability to recognize thirst and are more likely to become dehydrated. Drink even when you don't feel thirsty—at least eight 8-ounce glasses of water daily.

Asthma

During an asthma attack, breathing passageways narrow, and spasms in the bronchial tubes can cause chest tightness and wheezing. In many cases, daily exercise can decrease the severity of attacks by making breathing easier and reducing stress, which can worsen asthma. Plus, women over 40 who are taking oral corticosteroids or high doses of inhaled corticosteroids for asthma are at increased risk for osteoporosis. Exercise—especially strength training and running—can help prevent this bone-depleting condition.

Although exercise commonly triggers an attack, it happens only rarely, says Sally Wenzel, M.D., professor of medicine at the University of Colorado Health Sciences Center and the National Jewish Medical and Research Center in Denver. Overall, exercise is a healthy, safe way to manage asthma. Talk to your physician about your plans to exercise, and find out if you need to adjust any medication.

Your Fitness Prescription

To decrease the likelihood of your having an asthma attack and overcome any wheezing and discomfort that may occur during exercise, follow these precautions.

Drink up. Hydrating with water before, during, and after exercise can improve breathing.

Say "no thanks" to salt. One study found that a low-sodium diet enhanced breathing and decreased exercise-induced asthma, so watching your salt intake may help prevent attacks. *Prevention* magazine recommends no more than 2,000 milligrams a day.

Get lots of vitamin C. If you consume high amounts of vitamin C before exercise, you may be one of the 80 percent of people with exercise-induced asthma who have no symptoms. *Prevention* magazine recommends getting no more than 2,000 milligrams daily from food or supplements.

Use your inhaler. If you use a short-acting beta agonist inhaler, take a puff 15 to 30 minutes before exercising. Carry it with you and use it as needed.

Do a double warmup. Thirty to 60 minutes before you begin exercising, do a short warmup to increase protective compounds in your body that help guard against an asthma attack. Choose a low-intensity activity—such as jogging in place—that makes you break a light sweat and raises your heart rate slightly, then rest until you're ready for your workout. Just don't forget to do your regular warmup then.

Leave the cold behind. When the temperature dips, head indoors because exercising in cold, dry air can aggravate asthma. If you must work out outdoors, wear a face mask or put a scarf over your nose and mouth to warm the air before it reaches your lungs.

FIT FLASH

Strength Training Builds Your Resistance

Research shows that pumping weights can help strengthen your defenses against free radicals, those rogue molecules that zip through your body and damage cells and tissues.

A recent study found that a group of 62 people, average age 68, who had lifted weights three times a week for 6 months had only a 2 percent increase in free radical damage. The normal amount would have been a 13 percent increase—which is what the researchers found in a similar group of people who hadn't exercised during that time.

The group that strength trained got the same amount of protection whether they lifted heavy weights or light weights.

Get wet. Indoor water workouts offer the greatest benefits because the warm, moist air near the pool allows for easier breathing.

Beware pollen, molds, smoke, and pollution. If allergens are lurking in the air, it's best to skip outdoor workouts. If you must exercise outside, talk to your physician about adjusting your medication. Also, since lots of pollen floats through the air in the morning, do your outdoor workout later in the day, when pollen counts are lowest.

Don't ignore your body. If you've had a cold or the flu, or if your asthma isn't under daily control, avoid aerobic workouts until you feel better.

End easily. Finish each workout with a 10-minute cooldown that includes stretching.

Bone Spurs, Fractures, and Tendinitis

After age 40, wear and tear may cause your body to develop weak links, and your joints and muscle tissues may be more vulnerable to injury. As a result, you may be more likely to experience bone spurs, fractures, or tendinitis, all of which are treatable.

You can stay active and fit despite your injury. You just have to modify your exercise routine accordingly, says Nicholas A. DiNubile, M.D., orthopedic consultant for the Philadelphia 76ers basketball team and a former special adviser to the President's Council on Physical Fitness and Sports. "It's absolutely possible to keep yourself fit while you heal," he says. "You just have to be creative." (Consulting a sports medicine physician or other doctor accustomed to treating sports-related injuries, if possible, can make a big difference in your recovery.)

BONE SPURS

The small, sometimes painful projections known as bone spurs can occur anywhere on the body, but they appear most commonly on the heel. You may not even know you have one until it's aggravated by overuse or a change in shoes.

To treat a heel spur, avoid activities that require standing or place stress on your feet. Try cycling, water exercise, or exercising on an elliptical machine. Wear sneakers or shoes that offer adequate arch support. Since people with tight calf muscles and tight arches are predisposed to heel pain, stretch your calf muscles three or four times a day. A gel heel cup or cushion may provide comfort during the healing process. Your doctor may also prescribe a night splint that stretches your heel. Once the pain resolves, you can continue your regular activities.

FRACTURES

There are two types of fractures. In an acute, or sudden, fracture, an otherwise healthy bone breaks as a result of a fall or other impact, while a stress, or hairline, fracture most commonly occurs in the shin, foot, or ankle and gradually develops over a period of time from overuse. Simply put, if your bones are subjected to more force and activity than they can handle, they can break down. Either type of fracture should be a red light to evaluate your bone health and, if appropriate, request a bone-density test.

An acute fracture generally takes 6 to 8 weeks to heal. During that time, learn to exercise around the injury and protect the injured part. Ask your physician for advice. If you fractured your arm, for example, consider walking, instead of running, because the high velocity of running could put you at greater risk for falls.

If you've broken your leg, try exercising on an upper-body ergometer, which is similar to a stationary bike except that you use hand cranks instead of pedaling. If you have a waterproof cast and your doctor okays it, you can also do water workouts. Continue to strength train your upper-body muscles.

Exercise options for stress fractures are slightly different. First, stop doing the activity that caused the fracture. If you're a runner, for example, take a break until the bone heals. If you don't, the bone will continue to weaken and may even break completely. Switch to cycling or water exercise. You may continue weight training, but be cautious about how you use the injured limb.

TENDINITIS

Tendinitis in the rotator cuff is one of the most common ailments in active women over 40, Dr. DiNubile says. The muscles in

FITNESS MYSTERIES

Why do I feel sore after shoveling snow or digging up my garden in the spring, even though I take aerobics three times a week?

When you do a particular type of exercise, your body becomes accustomed to it, but these improvements don't necessarily extend to other kinds of exertion, explains Kathy Sward, Ph.D., clinical assistant professor in exercise physiology and programming director for the Health Enhancement Program of the University of Pittsburgh Medical Center. This kind of muscle adaptation is called *specificity*.

So, while your cardiovascular system might be great at doing aerobics, your muscles might not be ready for shoveling. If your muscles got accustomed to using the shovel, they would probably get sore after you painted your ceiling. To stay in shape for everyday activities, you should cross-train, or do different types of exercise that use different muscles. One day you may feel like walking, another day you may cycle, and still another day may be strength training. All these activities are very beneficial on their own, but when combined with other activities, an overall body conditioning results.

the rotator cuff, part of the shoulder joint, weaken and lose elasticity with age.

During recovery, avoid raising your arm over your head in movements such as serving a tennis ball (you can work on your ground strokes if you like, but take about 2 weeks off from doing overhead shots). Don't do strength-training moves, such as overhead presses, that require you to lift overhead. Stick to activities that keep your arms at or below chest level, and talk to a qualified fitness professional about exercises you can do to strengthen the rotator cuff.

Achilles tendinitis is a common problem for runners and dancers. Don't ignore it; rather, stop the offending activity until the tendinitis subsides. If you continue to exercise, you could tear the tendon. If you normally walk or run, exercise instead on an elliptical trainer or a stationary bike. If those activities aggravate the condition, you can exercise in water or on an upper-body ergometer. Because Achilles tendinitis often comes from having tight calf muscles, stretch your calf muscles regularly.

Above all, don't be discouraged. "You can always find ways to work safely around your injury," says Dr. DiNubile.

Breast Cancer Recovery ———•

Women recovering from breast cancer can be as active as women who haven't had breast cancer, and just as active as they were before their diagnosis. In fact, exercise can help you make a successful recovery, both mentally and physically.

Perhaps you feel that your body has betrayed you, and that's normal, says Susan Love, M.D., adjunct professor of surgery at UCLA and author of *Dr. Susan Love's Breast Book*. Through exercise, you can reclaim and redefine your body. "Exercise will improve your quality of life," she says.

Physically, exercise can speed your recovery by stimulating the healing process. Physical exercise can decrease stress, pain, nausea, fatigue, and depression. Regular exercise affects your hormonal balance as well as most of your body systems. Also, women who are overweight have higher rates of breast cancer recurrence, and exercise is one of the best ways to lose weight or keep it at a healthy level.

In addition, exercise can prevent a stiff or frozen shoulder, a common occurrence after breast cancer surgery. You may have pain and soreness in your chest, especially when reaching overhead, and the shoulder on the affected side may be tight. Although you may be tempted to baby the shoulder, doing that lets the muscles weaken and the tendons tighten.

Before you begin an exercise program, talk to your physician about any recommendations she may have. If you're undergoing chemotherapy and have never exercised, Dr. Love recommends that you start your program after you finish treatment. If you previously led an active lifestyle, however, you can continue exercising during treatment. In fact, physical activity may help diminish the side effects.

Your Fitness Prescription

Plan to include cardiovascular activity, strength training, and range-of-motion and stretching exercises. Do cardiovascular exercise, such as walking, three or four times a week for 30 minutes at a time. You might also try water exercise, such as swimming or aqua aerobics, which is less stressful for a tight, sore shoulder and may even help loosen it. Also do two sessions of strength training each week.

Do range-of-motion and stretching exercises daily. Your focus should be your shoulder muscles. Dr. Love recommends climbing walls and arm circles (see page 276).

Watch for swelling. As you exercise, keep an eye out for any swelling in your arm, which could indicate a common condition called lymphedema that often occurs after surgery. Lymphedema may be a sign that you're overdoing it or doing the wrong type of activity. Talk to your physician or physical therapist about modifying your exercise program.

Consult a physical therapist. If you're uneasy about exercising on your own, consult a professional to help you set up a program. Or check with your local YWCA for a program called Encore Plus, which is designed to help women recover from breast cancer. You can

reach the YWCA directly by calling, toll-free, (800) 95-EPLUS to find out if it offers programs designed to help women with recovery.

Cellulite

Cellulite has a dirty reputation among women. Its undesirable appearance has forced thousands to slather their bodies with expensive creams, follow trendy, dangerous diets, or undergo cosmetic procedures. But there's a less expensive, more effective alternative to diminish cellulite: exercise.

Cellulite, the common term for puckered, lumpy skin, is nothing more than a fancy word for fat. "It's a normal abnormality that's typical of women's skin," says Jerome Z. Litt, M.D., assistant professor of dermatology at Case Western Reserve University in Cleveland and author of *Your Skin from A-to-Z*.

As you age, your skin becomes thinner and looser. Clusters of fat cells, what many call cellulite, replace this lost skin. Although it can be found anywhere on the body, it's most commonly seen in the buttocks, thighs, lower abdomen, and upper arms.

No massages, creams, surgery, or diet can get rid of this fat, Dr. Litt says. Although exercise won't zap the fat completely, it can help, so preventing cellulite involves exercising and controlling your weight.

Your Fitness Prescription

The recommended regimen sounds like a traditional fitness program: cardiovascular

FITNESS PRESCRIPTIONS FOR **BREAST CANCER RECOVERY**

• Climbing wall

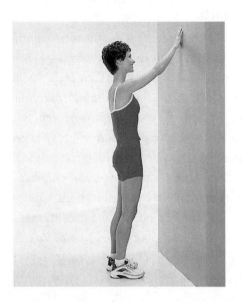

Stand facing a wall about an arm's length away. Place your hand on the wall and "walk" up it with your fingers, trying to stretch a little farther each time. As you "walk" higher, you will have to move closer to the wall. Do this five times and then repeat, standing perpendicular to the wall. You can do this once or twice a day.

Arm circles

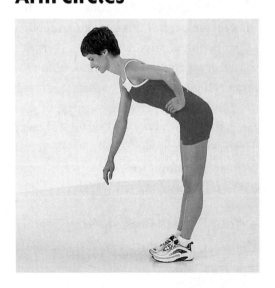

Lean forward from your hips, let your arm hang down naturally, and relax your hand. With one arm at a time, begin to make small backward arm circles, gradually increasing the size of the circles. Repeat 10 times with each arm.

activity, strength training, and flexibility work. But it's how you do each activity that makes the difference, says Michael Youssouf, the 2000 IDEA/Life Fitness Personal Trainer of the Year and manager of trainer education at the Sports Center at Chelsea Piers in New York City.

Sweat hard. In other words, if you want to blast that cellulite, you're going to have to really work. And that doesn't mean doing 500 leg lifts or 100 abdominal crunches every day. Spot reducing doesn't work.

Establish a solid base of cardiovascular endurance. Exercise regularly at a moderate intensity, then, after about 3 months, graduate to a higher intensity.

Choose your activity for intensity and interval training. Jogging, walking, or biking will let you work hard. (To make a walking workout more intense, add an incline or find a hilly area to walk in.) After you warm up, do an interval program, in which you alternate between periods of work and periods of rest. But *resting* doesn't mean that you get to sit down and relax. The idea is to exercise continuously. For example, Youssouf recommends jogging three telephone pole lengths, then walking one telephone pole length.

First, do 30 seconds of intense activity to a point where you're breathless (on a scale of 1 to 10, with 10 being the hardest, work toward a 9). Then recover for 60 seconds by doing a different activity. After you complete a sprint, for example, slow to a walk. After pedaling hard on a stationary cycle, stop and do some triceps dips or abdominal crunches. Add this workout once a week to your regular routine and work up to two or three times a week.

Eventually, make the workouts harder. Rather than doing 30 seconds of tough work, do 60 seconds and follow with 30 seconds of recovery activity.

Alternate with "regular" aerobics. On the days you don't do a high-intensity workout, Youssouf recommends doing regular aerobic conditioning, what he calls base training, such as walking or jogging at a comfortable pace. He suggests base training three days a week for 30 to 40 minutes at a time.

Make your strength training more intense. Do more multijoint, full-body moves such as squats and lunges rather than isolating single muscles with exercises such as leg extensions or leg curls. Work hard enough that you're fatigued after 8 to 12 repetitions. Think about varying each set, and find two or three different ways to do an exercise. For example, if you're doing a lunge, perform a front lunge, a side lunge, and a back lunge. If you're working the chest, do it on an incline, decline, and flat bench.

Stretch daily. Youssouf also recommends practicing yoga or Pilates to create a sinewy, lean look for your muscles.

Chronic Fatigue Syndrome

Busy women often complain of tiredness, yet day-to-day fatigue is much different from the

Resistance Bands

Elastic exercise bands, also called resistance bands, increase strength—and therefore tone muscles—by providing resistance, but without the use of gravity, which heavy dumbbells or weight machines use.

WHAT THE EXPERT SAYS: "Using resistance bands imitates how your muscle formulates the 'pushing' movement seen in the chest press or shoulder press," says Wayne Westcott, Ph.D., fitness research director at the South Shore YMCA in Quincy, Massachusetts. So they're particularly useful for "pushing" exercises, which help shape and tone your arms, bustline, upper back, and shoulders.

"As you stretch the resistance band, you increase the resistance," says Dr. Westcott. The biggest benefit? Your increase in so-called eccentric strength, the lengthening contraction of a muscle. And using resistance bands forces you to control movement—the key to gaining strength.

"With a dumbbell you might feel like dropping your arms after each biceps curl," says Dr. Westcott. "The resistance band forces you to go slower so you don't snap yourself in the eye."

Dr. Westcott suggests these resistance band exercises for women who want to tone their upper body.

Chest press: Sit in a chair with a back that's wider than your shoulders. Wrap the resistance band around the back of the chair and pretend you're doing a pushup by straightening your arms in front of you.

fatigue experienced by women with chronic fatigue syndrome. Their bodies ache, and they have trouble with concentration and short-term memory, adding mental fatigue to physical weariness.

If you struggle with chronic fatigue, therapeutic exercise will make you feel better, says Mark VanNess, Ph.D., professor of exercise science at the University of the Pacific in Stockton, California. Being active can help preserve range of motion in your joints,

maintain muscle mass (which helps battle atrophy), reduce joint pain, boost mood and self-esteem, and improve or maintain cognitive functions. Most important, it can increase your stamina so you can do daily activities such as vacuuming or gardening. The fitter you are, the more you can do before exhaustion overcomes you.

Understand, though, that you won't be as active as you were before you were diagnosed with chronic fatigue syndrome. "You have to

Overhead press: Sit in a chair with a seat that's wider than your shoulders. Wrap the resistance band under the seat of the chair. Raise your arms over your head.

Seated row: Sit on the floor. Wrap the resistance band at least once around your feet (so it doesn't snap back and hit you in the face). Pretend you're rowing and pull toward your chest.

PURCHASING TIPS: Bands come at different resistance levels for higher or lower intensity. Select what's most comfortable for you. Look for resistance bands with easy-to-use detachable handles. (While not as small or painful as a slingshot, the resistance band can hurt if you accidentally let go at the wrong time.) You can also purchase bands called Bodylastics, with clips that attach to door frames for easier use. Bands are available at sporting goods stores.

To order a complete set of Bodylastics bands, call (800) 500-1979 or visit www.bodylastics.com. The set includes four bands at different resistance levels, removable handles, ankle straps for leg exercises, a door anchor, a travel bag, a user manual, and an instructional video. The set costs $49.95 plus shipping and handling. Or you can order bands individually at regular prices.

redefine what exercise is for you," says Dr. VanNess. Be realistic, setting your sights on increasing your capacity to do everyday activities.

Your Fitness Prescription

Your best bet is to alternate short bursts of effort with rest periods of recovery. For example, a work period might involve walking on a treadmill or riding a stationary bike, or you could choose to walk around your garden. (It's best to exercise in an area where you can rest for several minutes.) You might stretch or do resistance exercises, such as 10 to 12 biceps curls, with little or no weight.

Conserve energy. Opt for resistance exercises that let you sit rather than stand. Work for 30 to 60 seconds, then sit and wait until you've recovered fully before beginning another work period. Your rest period should last at least a minute, but it may be several minutes.

Limit yourself to 20. Your entire exercise session should be no longer than 20 minutes. At first, you may not be able to do more than one work period, and that's okay. Allow your body to progress slowly. If you try to do too much, you'll increase your fatigue, and it may take you several days to recover. Progress to longer exercise sessions once you can complete five or more sessions without prolonged fatigue.

Start small. How many days a week you do this program depends on how you feel. Start with 2 days a week and work up to 4 days, if possible. Just remember that any amount of exertion may drain your energy bank. If your day includes other activities, such as going to the doctor or shopping, you'll tax your energy supply and will may have little left for exercise. Schedule workouts for less hectic days.

Fuel your body throughout the day. Eating small, carbohydrate-rich snacks of bagels, breads, cereals, and meal replacement bars can give you more energy to exercise and maintain cognitive function. You can even spread the snack out so that you're eating before, during, and after exercise. For example, nibble a third of a meal replacement bar before exercise. During exercise, nibble another third, and finish it afterward.

Try tai chi and meditation. They will improve your focus and memory and make you feel more relaxed. (For details on tai chi, see page 162).

Diabetes ━━━━━━━━━━●

Although exercise won't cure diabetes, it will help you lower blood pressure and blood glu-cose levels, increase insulin sensitivity, maintain healthy levels of cholesterol and other blood fats, reduce the risk of heart disease, and maintain or lose weight.

"Any woman with diabetes can benefit from regular exercise," says Joel B. Braunstein, M.D., a clinical cardiologist and Robert Wood Johnson National Clinical Scholar at the Johns Hopkins Medical Institutions in Baltimore. "People with diabetes who regulate their blood sugar, recognize their limits, and understand how activities influence their bodies can do virtually almost the same activities as someone without diabetes."

Before you begin, have a stress test if you are older than 35, have had type 2 diabetes for more than 10 years or type 1 diabetes for more than 15 years, or have one or more risk factors for heart disease, including high blood pressure, a family history of heart disease, or a current smoking habit. In some circumstances, your doctor may want you to have a stress test even if you don't fit these characteristics. And since exercise influences the rate at which your body metabolizes glucose, which in turn affects your blood sugar levels, talk to your physician about adjusting any of your medications to keep your blood sugar levels well-controlled.

Your Fitness Prescription

With your physician's go-ahead, do your favorite aerobic activities at least, but preferably more than, three or four times a week for 30 to

40 minutes. If you have any loss of sensation in your joints or muscles, do low-impact activities such as walking or swimming. Take 5 to 10 minutes to warm up, and spend another 5 to 10 minutes cooling down. In addition, do two or three strength-training sessions and two or three sessions of flexibility training a week.

Be aware of retinopathy. If you have retinopathy (tiny hemorrhages in the eye, a common effect of long-standing diabetes), discuss with your doctor which activities are safe for you. In more advanced cases, it is especially important to avoid activities that cause sudden increases in blood pressure, such as weight lifting and sprinting, and any activity in which you lower your head below your waist. Also, avoid sports that involve rapid, jarring movements, such as racquetball or jogging. Extra pressure built up behind the eyes during these kinds of exercises can damage the fragile blood vessels of your retina.

And also neuropathy. With neuropathy (nerve damage associated with diabetes), focus on low-impact activities such as walking, stationary cycling, or swimming. If you suffer from autonomic neuropathy (a related form that affects balance), avoid activities that encourage rapid position changes and upright activities, such as step aerobics or running. Such activities may lead to dizziness or a loss of balance and possible injury.

Wear a medical ID tag. This lets medical personnel and others know that you have di-

abetes, so in case of emergency, you get proper care if you're unable to speak.

If you rely on injected insulin, don't inject into the main muscles used in exercise, such as your quads or upper arms. If you typically inject insulin before exercising, an excellent site to do this is in your abdomen.

Exercise with a buddy. If that's not possible, join a fitness facility that's equipped to handle medical emergencies.

Treat your feet well. Wear properly fitted shoes; look for a wide toe box and a cushion of air or gel underneath the midsole. Avoid wearing cotton socks, which absorb moisture and can cause skin irritations and blisters. Instead, opt for socks made of moisture-wicking materials, such as CoolMax. Check your feet before and after your workout for signs of blisters, cuts, or other irritations.

Monitor your intensity. Pay attention to how you feel. If you think you're exercising too hard, you probably are.

Check your blood sugar before, during, and after you exercise. If you have type 1 diabetes, consider checking your blood sugar every 30 minutes during activity. If it's lower than 100 milligrams/deciliter (mg/dl), it is recommended that you consume 10 to 15 grams of carbohydrate, such as 8 ounces of orange juice—diluted with 4 ounces of water—four peanut butter crackers, or half a banana. If it's higher than 250 mg/dl, check your blood levels for ketones, by-products of metabolism produced in abnormally high

She Put Supports in Her Sneakers and Walked Away the Pounds

One day 20 years ago, New York City podiatrist Suzanne Levine couldn't find a cab, so she chose to walk to her meeting, foot pain and all. Walking became her best weapon for weight loss, good health, and greater self-esteem. Today, she's more than 50 pounds lighter.

My weight has always been influenced by foot issues. As a child, I had foot problems and had to wear special shoes that made it difficult to walk. While other kids were running and playing, I was usually reading and eating—*overeating*, in fact.

Through my teens and twenties, my weight fluctuated wildly—sometimes 10 to 15 pounds in a week—from all the crazy diets I tried, only to abandon with a craving and a binge. I'm sure those wild fluctuations contributed to my developing hypoglycemia.

My turning point came when I was leaving the hospital after delivering my second child. Someone asked me when my baby was due—another blow to my already low self-esteem. At age 29, I was 5 feet 4 inches tall, 180 pounds, and knew I had to finally change; I just wasn't sure how.

One day, I couldn't hail a cab and decided to hike it. I arrived at my meeting glowing and energized. I felt great. So I started walking three times a week, gradually increasing to over 4 miles, up to five times a week. Because I had always had pain in my heels and arches, I put arch supports in my walking shoes. After that, nothing could stop me from enjoying the wind blowing against my hair as I walked. For the first time in my life, I felt comfortable with my body. I adopted healthy eating habits (low-fat foods, more complex carbohydrates, portion control) and used nonfood rewards (such as pedicures).

That was over 20 years ago. I eventually lost 52 pounds and felt great. By my not carrying around so much weight, my foot pain and hypoglycemia disappeared. I felt really comfortable with who I was.

With a flourishing podiatry practice and three kids to raise solo, I seem to have less free time these days, but I still walk a lot plus do other aerobics three or four times a week. I limit my wheat and sugar consumption because they set off my cravings. When I do have a piece of cake or chocolate, I eat protein with it—such as soy nuts. It sounds odd, but it works for me. It stabilizes my blood sugar levels so that I don't end up craving more an hour afterward.

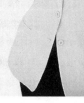

Foot pain kept Suzanne from exercise.

And I pamper myself. When I've had a stressful day, I don't head for the fridge—I hit the tub for an aromatherapy soak. The dog and kids can wait a bit.

I weigh 125 pounds now—and I'm happy and on track.

quantities in uncontrolled diabetes. If they are present, you may need insulin, and you should not exercise, says Dr. Braunstein.

Exercising when blood sugars are in this range and ketones are present may cause your already dangerously high blood sugar levels to rise further. If, however, your reading is higher than 250 mg/dl and there are no ketones, usually several units (one to three units, for example) of short-acting insulin will safely bring down your blood sugar levels. Despite all warnings, if you decide to exercise with blood sugars in this range, use caution and monitor yourself frequently, advises Dr. Braunstein.

Hydrate well. Drinking 8 to 16 ounces of water 1 to 2 hours before exercising, then having about 8 ounces of fluid for every 30 minutes of activity, is sufficient. Unless you're exercising for more than an hour, drink water instead of juice, sports drinks, or other fluids high in concentrated carbohydrates.

Watch the timing. Avoid activity when your insulin levels are likely to be highest, such as late in the day or 1 to 2 hours after your last dose.

Replenish carbohydrates. Within the first 2 hours after exercising, have 10 to 15 grams of carbohydrate. Again, during exercise, avoid highly concentrated carbohydrates, such as sports drinks. However, if diluted with equal parts of water, they may be a sufficient source of energy during exercise.

Carry snacks. If you feel faint or dizzy, stop exercising, hydrate, and check your blood sugar. If necessary, have a rapid-acting form of carbohydrate such as orange juice or glucose tablets.

Communicate. Discuss your exercise routine with your doctor. If things don't feel quite right, let your doctor know.

Fibromyalgia

Aerobic exercise might seem impossible if you have fibromyalgia, but physical activity is essential for managing this condition. Its cause is unknown, but millions of women are affected by its muscle pain and stiffness and fatigue.

"You have to find a way to exercise if you want to get better," says Dr. Harden.

Preliminary studies conducted by Dr. Harden indicate that there may be a link between aerobic conditioning and pain from fibromyalgia. Women who are in good aerobic condition may suffer less pain, while those who don't exercise may have more. Plus, doing aerobic exercise gives you an immediate boost of serotonin, a brain chemical that regulates mood, improving your mood without medication.

Your Fitness Prescription

Your long-term goal should be to exercise for 30 to 40 minutes every day. For about 20 minutes of that time, you should work at your target heart rate. (For instructions on determining your target heart rate, see chapter 9.) But don't expect to work at this level immediately. Get your physician's okay, then start slowly. If you do too much at once, your body will ache from the overload. Instead, take baby steps.

Allow yourself 3 to 6 months to progress. If you can do 1 minute of exercise, then do 1 minute, perhaps only walking to your mailbox at first. Gradually, increase your time so that after 2 weeks, for instance, you're exercising for 5 minutes at a time.

Choose swimming or walking. These are the two best forms of exercise if you have fibromyalgia. Both are low-impact activities that put little stress on your body. In water, of course, you weigh less, so swimming takes stress off your joints and muscles.

Warm up. At the start of your workout, start off by doing light aerobic activity. If you're walking, for example, spend a few minutes walking slowly. For extra warming of the muscles, take a hot shower or put heating pads on any tight spots before you begin exercising.

Cool down. After you've been working at your target heart rate, cool down by exercising for the last few minutes at the same pace you used to warm up.

Avoid becoming chilled. Many people with fibromyalgia claim that pain increases as their body temperature drops, so put on a jacket or sweatshirt as soon as you get out of the pool or during the cooldown portion of your walk.

Ice can be nice. To minimize discomfort after your workout, ice any swollen or inflamed areas around your muscles for 15 minutes. Use an ice pack or ice wrapped in a washcloth or small towel; don't apply ice directly to your skin.

Stretch regularly. This is especially important right after aerobic activity. Performing gentle stretches will help decrease muscle soreness. To help relieve pain, several times a day do easy range-of-motion exercises such as rotating your ankles or shrugging your shoulders.

Keep your chin up. Most important, try not to get discouraged. Exercising with fi-

---

FIT | FLASH

Mild Exercise Reduces Fibromyalgia Pain and Boosts Mood

Here's more evidence that people with fibromyalgia, a condition causing pain, joint stiffness, and fatigue, need to move. When 22 women with fibromyalgia participated for 10 weeks in a 60-minute, twice-a-week program of mild aerobics, strengthening, and stretching, they had significantly less pain, felt happier, and were able to walk more comfortably at faster speeds.

"Any movement increases mobility," says study author Kimberley Dawson, Ph.D., associate professor in the department of kinesiology and physical education at Wilfrid Laurier University in Waterloo, Ontario. "Do something today," she says.

bromyalgia takes patience. Know that you'll have good days and bad days. If you have a bad day, shorten your exercise session or do an easier workout. As time progresses and your ability to exercise increases, the good days should outnumber the bad.

Hay Fever

You know allergy season has returned when you begin battling puffy eyes, frequent sneezing, and a drippy nose. None of that has to stop you from exercising, though. In fact, exercise can provide temporary relief from symptoms and help prevent further complications from hay fever, says Betty B. Wray, M.D., interim dean of the school of medicine at the Medical College of Georgia in Augusta.

When you exercise, you stimulate the flow of adrenaline, which in turn opens airways in your body. As a result, nasal congestion clears, and you receive temporary relief from hay fever symptoms.

Women with hay fever stand an increased risk of developing asthma. By keeping yourself as active as possible, you'll increase your lung capacity, which will allow for better breathing. If you develop asthma, your fitness conditioning will enable you to manage your breathing more effectively.

Your Fitness Prescription

Keeping your hay fever under control is especially important if you're exercising outdoors when allergens are high. Complications from hay fever can lead to headaches and sinusitis. If those symptoms occur, take a decongestant and skip exercise until you feel better. Otherwise, talk to your physician about using an antihistamine before you exercise. Here are more tips.

Take action before a flare-up. If you know your hay fever is going to act up, you can help minimize symptoms by using allergy-relieving eyedrops, such as Naphcon or Vasocon, beforehand. Both are available over-the-counter (OTC). Nasalcrom, a preventive nose spray also available OTC, can provide relief from hay fever symptoms and other nasal allergies. Just avoid using a decongestant nose drop on a daily basis because it can cause rebound symptoms, advises Dr. Wray.

If you wear contacts, don your glasses when exercising. Or ask your optometrist to prescribe eyedrops that can be used with contacts, to decrease itching. Carry your glasses with you in case the itching becomes unbearable.

During allergy season, exercise later in the day. Pollen counts often peak in the morning and diminish as the day progresses. Perhaps one of the best times to exercise outdoors is after a rainstorm, Dr. Wray says. Unless heavy winds accompanied the storm, rain will have washed pollen out of the air.

Keep it clean. If you exercise indoors at home, close the windows in your house during allergy season. Pollen and other allergens settle quickly into furniture and drapes and often take days to be removed.

Carpeting can harbor allergens, so vacuum and steam clean carpeting and rugs frequently. If your home gym is in the basement, check for mold or dampness and control the humidity. You may need to put a dehumidifier in the basement.

Keep any pets out of your home gym, especially if they go outside. Pollen and other allergens can accumulate in their coat.

Head to a pool. The moist air allows you to breathe easier, but if the pool's outdoors, check the pollen and mold counts, as well as ozone and other air quality markers, in your local newspaper or on the Internet at www.epa.gov/airnow. Also, mold and mildew may lurk near showers, hot tubs, saunas, and indoor pools. To avoid an allergy flare, give the facility a thorough checkup before exercising.

Finally, if you experience abnormal shortness of breath or coughing when exercising, schedule an appointment with an allergist to rule out asthma (or treat it, if it's diagnosed).

Heart Disease and High Cholesterol ●

Your level of physical activity directly influences your cholesterol levels and heart health. Keeping active helps decrease the risk of heart disease and symptoms while increasing HDL, or good, cholesterol levels and lowering total cholesterol. It also allows you to perform more daily activities with less effort, says Richard Stein, M.D., chief of cardiology at Brooklyn Hospital Center in New York and spokesperson for the American Heart Association.

Consult your physician before you engage in exercise, especially if you are over 60, have elevated risk factors for heart disease, or have been inactive for the past several years. Then focus on aerobic exercise, the key to improving cardiovascular health. Think about doing sustained activities such as biking or swimming. Walking is perhaps one of the best heart-healthy exercises because it requires no training, lets you control how long and how hard you work, allows you to start and stop when you want, and carries a low risk of injury.

Your Fitness Prescription

Doctors advise women who want to protect their heart health to spend at least 30 minutes 5 or 6 days a week doing aerobic activity. Warm up for 5 minutes, slowly increasing your intensity. After your workout, cool down for another 5 minutes. Stretch before and after exercising.

Keep a check on your intensity. Dr. Stein advocates using a scale of 1 to 10 (1 being easiest, 10 hardest). After your warmup, try to keep your intensity between 6 and 8. That might be difficult at first, so work at a lower intensity for a few weeks and gradually increase the intensity as you get fitter. Continually assess how you feel during exercise. If you feel unusually dizzy or have abnormal shortness of breath, stop exercising and see your physician.

Build muscles. Strength training also may benefit heart health and cholesterol levels. Do strength training 2 days a week. Perform one set of 10 to 12 repetitions for each major muscle group. Work to the point where you can do only one more repetition. Don't hold your breath when using weights. Exhale during the strenuous part of the exercise, and inhale as you release the contraction.

Know your special precautions. Most important, be careful about any exercise that requires you to work with your arms above your head. Raising your arms to that height will increase oxygen demands on your heart and elevate your heart rate and blood pressure, Dr. Stein says. Instead, modify the movements. If you're in an aerobic class and the instructor cues you to lift your arms overhead, simply move your arms at or below chest level.

Similarly, avoid any strength-training exercises that require your arms to go above your head or your head to go below your heart. Simple modifications can make moves safe. An overhead press, for instance, a popular exercise for the triceps, requires you to lift a weight over your head. To modify the move, hold a weight in your right hand and stand in a lunge position with your right leg and foot in front about one step. Bend your knees slightly. Your body weight should be balanced evenly over both feet. Lift your right elbow alongside your body until it's slightly behind you. Hold your elbow in place as you extend the lower half of your right arm behind you. Return to starting position without moving your elbow and repeat, performing equal sets and repetitions on each arm.

Whenever in doubt about a particular exercise, talk to your physician or work with a qualified fitness professional.

High Blood Pressure

The American Heart Association defines high blood pressure as 140/90 mm Hg. Normal blood pressure is less than 130/85 mm Hg, while optimal blood pressure is below 120/80 mm Hg. Left untreated or uncontrolled, high blood pressure increases the risk for cardiovascular disease and strokes.

Medications and a change in diet are your first defense against high blood pressure, also known as hypertension. But exercise also can be a potent remedy for lowering blood pressure.

Through exercise, you can lose weight. A drop in blood pressure often accompanies weight loss. Exercise also strengthens your heart, which means it can pump more blood with less effort. In some individuals, blood pressure may respond to exercise in as little as 4 to 6 weeks, says Gerald Fletcher, M.D., cardiologist at the Mayo Clinic in Jacksonville, Florida.

Your Fitness Prescription

Before you begin any exercise program, talk to your physician. Learn to use a home blood pressure kit, and check your pressure occasionally before and after exercising. Be on the lookout for sharp drops or increases in your blood pressure. If you notice anything unusual, consult your physician. Your workout routine may need to be modified.

Make activity part of your daily routine. Your activity should be moderately intense, and the best exercise prescription to combat hypertension is aerobic activity. Walking is a favorite since it requires no training. Even household chores, such as gardening and mowing your lawn with a push mower, count as exercise. Ideally, you should do aerobic exercises 5 or 6 days a week for 30 to 40 minutes.

Know the warning signs. If you notice side effects such as headaches, excessive perspiration, or faintness, slow down and check your heart rate. When you're exercising, your heart rate should fall within the range of 130 to 140 beats per minute. If it's above this range, stop exercising, and rest until your heart rate returns to normal.

Temper your arm activity. Be careful about doing too much with your upper body, Dr. Fletcher warns. Using your arms to exercise aerobically, as you do on a cross-country ski machine or while performing certain steps in an aerobics class, can cause a temporary increase in blood pressure. If you're new to exercise, avoid these activities until you're in better shape. Or use just your legs. For example, on a cross-country ski machine, hold your arms to your side while you swish your legs forward and back.

Don't forget the weights. Although there's no guarantee that strength training can help decrease blood pressure, women who strength train can increase bone density and ward off osteoporosis. If you would like to participate in strength training, remember that upper-body exercises may also cause blood pressure to rise, especially when you lift your arms above your head. Rather than lift your arms over your head while exercising, keep them at or below the level of your heart. Also, avoid exercises, such as an incline situp, where your head drops below your heart.

When strength training, use light weights and do high repetitions. Start with 5-pound weights and work your way up to 10 pounds. And remember to breathe—holding your breath may cause your blood pressure to rise. Exhale through your mouth on exertion.

Try alternative exercise. Because stress can also contribute to high blood pressure, relaxation techniques such as meditation, yoga, and tai chi can often benefit hypertensive individuals.

Keep an eye on the pounds. Although exercise certainly helps lower blood pressure, the benefits may be reversed if you gain weight or quit exercising. Control your weight, exercise regularly, and follow your physician's advice about medications, and you should be able to see a change in your blood pressure in as little as 4 to 6 weeks, says Dr. Fletcher.

Hot Flashes

If you're approaching menopause and experiencing hormone-related hot flashes, exercise can help you cope. Here's why.

Hot flashes are a sign that your body's progesterone and estrogen are waning. There are several factors involved. For starters, estrogen is involved in the metabolism of norepinephrine, which is produced when you exercise and when you experience stress. The body responds to exercise and stress by sweating. When your estrogen is low, less norepinephrine is metabolized in the brain, and your body responds as it does when you exercise or are stressed. In other words, you feel hot, and you sweat. In addition, when you are perimenopausal, you typically have high levels of follicle-stimulating hormone (FSH), which is normally released just before ovulation and which raises your internal temperature set point. Because you are no longer ovulating regularly, FSH may remain at high levels, contributing to your body's temperature troubles.

Keeping physically active allows your body to maintain better control of your internal temperature. Regular, vigorous exercise can ease stress-related tension and help you cool more efficiently as your body learns to perspire sooner after the onset of exertion. But because vigorous exercise also releases the hormone norepinephrine, which is responsible for accelerating the heart rate, constricting blood vessels, and raising blood pressure, consider avoiding highly stressful exercise settings—those where competition or physical appearance is overemphasized.

Your Fitness Prescription

Perimenopause means not only a switch in your hormones but also changes in your exercise needs. "This is a time to make the transition from being an aerobic animal to having a more balanced exercise program," says Ann Cowlin, assistant clinical professor at the Yale University School of Nursing and movement specialist with the Yale University Athletic Department.

Balance your exercise program. Aerobic exercise and strength training both contribute to heart and bone health. Aim for doing aerobic activity three to five times a week for 20 to 30 minutes, and strength training 2 days a week. Just watch out for activities that require you to suddenly change position and level, such as a dance step that goes from a high-reaching motion to the ground in one or two counts, or a racquetball game that requires similar motion, which could trigger a hot flash, Cowlin says.

Strengthen and tone. After you've been doing aerobic activities comfortably for a few weeks, add strength training to your program. Exercises to strengthen your rotator cuff, upper back, abdomen, gluteals, hamstrings, and pelvic floor muscles are important, along with leg presses, which strengthen all the muscles of the legs and hips and are important for bone strength and avoiding falls.

Don't forget stress reduction. You don't need to join a class to do this. You could practice deep breathing and relaxation techniques such as guided imagery—mentally seeing yourself relaxing on a warm beach. Simply take 5 or 10 minutes before or after your workout to do these activities. If you want formal instruction, check out classes in yoga, tai chi, or meditation.

Keep your cool. If you have a hot flash while you're exercising, lower the intensity of your activity and take several deep breaths.

You can make adjusting to temperature changes easier by dressing in layers—tank tops, T-shirts, cardigan-style warmup jackets, fleece vests, and windbreakers. If a hot flash hits, peel off an outer layer to help your body cool. As you get chilled, bundle up again.

If the air is hot and muggy, skip the outdoor workout and head indoors. Heat typically decreases performance and can contribute to hot flashes.

Keep yourself well-hydrated. Hot flashes may cause sweating, which can lead to dehydration, especially during exercise.

Know when to take it down a notch. If hot flashes persist while you're exercising and you're doing all that you can medically and nutritionally to control them, you may have to modify your exercise program. Perhaps your workouts have become too intense or competitive. Intense activities can often load the body with extra stress and norepinephrine. Lower the intensity, or find an activity that's less competitive.

Speak with your doc. If your hot flashes occur in the aftermath of a hysterectomy, with certain medications, or during postpartum or pregnancy, or from other medical conditions, Cowlin advises talking to your physician about exercising. He may prescribe a slightly different exercise program.

Hysterectomy

After having a hysterectomy, many women are scared to start moving, afraid they'll tear something. But in fact, done prudently, exercise can help speed recovery.

"The sooner women are out of bed and moving around, the faster the healing process is put into motion," says Dwight Im, M.D., associate director of the Gynecologic Oncology Center at Mercy Medical Center in Baltimore. "The worst thing they can do is lie around and do nothing."

When should you start moving? It depends. Physicians differ on when women who have had a hysterectomy should start activity. Talk to your physician, who is familiar with your medical background and case history, and follow her advice.

Dr. Im offers general guidelines for activity. The day after your hysterectomy, get up and move around a little. You'll probably feel great: You'll probably be on pain medication, and any presurgery anxiety is likely to be gone.

The toughest time is 2 or 3 days after the surgery, when the pain returns. You may think you'd be better off resting comfortably in bed. But if you want your body to recover more quickly and effectively, then do light activity.

Your Fitness Prescription

Take a casual stroll around the block or be more active with chores around the house. Let your body be your guide. "Some women can walk a mile after surgery, while others can barely walk half a block before they get tired and sore. Just try to avoid doing anything strenuous," says Dr. Im.

Stay away from weights. That goes for lifting anything heavier than 5 pounds. If you've been doing strength training, keep the resistance to 5 pounds or less. Get clearance from your physician before you lift heavier items.

Don't skimp on the Kegels. Dr. Im also recommends doing Kegel exercises immediately after surgery. After a hysterectomy, the pelvic floor muscles may be weakened. By doing Kegels, you'll keep your pelvic floor muscles toned and be better able to void urine and perform other functions. Do Kegels several times

a day to build those muscles. (For details on how to perform Kegels, see page 304.)

Hold off on crunches. Getting your abdominal muscles back in shape is another important part of recovery, but wait about 4 to 6 weeks before you do any kind of abdominal exercises. Again, this will vary from one woman to another. Check with your doctor first. Once you've received your doctor's okay, begin strengthening and firming the abdominal muscles with crunches and other abdominal exercises. (For more information, see chapter 10.)

Be proactive. The women who recover most quickly from hysterectomy are those who were in good shape beforehand. If you know you're going to undergo a hysterectomy at some point, start an exercise program immediately. Build your aerobic endurance and strength train, paying particular attention to your abdominal muscles.

Menstrual Cramps

Popping over-the-counter medications isn't the only way to combat menstrual cramps. Exercise regularly, and your cramps may even disappear.

Cramps occur when the tissue that lines the uterus contracts to rid itself of debris and blood. After all, the uterus is a muscle, and like any other muscle in the body, it can contract and relax. In some women, cramps can be debilitating. Even worse, women over 40 may experience more painful cramping, often linked to either fibroids, which are benign growths that in some cases can intensify uterine contractions, or endometriosis.

Your Fitness Prescription

If your doctor has ruled out an underlying medical cause for cramps, regular aerobic exercise may bring some relief. During vigorous exercise, your body secretes endorphins and enkephalins, naturally occurring opiate-like chemicals in the brain that blunt pain. And like morphine or other opiates, endorphins triggered by exercise increase pain tolerance.

Pick an activity you enjoy. Commit to doing it regularly—5 days a week for 45 minutes at a time. If you don't have the time or the stamina for 45 minutes, exercise for 5 to 15 minutes to stimulate the release of endorphins. The point is to make your commitment to exercise as regular as possible.

"If you can do this, you won't have menstrual cramps, or if you do, they'll be diminished," says Susan C. Fox, M.D., a New York City internist who specializes in women's health and hormonal problems. Dr. Fox prescribes exercise for all of her patients, especially women suffering from menstrual cramps. Walking is a favorite because of its accessibility.

Take preventive medicine. To prevent menstrual cramps from occurring during exercise, take a nonsteroidal anti-inflammatory drug (like ibuprofen) with food 1 hour ahead of time. If you experience a cramp while you're exercising, stop activity and rest until the cramp vanishes. As your body relaxes, so will the uterine muscle, Dr. Fox says. When the cramp is gone, resume activity at a lower intensity. A menstrual cramp during exercise may indicate that you're working too intensely during this time in your cycle.

Know when to take it easy. When menstrual cramps are at their worst, though, even walking may be too difficult. If that happens, do gentle stretches, focusing on those that elongate the abdominals and lower back. You'll help the uterus relax and ease the lower-back pain that often accompanies menstrual cramping. "You're almost trying to squeeze the uterus like a sponge to promote fluid drainage," Dr. Fox explains.

To help relieve stress in the uterus, try the cobra pose, seen on page 261, and the baby pose, seen on page 249.

Migraine Headaches

Migraine headaches occur when the blood vessels that cover the brain dilate and release neuropeptides, such as substance P and neurokinin, that cause a pain response. These headaches are debilitating and frustrating, but regular exercise can control and prevent painful episodes in the same way it relieves menstrual cramps—by stepping up production of pain-relieving compounds: endorphins and enkephalins. When the levels of those compounds decline, often because of stress, your head may begin hurting.

Your Fitness Prescription

Regular exercise boosts the amount of endorphins and enkephalins in your body. So if you exercise regularly, you'll suffer less frequent and less severe migraines. "The more chronic the headaches, the more important exercise becomes," says Fred Freitag, D.O., associate director of the Diamond Headache Clinic in Chicago. Plus, you'll respond to a lower dosage of medication.

How much exercise is needed to combat migraines varies according to the individual. Freitag recommends a baseline of 3 or 4 days a week of 20 to 30 minutes of exercise. Before you begin, be sure to take a few minutes to warm up—with cycling, for example—just enough to work up a light sweat before you begin your exercise routine. Choose an activity you enjoy—such as gardening, ballroom dancing, swimming, water aerobics, walking your dog, or strength training.

Don't double up. Instead of doing hour-long workouts twice a week, try exercising more regularly—it's a more effective strategy to manage migraines. Find ways to work more activity into your daily routine. Walk to your neighbor's house rather than call her on the telephone. Or slip on your sneakers during your lunch break and go for a quick walk.

Avoiding migraine triggers. Be aware that certain types of exercise can trigger a migraine. Jarring activities, such as running and tennis, can provoke headaches and aren't recommended for people who are prone to migraines. Experiment with different activities to find those that allow you to exercise without pain.

Protect yourself. If you bike or go inline skating, be sure to wear a helmet to protect your head if you fall. Even if you're not injured, a blow to your head could cause a migraine.

Approach weights with caution. Weight lifting also may trigger a migraine, which is unfortunate because strength training plays a crucial role in helping women combat both weight gain and osteoporosis. If you find that strength training brings on a migraine, spend several weeks improving your general fitness. Once you're in better shape, you may be able to strength train without a problem. Use light resistance to begin.

Don't work through pain. If a migraine strikes while you're exercising, stop activity immediately. Apply ice for 15 minutes to the back of your neck and the area where you feel the most intense pain.

Beware headaches that begin lower. Many individuals who are prone to migraines also experience related pain in their neck and shoulders. To decrease the frequency and severity of these headaches, work on improving the strength and range of motion in your neck, shoulders, and lower back.

Try yoga. Allow your mind to relax by doing yoga. Yoga allows you to focus—and, in doing so, reset your brain chemistry, which may just chase those migraines away.

Check with your doctor regularly. If you consistently get headaches when you exercise, check with your physician to make sure everything's okay. In rare cases, persistent headaches can signal more serious problems, such as a brain tumor or an aneurysm, Dr. Freitag says. Chances are you may just be prone to getting migraines while exercising and will have to take precautions.

Mitral Valve Prolapse ———————•

Mitral valve prolapse syndrome occurs when the leaflet of mitral valve of the heart flutters harmlessly. However harmless, mitral valve prolapse sometimes causes truly uncomfortable symptoms, including chest discomfort, heart palpitations, racing pulse, shortness of breath, panic attacks, fatigue and mood swings, as well as dizziness when changing positions.

Women who have been diagnosed with mitral valve prolapse are often afraid to exercise, which explains why many of them are out of shape. Yet regular exercise can be the key to dealing with this condition, says Phillip Watkins, M.D., medical director of the Mitral Valve Prolapse Center of Alabama in Birmingham.

Your Fitness Prescription

Once your doctor gives you the go-ahead, start with cardiovascular activity such as walking, cycling, or swimming. Avoid working with weights until you're more phys-ically fit, perhaps after 4 to 6 weeks of regular exercise.

Shoot for 150. Try to do 150 minutes of cardiovascular activity every week, Dr. Watkins advises. Break up that time to fit your schedule and fitness level. Some women may be able to start with five 30-minute sessions. If you're extremely out of shape, break that time into smaller increments—perhaps 10-minute sessions performed 15 times each week. Those smaller workouts may even be something as convenient as walking up and down stairs in your office building or strolling through a shopping mall. (For more ideas for how to build small increments of exercise into your routine, see chapter 14.) If doing 150 minutes a week is still too difficult, do what you can at first, then build up to 150 minutes over the course of several weeks.

Exercise safely. As you exercise, ask yourself how hard you feel you're working. Your goal should be to work at a moderately hard level.

Warm up before exercising, and cool down when you're finished. Also, stretch before and after exercise. Many women with mitral valve prolapse experience muscle spasms, which can lead to tight, sore muscles. Stretching will help relieve that tension.

Add in weights. Once you've devoted a few weeks to aerobic activity, which should make up more than half of your exercise time, add strength training to your workout program. Use light weights, and do high repetitions.

Pay special attention to your upper body. Women with mitral valve prolapse often have decreased upper-body strength, making it hard to reach cabinets or use a hair dryer. Use dumbbells and do exercises such as chest presses and biceps curls. (For details on how to do these exercises, see chapter 10.)

Keep yourself hydrated. Drinking water before, during, and after exercise can help regulate your blood volume and blood pressure. In a day's time, try to consume at least 64 ounces of water. If you're exercising outdoors or if you're involved in a recreational sport such as tennis where exercise sessions may last more than an hour, chug a sports drink that contains sodium.

Bliss out. You may also want to do some relaxation activities, such as yoga, tai chi, or meditation, to help ease anxiety and decrease panic attacks.

Obesity

Move it, and you *will* lose it. That's the message that physicians offer women who weigh up to 100 or more pounds than they should. "The more you move, the more you'll lose," says Sharonne Hayes, M.D., director of the Mayo Clinic Women's Heart Clinic. Women who carry extra pounds jeopardize their health by increasing their risk for certain diseases, including type 2 diabetes, which in turn is also a risk factor for cardiovascular disease. Obesity can increase cholesterol and blood pressure, boosting the risk for heart

disease and stroke. Many extremely overweight women also have sleeping problems, depression, and low self-esteem. Overall, they just don't feel well. Losing weight is critical to improving their health.

Successful weight loss comes from combining more activity with better nutrition—essentially, following this book's Fit Not Fat Plan for food and exercise, which will enable you to burn more calories than you eat. The payoff? "Exercise will make you feel better," says Dr. Hayes. Don't expect immediate results, though. It may be 4 to 6 weeks before you begin to notice a difference.

Make it your goal to burn 1,000 to 2,000 calories a week, which means doing some type of exercise for 30 to 60 minutes every day. Forget about whether you're losing weight. Instead, focus on how good exercise makes you feel and how much more energy you have.

Your Fitness Prescription

Start with 30 minutes of activity a day. Doing anything is better than doing nothing, but the more you do, the better. Garden, walk your dog, clean the house, walk several flights of stairs. If you've been inactive, walk 5 minutes a day. Gradually, increase your time in increments of 5 minutes until you reach 30 minutes. (For more ideas, see chapter 14.)

Go low-impact. You might also do aqua aerobics or walk in the shallow end of a pool. Water workouts are easy on your joints, an important consideration if you have any pain in your knees or back. Classes are often offered through local Y's or health clubs. Riding a recumbent bike also places little stress on your body; plus, recumbent bike seats are usually more comfortable than seats on a regular bike. Just avoid high-impact activities such as jogging, which can stress your joints, or vigorous activities such as shoveling snow. If standing is difficult, wheel yourself in a wheelchair or do chair aerobics.

Take your breath away—slightly. Your sessions of activity don't have to be intense, but they should leave you a little breathless, so that you could have only a brief conversation with a friend. And don't worry about slight shortness of breath; it's a natural by-product of exercise. If you feel faint or experience extreme breathlessness or chest discomfort, though, stop exercising and immediately get medical help.

Invent reasons to walk. Adopt a dog, if possible, or walk with a friend rather than meeting for coffee.

Set realistic goals. Don't concentrate on weight loss, only on increasing activity. For example, aim to walk for 20 continuous minutes each day for a week, an increase of 5 minutes from last week.

Reward yourself—but not with food. When you meet a goal, do something nice for yourself. Buy some perfume you've always wanted, treat yourself to a movie, or get a manicure.

Exercise with your family. Be a good role model and encourage your family to join you.

Use the buddy system. You're less likely to skip a workout if you know someone's waiting for you.

Seize the opportunity. Sneak activity into your schedule whenever you can. Pace the room when you talk on the phone. Do your stretching as you watch your favorite television show.

Osteoarthritis

If your joints feel stiff and achy due to arthritis, the last thing you might feel like doing is exercising. But, in fact, inactivity can cause further discomfort, while exercise has multiple benefits. Exercise can decrease pain and stiffness; prevent further deterioration of joints and muscles; improve your ability to do daily activities; increase the range of motion of your joints; keep your muscles, bones, and cartilage strong and healthy; combat depression; and boost your self-esteem and feelings of well-being.

"Exercise is an important part of dealing with arthritis," says Bernard Rubin, D.O., chief of the division of rheumatology at the University of North Texas Health Science Center in Fort Worth.

If you have arthritis, start slowly and work toward the future, knowing that each time you exercise, you do a little more to improve your life. And be patient; you may not experience relief until you've been working out regularly for several weeks. Try to do some activity daily, advises Dr. Rubin.

COOL TOOL

Lei Weights

Invented by a onetime resident of Hawaii, Lei Weights are soft, sand-filled nylon weights that easily drape and form-fit to your body, similar to the flower necklaces for which they are named.

"The day I left Hawaii, friends and family members each brought me a beautiful Hawaiian lei," says Lisa Dereszynski, the inventor of the weights. "I had so many around my neck and arms that they were actually heavy, yet soft and comfortable." Lei Weights hark back to the leis Dereszynski wore that day.

WHAT THE EXPERT SAYS: Lei Weights stay in place, can go anywhere, and are versatile. "You can use Lei Weights for any exercise that you'd use free weights for," says Wayne Westcott, Ph.D., fitness research director at the South Shore YMCA in Quincy, Massachusetts. That versatility translates to a number of benefits. Lei weights:

▶ Are an easy way to add resistance to exercises like crunches, back extensions, and pushups

▶ Require no straps or wraps to use

▶ Provide varying levels of intensity (the farther away you place the weight, the more difficult it is to lift)

▶ Are easier to hold than dumbbells, especially for people with arthritis

▶ Require slow movement, which provides more strength-training benefits and reduces risk of injury

PURCHASING TIPS: Sold by Akua, Lei Weights are available in 1-pound increments (in 2- to 12-pound sets) and start at around $28 plus shipping and handling. To order, call (800) 691-4427, or go online at www.leiweights.com.

Your Fitness Prescription

Your regimen should include endurance or cardiovascular activities, strengthening exercises, and range-of-motion or flexibility exercises. You may also want to check out PACE (People with Arthritis Can Exercise) classes at a Y or community center.

Cardiovascular exercises include walking,

riding a stationary bike, and swimming. Swimming is considered one of the best activities, especially if you have osteoarthritis in your hips, knees, neck, or hands. Water keeps you buoyant, takes weight off your joints, helps your muscles relax, decreases pain, and allows you to move your joints through a greater range of motion without injury. Build up gradually to doing endurance activities 3 days a week for 20 to 30 minutes per session. (For information on exercising with rheumatoid arthritis, see page 301.)

Try isometric and isotonic exercises. Exercises that can help maintain and increase muscle strength are equally important. The Arthritis Foundation recommends two types. One is isometric exercise, in which you build strength by contracting, though not moving, specific muscles. For example, to strengthen your quadriceps, the muscles in the fronts of your thighs, you can just sit in a chair and tighten them while holding your legs straight.

The other type is isotonic, which means using your muscles to move your joints, perhaps by doing exercises in which you lift and lower a weight. You can do isotonic activities when your arthritis isn't flaring up. Twice a week, on land or in water, use light weights or resistance, and do a high number of repetitions. If you have trouble gripping objects, consider using weights that strap around your wrists and fasten with Velcro. Talk to a physical therapist or a qualified fitness professional about the right exercises for you.

Build the muscles around the joints. If your hands are affected, for instance, you can build their strength by squeezing Silly Putty or a flexible rubber ball.

Increase flexibility and range of motion. Do stretching exercises and consider trying the gentle movements of tai chi. Yoga or Pilates can also offer further improvement.

Find the best time. To make exercise more enjoyable, experiment with the times you work out. Many women with arthritis feel better exercising later in the day, after stiff joints have had time to loosen up through use.

Be sure to warm up. Make it a habit to spend time before any activity doing easy exercise, such as walking slowly or marching in place. To warm your tissues even more, you can use a heating pad or hot, moist towel on particularly sore areas or take a hot shower before you exercise.

Always stretch. After warming up, spend a few minutes stretching. At the end of your workout, cool down with more easy exercise, then stretch again.

Watch your form. Concentrate on using good posture when you're active because poor posture may aggravate your aches and pains.

Listen to your body. If you experience sharp pain or more pain than normal during exercise, stop. If pain persists for an unusually long time after a workout, you may need to make changes in your exercise program. You should also evaluate your everyday activities and chores to determine if they are contributing to your pain.

Osteoporosis

Exercise does your bones good. More active people have stronger bones.

As explained in earlier chapters, physical activity slows or halts bone loss, increases bone density, and improves muscle strength and balance, crucial factors in preventing falls and their serious consequences. Of course, a diet high in calcium and vitamin D, a healthy lifestyle with no smoking or excessive alcohol intake, bone-density testing, and medications, if necessary, also can help prevent and manage osteoporosis.

Because building bone requires time, your commitment to exercise must be long term, says Christine Snow, Ph.D., professor of exercise and sports science and director of the bone research lab at Oregon State University in Corvallis. The research by Dr. Snow and her colleagues shows significant gains in bone density from regular physical activity after 12 or more months. To keep yourself motivated, find a workout buddy.

Your Fitness Prescription

The best bone-building activities overload the body. In other words, you need to put more force or load on your bones than they're used to from daily activities. To accomplish this, do a combination of weight-bearing cardiovascular activities and strength training.

Go beyond walking. In weight-bearing activities, your feet bear most of your weight. Walking, jogging, and standing strength exercises all count; swimming doesn't. Yet if walking is your only cardiovascular activity, you may not be doing enough for your bones. Although women who have walked for exercise their entire lives have a higher bone den-

sity than inactive women, walking doesn't provide enough overload to your bones. "Walking can help maintain bone mass in premenopausal women," Dr. Snow says, "but no evidence suggests that it can improve bone mass if you're normally active."

In addition, try jogging, stair stepping, and step aerobics. Even hiking several times a week with a backpack—true "weight-bearing" exercise—can contribute to bone mass. Do these activities three times a week. If you're a walker, alternate every few minutes between walking and jogging or running.

Make time each week for two or three strength-training sessions. Focus on building the muscles attached to the bones of your wrists, hips, and spine, the three areas that osteoporotic fractures most often strikes. Gain wrist strength, for example, by doing pushups (page 69), or biceps curls with weights (page 213). Exercises such as squats (page 191) can improve hip strength, while almost every upper-body strength exercise increases spinal strength. Stand, rather than sit, for most of your strength exercises.

Start with two or three sets of 10 to 12 repetitions. As you get stronger, increase the demand placed on your bones by decreasing to 8 to 10 repetitions but increasing the weight.

Don a weighted vest. As an alternative to weight machines, a weighted vest allows you to exercise in a standing position, which puts more weight on your bones, and also challenges your postural system and improves balance; thus, it can help reduce falls. Buy a weighted vest at a local sporting goods store.

Jump around. After a minimum of 3 months of lower-body strength exercises, add jumping activities such as jumping in place. Jump about 4 to 5 inches in the air and land fairly flat-footed. Dr. Snow cautions, though, that you should do such exercises at least 3 to 4 months after developing strength in your hips, knees, and ankles. As a bonus, you'll improve your balance by doing these activities.

Do yoga—carefully. You can also do yoga to boost your balance skills and help prevent falls. Just watch out if you're doing yoga; it can put excessive force on your spine. If you have severe osteoporosis in your spine or have had fractures, avoid more advanced yoga poses that require extraordinary balance and flexibility.

Protect your back. If you have severe osteoporosis, especially in the spine, avoid exercises that require bending and twisting at the waist while lifting objects that weigh more than 10 pounds. And make sure to keep your trunk straight as you exercise.

Remain upright. Finally, be careful to minimize your risk of falling during exercise. Avoid potentially risky activities, and be sure to hold on to stationary objects for support as you exercise.

Raynaud's Phenomenon ———•

Cold temperatures and emotional stress can often trigger Raynaud's phenomenon, a condition that causes fingers and toes to turn pale and white.

When an episode occurs, blood vessels narrow in the affected area—usually the fingers or toes—preventing blood from flowing there, says Dr. Rubin. If you're prone to Raynaud's, be aware that you could trigger an episode anytime you decrease circulation in your hands. For example, gripping a golf club slows bloodflow temporarily, making your hands more prone to becoming cold, especially if the air temperature is chilly.

Your Fitness Prescription

Women with Raynaud's phenomenon should take extra precautions when exercising outdoors. Depending on how sensitive you are to temperature, wear gloves or mittens. Because you lose much of your body heat through your head, thereby diverting it from your extremities, don a hat in cold weather. Wrap a scarf around your face and ears. Also, wear layers of loose-fitting clothing, and make sure you have good shoes to avoid problems such as blisters.

Poor bloodflow may cause dry skin, which can lead to cuts, cracks, and sores. If you play golf or softball outdoors in chilly weather, wear gloves. If you play tennis in the cool air, stick your hands under your arms between points or wrap them in a towel between changeovers.

Think twice before swimming. You may also want to avoid working out in water. Unless the pool is well-heated, the water may trigger an episode.

Don't ignore symptoms. If, despite these precautions, you experience an episode while you're working out, don't try to tough it out—go indoors to warm up or put on additional clothing. Then place your hands under your armpits for warmth. Wiggle your fingers or toes; walk around as much as you can to generate heat. Finally, place your hands and toes under warm, not hot, water until your skin color returns to normal. Avoid using a hot water bottle or a heating pad, which could burn your skin without your realizing it because the Raynaud's may decrease sensation, making it more difficult to feel pain.

Rheumatoid Arthritis ————— •

Rheumatoid arthritis (RA) is very different from osteoarthritis (page 296). In RA, the immune system somehow goes awry and attacks the body's connective tissue. During flare-ups, women with rheumatoid arthritis experience pain, hot swelling, possibly fever, sweating, and weakness in the muscles connected to the affected joints. RA can cause joint deformity and a loss of mobility.

Women with rheumatoid arthritis are caught in a vicious circle. Because of their joint pain, many aren't physically active. Yet without exercise, their muscles weaken further. In many cases this actually worsens pain.

The right kind of regular activity, however, can enable you to go about your day per-

forming your usual activities with less pain and less fatigue. You'll also increase muscle mass—which will support and protect your joints—and you'll improve your mood.

Your Fitness Prescription

Exercise programs for rheumatoid arthritis resemble general exercise programs for arthritis. You should do endurance or cardiovascular activities, strength exercises, and flexibility and range-of-motion exercises. Consult a physical therapist to help you set up an exercise program.

Start gently. If you're new to exercise, start with gentle range-of-motion exercises, often the least painful and easiest activity to do, says Lisa Geyman, physical therapist at the National Jewish Medical and Research Center in Denver. Examples include lifting your arms overhead, bending and straightening your elbows, and opening and closing your hands. Do these exercises once or twice daily, as tolerated. ("As tolerated" means the activity should not cause or increase pain, especially pain that lasts more than 2 hours after exercise.)

Eventually, add aerobic activity. Working three times a week for up to 20 minutes is enough. But do what your body will allow, even if that means starting with 5 minutes. On a scale of 1 to 10, 10 being the hardest, work at a level of between 2 (very easy) and 5 (feeling a bit winded).

Choose the best exercise for you. Water exercise is a good choice for aerobic exercise since the water supports your joints and allows you to move your muscles through a larger range of motion with less pain. Just make sure the temperature is right. Find a pool with water close to the temperature of your skin. Colder water may increase your pain.

Walking and stationary biking also may appeal to you. Wear supportive shoes when you walk. Evaluate how you feel on the bike; if riding increases your joint pain, discontinue biking and find another activity.

Add strength training. You should do strength exercises two or three times a week. If you're having an acute flare-up, do isometric exercises, which require no movement. Instead, you contract your muscles on your own and release the contraction. For example, you might push against a wall to increase arm strength.

If you're not experiencing a flare-up, do isotonic exercises, such as biceps curls, that involve movement around a joint. When you begin, use only your body weight as resistance. Start with one set of two or three repetitions, then increase weekly by one to three repetitions until you can do one set of 10 to 12 repetitions. Eventually, add light resistance by using dumbbells or elastic bands. If you have trouble gripping objects, use weights that strap on to your wrist and fasten with Velcro.

Fight pain with NSAIDs. An hour before exercising, take an aspirin or other non-steroidal anti-inflammatory drug (if your physician approves it).

Take it easy. Spend 3 to 5 minutes warming up. After exercising, cool down for a few minutes and end with stretching and range-of-motion activities. (For more detail, see chapter 11.) Keep your stretches light, and go only to the point of mild tension. Most important, avoid high-impact, high-resistance exercise such as running, vigorous stair stepping, and lifting heavy weights (more than 5 pounds), or doing more than 12 repetitions of a strength exercise.

Tune out pain. Music may help you stay active longer. Researchers at Glasgow University in Scotland found that women with rheumatoid arthritis could walk 30 percent farther when they listened to the music of their choice than when they walked in silence. "The music didn't make their pain disappear," says lead researcher Paul MacIntyre, M.D. "But it took their minds off it, so they could walk farther without needing to stop."

Remember your form. Always focus on using good posture to protect your joints. Don't put them in any awkward positions.

Geyman also recommends sessions of yoga or tai chi two to three times a week to help restore flexibility and range of motion to the joints, improve circulation to the joints, and trigger endorphins, your body's own feel-good "medication." While you release muscle tension, you'll also release mental tension. Just watch out for extreme positions, Geyman warns. And if you're having trouble standing, sit in a chair and modify the moves.

Mind the intensity. If you feel pain when you're exercising, reduce the intensity. If that eases your pain, continue exercising. If pain persists, consult your physician or therapist, especially if your joints become red or inflamed. Also, if you experience pain that lasts 1 to 2 hours after exercise, increased weakness, decreased range of motion, or increased joint swelling or pain, modify your exercise program.

Smoking Cessation ●

The same exercise-induced endorphins that relieve migraines and menstrual cramps (page 292) can help women who smoke quit, once and for all. Combining vigorous exercise with a smoking cessation program can considerably increase your chances of success. And when you quit, you'll breathe better, feel better about yourself, and reduce your risk of dying from heart disease.

And if that's not enough, exercise is a powerful weapon against one thing women dread most when they quit smoking—weight gain. On average, people gain 5 to 7 pounds when they quit smoking, says Norman Edelman, M.D., medical consultant for scientific affairs for the American Lung Association. Burning calories through exercise can counteract that weight gain.

Before you begin an exercise program, talk to your physician. Find out if you suffer from any health conditions that would require modifications to an exercise program. Smokers, after all, are at risk for such conditions as asthma, heart disease, and lung disease.

Your Fitness Prescription

When you get the doctor's okay, focus your efforts on aerobic activities such as jogging, walking, biking, swimming, and cross-country skiing. To improve your cardiovascular health and prevent heart disease, do

FIT|FLASH

Try Yoga for Rheumatoid Arthritis

For women suffering with rheumatoid arthritis (RA), yoga can help from both a physical and a mental aspect. Physically, yoga provides all the benefits of range-of-motion exercises. It helps restore flexibility and improves circulation to the joints, allows more healing nutrition to reach them, forces more oxygen into those joints, and triggers the release of endorphins, which are the body's own natural painkillers. Yoga also relieves pain by reducing muscle tension. Mentally, yoga has a calming, relaxing effect. Have your doctor or rheumatologist monitor your progress, then learn yoga. Some women fare best in a group setting; others, one-on-one with an instructor. Start out slowly, two or three times each week. RA is a serious disorder, so try to do yoga every day.

these activities four or five times a week for 30 minutes at a time.

Ease into an exercise program. Many women begin an exercise program overenthusiastically, suffer an injury, and then quit exercising, says Dr. Edelman. Plus, breathing may be a little difficult at first. Work at lower intensity levels during the first few weeks of exercise, then gradually pick up your intensity so that you're working moderately hard. Also, if half an hour seems difficult, then start with 10 or 15 minutes of exercise and build from there.

Really commit. Although exercise can certainly help you make a successful transition from smoker to nonsmoker, you should look at exercise as a long-term commitment. Says Dr. Edelman, "Exercise should be an activity that you enjoy for the rest of your life."

Urinary Incontinence

As they age, some women face incontinence problems, making it difficult to exercise without leaking. There's a simple solution to that problem: strengthen the pelvic floor muscles.

The pelvic floor muscles stretch from the pubic bone to the tailbone. They're responsible for supporting the bladder, urethra, and other organs. As women age, those muscles can weaken, causing bladder control problems. Weakening may be even more pronounced in women who have given birth.

Your Fitness Prescription

The best way to strengthen the pelvic floor muscles responsible for bladder control is to do Kegel exercises regularly.

Unfortunately, these muscles are difficult to isolate, so many women do Kegels incorrectly. Many mistakenly contract the abdominal and gluteus muscles, which does nothing for the strength of the pelvic floor. One way to be sure you're contracting the correct muscles is to stand naked in front of a mirror and do Kegels. "You should see nothing on the outside moving," says Elizabeth W. Bozeman, M.D., a urologist in South Carolina who specializes in women's health and a member of the Project Advisory Council for the National Association for Continence.

To do Kegels correctly, be as relaxed as possible. Without tightening your abdominals or buttocks, squeeze your pelvic floor muscles. Watch yourself in a mirror to make sure you don't spot movement in your hips, abdominals, or buttocks. One way to check if you've isolated the pelvic floor muscles is to stop your flow of urine in midstream, although doing this isn't a substitute for Kegel exercises.

If you're still having trouble doing Kegels, talk to a urologist, who may use biofeedback or electrical stimulation to help you feel your pelvic floor muscles.

Do two or three sets of 10 repetitions daily. Vary the speed of your contractions. Occasionally, do what Dr. Bozeman calls quick flicks: Contract hard for 1 to 2 seconds and then repeat. The next time you do Kegels, you might focus on holding the contractions 5 or 10 seconds if possible.

Check into weights. Your urologist or gynecologist may also prescribe special weights or cones, available in progressively increasing resistances, which you insert into your vagina. As your pelvic floor muscles get stronger, you graduate to the next resistance level.

Stay dry. In addition to doing Kegels, you can take other precautions to keep dry when you exercise. Always go to the bathroom before you exercise. Avoid heavy weight lifting; instead, do high repetitions with light weights. Also, wear panty liners if you're still concerned about leaking.

Speak up. If you leak only when you exercise, talk to a gynecologist or a urologist about using a pessary, a doughnut-shaped device specially fitted to your body that compresses the urethra and prevents leaking.

Don't be embarrassed about seeking medical help for incontinence. As Dr. Bozeman says, "This is a problem that can be easily treated, and it's one that women don't have to struggle with their entire lives."

CHAPTER 14

CUSTOMIZING YOUR WORKOUT:

FITNESS PRESCRIPTIONS FOR WHEN YOU HAVE 10 MINUTES OR LESS

In chapter 9, experts recommended working out 45 minutes to an hour a day (30 minutes for beginners) for weight loss. That chapter offers a couple of dozen different types of exercise you can try, from aerobics classes to yoga.

Chapter 10, Sculpt and Strengthen Muscles, introduced a step-by-step program for building bone, toning muscles, and "de-fatting" your physique. But if you're like most women, you don't always have a block of 30 to 60 minutes a day to devote exclusively to exercise. But you can still exercise—you just need to sneak in the equivalent in resourceful ways.

Take fitness expert Ann Grandjean, Ed.D., for example. On the days when life sidetracks her exercise plans, the executive director of the International Center for Sports Nutrition improvises, squeezing workouts in 5- to 10-minute bursts.

To talk to a colleague, Dr. Grandjean walks to the coworker's office instead of picking up the phone. If she needs a book from the company library, she fetches it herself. Instead of using her out box, she hand-delivers documents.

Once, Dr. Grandjean wondered how far she really walked during a typical day at her office in Omaha, Nebraska. She strapped on a pedometer and was thrilled to discover she'd racked up 2 miles.

Her steadfast rule—at home or on the road—is that she cannot go to bed unless she's squeezed in some form of exercise. "If I had a set routine and couldn't get to do it because of a crazy day, I'd use it as an excuse to do nothing at all," Dr. Grandjean says.

"The idea is to keep moving," she says. "Get a cordless phone or put a long cord on your regular phone, and walk when you talk. Find whatever works for you and just move. Park half a mile from the mall and walk. Take the stairs instead of the elevator. Those little, itty-bitty things add up."

Stolen Moments Add Up

Lest you think that short bursts of activity have a negligible effect on your fitness pro-

BESTBET

Get Your Heart Rate Pumping

In order for a short burst of exercise to be an effective calorie-burner, it helps if you reach your target heart rate. To do that, try what exercise physiologist Glen Gaesser, Ph.D., calls the "super spark," in his book *The Spark*. "This technique can be used with all forms of exercise, including walking."

For the 1st minute: Hold yourself back so the effort is somewhere between "almost imperceptible" and "fairly easy."

For the 2nd minute: Increase to a moderate amount of effort.

For the 3rd and 4th minutes: Exercise at a reasonably hard pace, just shy of your all-out effort.

For the 5th minute: Exercise at a moderate pace again.

For the 6th minute: Downshift into a fairly easy pace.

For the 7th to the 9th minute: Ratchet back up to a reasonably hard effort, just shy of working your hardest.

In the 10th minute: Move back down to fairly easy effort, and finally an almost imperceptible effort.

HOW THEY DID IT

She Figured Out How to Eat Right While Traveling

With a husband, three kids, and two businesses to watch over, Rosanna Pitella of Iselin, New Jersey, was always on the fly. Life on the road took its toll on her weight until she took charge of herself. Now she's flying high without 103 pounds of excess baggage.

Spur-of-the-moment business trips across the country were routine; exercise and good nutrition were not. Whenever I got the call to leave town, my only concerns were for my family and staff: Did they have everything they needed to survive without me? The last thing I worried about was whether my hotel had a gym or served low-fat food. So I'd arrive wherever I was going late at night, and, as a vegetarian, my only options often were either french fries from room service or a candy bar from the vending machine. It was no surprise that I had a weight problem.

In 1998, I hit two landmarks: I turned 40, and my weight reached a lifetime high of 263 pounds. It was time to make a change. I started by taking the time to take care of myself.

I looked at my weight the same way I tackle a business problem: find ways around, under, or through the barriers to success. My major barrier to weight loss was traveling. My solution: pack my routine with me. Tiny cans of tuna fish; bags of oatmeal; and snack packs of fruit, raisins, and nuts became my standard emergency stash for a healthy snack or small meal. A jump rope, running shoes, and my unitard, good for either the gym or pool, lay next to the tuna and panty hose.

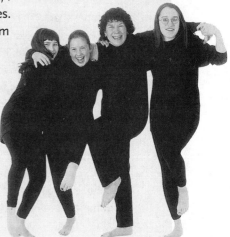

Rosanna's new organization and priorities meant more fun and fewer pounds.

Now I even fit my workout to my location. For instance, San Francisco has hills, so I tour the city by foot and power up those inclines. When the weather's bad, I turn on the radio and dance in my room for 15 minutes. If the hotel has a pool, I swim. I mix it up so boredom doesn't become another barrier.

Once I focused on the problem, the weight came off. Now I'm 103 pounds lighter and a lot smarter. Whenever I catch a plane, I have my emergency foods and workout clothes ready to go.

There are other benefits to my "selfish" ways. Organizing my personal life has made me more efficient at work. Plus, now "Mommy time" means my girls and I work out in fun ways, like swimming, beating a punching bag (big fun), and dancing. That's the best part: Losing weight helped me be even closer to my kids.

gram, think again. (After all, Ludwig van Beethoven composed his Seventh Symphony in less than 10 minutes at a time.) One study found that women who split their exercise into 10-minute increments were more likely to exercise consistently, and lost more weight after 5 months, than women who exercised for 20 to 40 minutes at a time.

In a landmark study conducted at the University of Virginia, exercise physiologist Glenn Gaesser, Ph.D., asked men and women to complete 15 10-minute exercise routines a week. After just 21 days, the volunteers' aerobic fitness was equal to that of people 10 to 15 years younger. Their strength, muscular endurance, and flexibility were equal to those of people up to 20 years their junior.

In yet another study, researchers at the Johns Hopkins School of Medicine in Baltimore found that for improving health and fitness in inactive adults, many short bursts of activity are as effective as longer, structured workouts.

"It would be useful for people to get out of the all-or-nothing mindset that unless they exercise for 30 minutes, they're wasting their time," says Dr. Gaesser.

"Instead of hiring a neighborhood kid to mow your lawn, you could cut it yourself, and in the winter a great activity is shoveling the driveway," says Ross E. Andersen, Ph.D., of Johns Hopkins School of Medicine, who gave volunteers pedometers and told them to build up to 10,000 steps a day.

"Rather than piling things up on the staircase to bring upstairs once a day, make several trips throughout the day," he suggests.

Keep in mind, though, that short bursts of exercise are meant to supplement, not replace, your regular fitness routine.

An Exercise in Time Management

Breaking exercise into small chunks on your overscheduled days can also keep your confidence up, says Harold Taylor, time management expert and owner of Harold Taylor Time Consultants in Toronto, who has written extensively on the subject.

"Skipping exercise altogether is 'de-motivational'—you feel depressed and guilty," Taylor says. "If you skip it, you tend to figure, 'What's the use? I can't keep up with it anyway.' Yet as long as you make some effort each day, that motivates you onward. Success breeds success."

Experts point to other benefits of short exercise bursts.

▶ You can do it almost anywhere—at the desk in your office, on the living room floor, at your child's soccer game.

▶ You trigger the release of growth hormone (mentioned in chapter 3), which boosts the immune system, strengthens bones, and makes bodies supple.

Beginning exercisers or very heavy people who want to ease into a longer program often find short bursts work well when they're getting started, says John Acquaviva, Ph.D., an exercise physiologist who is an assistant professor of physical education at Roanoke College in Salem, Virginia.

Here's a roundup of practical ways to work exercise into your day even when you "don't have time to exercise." (You don't have to do them all in one day; select what works for you.)

Around the House

▶ After you shower and apply moisturizer but before you get dressed and put on your makeup, perform the stretching exercises in the "Best Bet" sidebar on page 227.

▶ When you go outside to pick up your morning newspaper, take a brisk 5-minute walk up the street in one direction and back in the other.

▶ If you're housebound caring for a sick child or grandchild, hop on an exercise bike or treadmill while your ailing loved one naps.

▶ Try 5 to 10 minutes of jumping jacks. (A 150-pound woman can burn 90 calories in one 10-minute session of this calisthenic.)

▶ Cooking dinner? Do standing pushups while you wait for a pot to boil. Stand about an arm's length from the kitchen counter and push your arms against the counter. Push in and out to work your arms and shoulders.

▶ After dinner, go outside and play tag or shoot baskets with your kids and their friends.

▶ Just before bed or while you're giving yourself a facial at night, do a few repetitions of some dumbbell exercises (see chapter 10), suggests exercise instructor Sheila Cluff, owner and founder of The Oaks at Ojai and The Palms, in Palm Springs, California, who keeps a set of free weights on a shelf in front of her bathroom sink.

When Running Errands

▶ Walk around the block several times while you wait for your child to take a music lesson. As your fitness level improves, add 1-minute bursts of jogging to your walks.

▶ Walk around medical buildings if you're expecting a long wait for a doctor's appointment. "I always ask the receptionist to give me an idea of how long I have left to wait," Cluff says. "Most are usually very willing to tell you."

▶ When your son or daughter plays a soccer game, walk around the periphery of the field.

▶ Turn a trip to a park with your child into a miniworkout for you. Throw a ball back and forth and run for the fly balls.

Battery-Powered Belly Toners: Ab-Solutely Useless for Weight Loss

Push a button and get up to 700 multiple ab contractions in minutes—no pain, no work, no situps!"

So says the box for one of those "as seen on TV" abdominal exercise belts. But before you whip out your credit card, know what these gadgets can deliver—and what they can't.

Abdominal exercise belts—such as the AB Energizer, Ab-Tronics, and the Rio Ab Belt—employ electrical muscle stimulation (EMS). With EMS, muscles are "exercised" by being zapped with a weak electrical current, which causes them to involuntarily contract.

Most of these devices—which can also be used to "tighten" and "tone" the thighs and butt—work the same way. You swab a special gel on your skin, fasten the belt around the body part of your choice, turn on the unit, adjust the intensity of the stimulation, and sit back and relax.

EMS has a legitimate therapeutic use: It's long been employed to help preserve muscle tone in people who can't move after surgery or severe injury (such as a spinal cord injury). And exercise belts that use EMS technology probably do cause some muscle contraction, leading to some increase in muscle tone, says Mary O'Toole, Ph.D., an exercise physiologist at the Women's Exercise Research Lab at Saint Louis University in Missouri. "But you'd get a much stronger contraction by just squeezing and releasing your abdominal muscles while driving or sitting at your computer," she says.

Moreover, exercise belts won't help you shed extra pounds or burn fat. Researchers at the University of Wisconsin in La Crosse were commissioned by the American Council on Exercise to test the effectiveness of EMS (not the belts themselves). The researchers divided 29 volunteers into two groups. The first group underwent EMS three times a week for 45 minutes at a time. The second group didn't get EMS. After 8 weeks, those using the gadget experienced no significant change in their weight or the percentage of their body fat.

The manufacturers of some of these gadgets seem to be aware of their products' limitations. The instruction manuals that come with at least some of these devices note that they don't promote weight loss and recommend that they be used in conjunction with a healthy diet and regular exercise—which would probably do the job on their own!

Caution: Do not use these devices if you have recently given birth; have a pacemaker; have high blood pressure; have heart disease, epilepsy, or diabetes; or are recovering from an operation.

At Work

▶ Walk to work if you can. "I once walked to work for months, 1½ miles each way," says Mary Dallman, Ph.D., professor of physiology at the University of California, San Francisco, and she really saw results.

▶ To add oomph to your workout, use hand weights or use one or two walking poles, which help build body strength and increase your calorie burn.

▶ If you dine out on your lunch hour, walk to a restaurant on a route that takes you a little bit out of your way, Dr. Gaesser advises.

▶ If you have a meeting in another building, leave 5 or 10 minutes early (or take some time afterward) and do some extra walking.

▶ On breaks, spend 5 to 10 minutes climbing stairs.

▶ If you're pressed for time and must wait for an elevator, work your abdominal muscles. Stand with your feet parallel and your knees relaxed. Contract the muscles around your belly button. Then

COOL TOOL

Pedometers

Want to calculate exactly how many steps you take in the course of a day? Consider buying a pedometer.

WHAT THE EXPERT SAYS: Today's pedometers offer compasses, alarms, and radios. Some can even be programmed to help track your golf scores. But don't let these functions distract you from the device's most useful job: counting your steps.

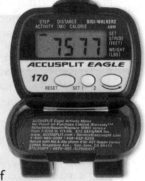

"Electronic pedometers are quite accurate in counting steps, but they are not quite as useful when it comes to estimating distance and calories," says David Bassett, Ph.D., professor of exercise science and sports management at the University of Tennessee–Knoxville.

So use your pedometer primarily to count the steps you take every day toward your fitness goals. "Wear it during all waking hours of the day, except in the shower or pool," Dr. Bassett says. "You should try to accumulate 10,000 steps a day." This typically means that you'll need to walk 2 or 3 miles in addition to your normal activities.

Hitting that number also requires at least 30 minutes of moderate activity, which many health authorities recommend you do at least 5 days a week.

PURCHASING TIPS: You can buy a good pedometer for about $30 or less at most sporting goods stores.

Why are food portions getting larger while airline seats are getting smaller?

While neither trend makes sense for customers, both practices help the industries' bottom lines.

Food vendors and restaurants compete for purchases by pushing larger and larger portions on consumers, says Melanie Polk, R.D., director of nutrition education at the American Institute for Cancer Research in Washington, D.C.

There are no "small," "medium," and "large" soft drinks, just "large," "super," and "mega," for instance. "It's always 'more food for less money,'" Polk says. One solution: share.

Meanwhile, the typical width of a coach seat on most domestic airline flights is 17 to 18 inches, says Ed Perkins, a syndicated travel columnist, an author, and former editor of *Consumer Reports Travel Letter*. That's 2 to 3 inches narrower than a standard office chair.

To make matters worse, airlines that once equipped 747s, DC-10s, and other aircraft with nine seats in each row often add a 10th seat and cut legroom, Perkins says. "They're squeezing us fore and aft," quips Perkins. If space is a problem for you, go to the airlines' Web sites or air travel Web sites and research the seat and aisle size of the aircraft you plan to fly on before you book, and choose your airline accordingly. If you'd be more comfortable in an aisle seat, book early.

elevate your upper torso, and release. Finally, contract your buttocks for a few seconds.

▶ Use a ringing phone as an excuse to stretch your back. Stand with your feet astride. Imagine that you are encased in a plaster cast from your waist to your head. Gently tilt the lower part of your pelvis backward. Contract your abdominal muscles. Then gently tilt your pelvis forward.

When You're Watching TV ———•

▶ Put away your remote and change channels the old-fashioned way—by getting up and walking to the television set.

▶ Dance as if you were 16 again. Put on a music program or MTV. Then dance like crazy, advises Peg Jordan, R.N., Ph.D., a fitness expert in Oakland, California, and author of *The Fitness Instinct*. "Free yourself to think of movement as something that you have a right to do," she says.

▶ During commercials, jog in place. A 150-pound woman can burn up to 45 calories in 5 minutes.

While Traveling ————————•

▶ Pack your sneakers and an exercise video. Call ahead to make sure your hotel has a videocassette player. If it doesn't, ask to rent one from the hotel.

FIT | FLASH

Fidgeting Can Burn Extra Calories

As more proof that small efforts add up, researchers at the Mayo Clinic discovered that people who tap their feet, squirm in their seats, and move a little bit all day can burn as many as 350 calories each day.

Scientists asked 16 normal-weight women and men to stop exercising and overeat by 1,000 calories a day for 2 months. Some of the individuals gained less than a pound; others gained nearly 10. Scientists found that those who gained the least weight moved the most—walking up and down stairs, strolling around the office, or simply fidgeting.

The lesson? Adhere to your regular exercise routine—but also make a conscious effort to move every chance you get.

▶ If you're traveling by car, stop twice a day for short, brisk walks and some stretching. (For stretches, see chapter 11.)

▶ During layovers at airports, avoid the mechanized "moving carpets" that transport travelers from concourse to concourse. "If you're in between flights, walk around the concourse as much as you can," suggests Cluff.

▶ Book a hotel room between the fifth and eighth floors, "then ignore the elevator," says Cluff. Better yet, take two stairs at a time. (Check with the hotel first because for security reasons some hotels do not allow guests to use stairs except for emergencies.)

▶ Do calf stretches while riding in elevators (see page 254).

▶ Do leg lifts with small weights while you watch the Weather Channel, cooking shows, movies, or news coverage. (For instructions, see page 186.)

CHAPTER 15

CUSTOMIZING YOUR WORKOUT:
FITNESS PRESCRIPTIONS FOR INCREASING YOUR ENERGY AND ENDURANCE

According to legend, the first marathon runner, a Greek messenger sent from the Plain of Marathon to Athens to deliver news of a battle victory, collapsed and died from exhaustion.

Some ambitious women want to run marathons after age 40. Most, however, have more modest goals related to quality of life. According to a *Prevention* magazine reader survey, women want to stay energized through the afternoon slump, spend more time being active with their families, and climb stairs without huffing and puffing, and they hope that getting in shape will give them the stamina they need.

It's common for women 40 and older to feel like they don't have the energy to do activities they've done all their life, says Betsy Keller, Ph.D., associate professor and chair of the department of exercise and sports sciences at Ithaca College in New York. And when they try to do even more—like add an aerobics class to their schedule—they don't have the stamina. Other women who work out moderately may find that more intense efforts—adding a long, steep hill to their walking route or a day-long hiking or biking excursion on vacation—leaves them exhausted.

The culprit behind low energy? Women's tendency to lose muscle, gain body fat, and become less physically active as they get older. With less muscle to power you through

demanding activities, your body gives out before you're ready to call it a day. It's a downward spiral: The less energy you have, the less you do, and the less conditioned you become.

Chronic conditions that tend to develop at midlife compound the tendency to do less. Simply being 45 or older increases your risk for arthritis, for example. What's more, doing less increases your risk for those very conditions. A weight gain of 11 to 24 pounds from the age of 18 increases your risk for type 2 diabetes. And any chronic condition can suck the energy right out of you.

The irony is, exercise protects you from some of these energy-draining conditions or improves the way you feel if you already have a condition. According to the American Institute for Cancer Research, 60 to 70 percent of all cancers are directly linked to lifestyle factors, such as inactivity.

If you don't exercise already, your first step toward losing weight, gaining energy and endurance, and lowering your risk for chronic conditions is to start an exercise program. Chapter 9 shows you how—15 minutes at a time. If you already work out but want to increase your endurance, work on exercising longer or slightly harder. You'll still benefit: A study of more than 72,000 female nurses ages 40 to 65 found that walking at a brisk pace, compared with a casual pace, substantially reduced risk of stroke. And activities you may struggle with—keeping up with

BEST BET

Take a Deep Breath

Sitting hunched over a keyboard all day, taking shallow breaths, deprives your blood and brain of rich, energizing oxygen. To reenergize during the workday, sit straight up in your chair, and let your arms dangle at your sides. Take 10 deep breaths, inhaling slowly through your nose as your abdomen fills with air and then gently releasing the air through your mouth as your abdomen empties. Follow that with a stretch of your arms and shoulders. Raise both your arms to your sides and move them in big circles forward as if you're doing the breaststroke in a pool.

your teenagers while sightseeing on vacation, for example—will become easier. The best part: You'll burn more calories, bringing your weight-loss goal even closer.

Nutrition, too, plays a role. "What you eat can make exercise easier or harder," says Ellen Coleman, R.D., nutrition consultant at the Sport Clinic in Riverside, California, and author of *Eating for Endurance*.

This chapter shows you how to transform your workout into one that will give you more energy, help you lose more weight, and show you how to eat to feel your best.

To Boost Energy, Work Harder

If you exercise for 10 or 15 minutes at a time, you're doing a lot to improve your health and lose weight. If you've been inactive, it's a great start. But if you can go 30 minutes, benefits like lowering your risk for heart disease, cancers, diabetes, and depression skyrocket, says David C. Nieman, D.P.H., professor of health and exercise science and director of the health promotion and human performance lab at Appalachian State University in Boone, North Carolina, and author of *The Exercise–Health Connection*. And if you exercise for even longer, benefits continue to rise moderately for up to an hour.

Ratchet up your intensity, and your heart pumps more blood, your lungs burn up more oxygen, and you multiply the calories burned. A 150-pound woman burns 102 calories when she walks for ½ hour. But she burns 238 calories when she jogs for the same amount of time.

As you begin, be sure to concentrate on increasing either distance or intensity, but never both at the same time. And don't work harder than you feel comfortable with, Dr. Nieman says. "Some people like pain and sweat," he says. "Others don't. Do what you feel comfortable doing."

Eventually, you should be able to gradually increase the amount of time you exercise or the intensity of your exercise. Who knows, you may even gain enough energy to hike a mountain summit, tour Provence or Tuscany by bike, cross-country ski in Yellowstone National Park, or dance the night away in the Caribbean.

The Best Ways to Increase Endurance

These six strategies will help you to condition you heart, lungs, and muscles so you can comfortably handle more effort for longer periods of time.

Find your own flow. Your heart, lungs, and muscles were designed to be used for and adapt to increased demands. If you aim for 30 minutes of moderate exercise, you'll find that your endurance will increase naturally. For example, if you walk the same route every day, you'll start to walk it faster without trying to increase your pace. Soon, a 40,000-square-foot superstore might not feel so huge—or traipsing through it, so exhausting.

Make a concentrated effort. After you feel comfortable going for 30 minutes, pick up your walking pace, add hills to your bike route, or kick higher in your kickboxing class. Try to keep a moderate to somewhat hard pace by rating your exertion on a scale of 1 to 10, with 3 being very, very light (such as sitting in a chair), 10 being very, very hard, and 6 to 7 your goal of moderate to somewhat hard.

Shorten your sessions. As you become accustomed to exercising for 30 minutes, go for only 15 or 20 minutes at a slightly faster pace after warming up. Expect to breathe harder, feel a little more uncomfortable, and be a little sore the next day, says Jack Raglin Jr., Ph.D., professor of kinesiology at Indiana University in Bloomington. Working harder—for a shorter amount of time—trains your body to be able to go longer than usual at a slower pace. But keep in mind that recovery is key. Take the next day off from vigorous aerobic exercise, and weight train or do something at a lower intensity, such as a moderate walk or an easy bike ride.

Train like a pro. "Twenty years ago, marathon runners looked like they were about to die after finishing 26 miles," Dr. Raglin says. "But now they barely look winded." Their secret, interval training, is one you can benefit from even if you never want to run a marathon. Intervals involve a 10-minute warmup, a mix of short bursts of high-intensity exercise and recovery, a 10-minute or longer cooldown, and a thorough stretch of all your major muscle groups.

The best way to do intervals is probably in a structured class outside or inside on a treadmill or stationary bike, Dr. Raglin says. An instructor will lead you to increase your pace for 30 seconds to a few minutes before you back off and go easy for a few minutes. At some gyms, it's called "trekking."

If you don't have access to a class, try intervals on your own. Wear a watch and time yourself as you increase your pace for 30 seconds before slowing down. When you pick up your pace, you should rate your intensity at 7 or 8 (out of 10) on a scale of perceived exertion, or hard to very hard. (For a structured walking interval plan, see page 136 in chapter 9.)

Expect to feel a little uncomfortable when you work harder, Dr. Raglin says. And because going faster involves different muscle fibers than you're used to, you'll probably be sore the next day. (Muscles have two kinds of fibers—so-called short-twitch muscles for explosive efforts, and long-twitch muscles for extended efforts.) To recover, take the next day off from exercise or do something at much lower intensity, such as walking at a moderate pace.

Keep lifting weights. Lifting weights won't necessarily help you walk longer than usual. But strength training *will* help you get through your day with less effort. Follow chapter 10's weight-training program, and you won't feel so tired after rigorous undertakings like helping your daughter move into her college dorm or rearranging the furniture in your living room. Just a few months of regular strength training can make up for 5 to 10 years of muscle loss. It can also lower your risk of becoming frail from osteoporosis later in life.

Stretch tired muscles. Whether you work out more intensely or not, make sure you stretch your muscles after doing exercise. Stretching helps your muscles stay flexible—to allow you to reach the spices on the top shelf of your pantry without strain—and keeps your muscles lose for the next day's activities. You'll find a complete stretching routine in chapter 11.

Eat for Endurance

If competitive athletes don't eat properly, they "hit the wall," or run out of energy, during an endurance event.

You may not be a professional athlete, but your food choices affect how well you feel throughout the day and during exercise.

"Many women think they should skip breakfast to 'lean up' for exercise because they think if they lose another pound, it won't be as hard to run another mile," says Diane Habash, Ph.D., R.D., a bionutritionist and nutrition research manager at the General Clinical Research Center at Ohio State University in Columbus. "Instead, you need to give your body the amount of fuel at the right time to get through the day." This is especially important as you increase endurance because your body relies more than usual on your fuel stores.

Reaching for a candy bar is not the best strategy. Though it may give you an initial burst of energy, your energy levels will eventually plummet, stopping you in your tracks.

Following the Fit Not Fat Food Plan (page 82) will give you perfect sustenance while you work out. Studies show that pre- and post-workout snacks, followed by a

---

FIT FLASH

Walking Can Aid Sleep

There's nothing like a good night's sleep to make you feel energized. But many women experience sleep disturbances—like waking in the middle of the night or having nightmares—that leave them feeling tired throughout the day.

Fortunately, the solution is just six blocks away. In a study of more than 700 men and women, researchers found that those who walked at least six blocks a day at a normal pace were one-third less likely to have trouble sleeping than those who didn't walk at all.

healthy meal, gives athletes the energy they need for up to 90 minutes of tough exercise. So the plan should leave you with unrelenting energy to get through your most intense workouts.

If you have diabetes or you're insensitive to insulin, it's especially important that you choose complex carbohydrates (whole wheat bread, whole grain cereal, oatmeal, peas, corn, rice, beans and pasta, fruits and vegetables) over simple carbohydrates (white bread, doughnuts, candy, sugar-filled cereal, and soda). It's also a good idea to talk to your doctor or diabetes educator about what to eat before and after you exercise.

Quench your thirst. Dehydration is a key factor in fatigue. You can't rely on physical signals to tell you when to drink because by the time you feel thirsty, you're already dehydrated. To know whether or not you're well-hydrated, monitor the color of your urine. If you're not taking vitamins or medications that change the color of your urine, it should be pale. If you're dehydrated, it will be more yellow.

"When I get women to start drinking more water, it's amazing how much better they feel," Dr. Habash says. Water helps rid the body of waste, delivers nutrients, and helps you feel more energized. According to

Sports Drinks Can Be Helpful

Packed with carbohydrates, minerals, sodium, and potassium, sports drinks supposedly restore energy and replace electrolytes (minerals needed for muscle function) quicker than plain water. If you've been exercising for more than 1 hour, they can definitely help, say experts at the American College of Sports Medicine.

Sports drinks can also provide energy for women who typically exercise without enough fuel, says Jackie Berning, R.D., Ph.D., assistant professor at the University of Colorado in Colorado Springs and nutrition consultant to the Denver Broncos, Colorado Rockies, Cleveland Indians, and the University of Colorado at Boulder department of athletics. Plus, you're likely to drink more—and avoid dehydration—if you like the taste. In one study, researchers evaluating 50 triathletes and runners found that they drank 25 percent more orange-flavored sports drink than plain water, diluted orange juice, or an orange-flavored homemade sports drink.

Sports drinks may in fact improve your performance. In one study, men and women exercising in high-intensity sports, similar to what a basketball or soccer player might encounter, maintained their high-intensity effort longer when they drank a sports drink than when they drank a similar-tasting placebo.

If you're following the Fit Not Fat Food Plan, bear in mind that a typical 12-ounce sports drink contains 125 calories, and plan accordingly.

FITNESS MYSTERIES

At *a dollar or more apiece—and about 250 calories each—are energy bars (also called sports bars or performance bars) any better than a bagel or other portable high-carbohydrate workout fuel?*

Not really. Some energy bars get more than 60 percent of their calories from carbohydrates. Others supply a mix of 40 percent carbohydrates, 30 percent protein, and 30 percent fat and 5 or more grams of fat. A bagel, on the other hand, has 157 calories and just 1 gram of fat.

The difference in performance may be negligible. In a small study, a researcher failed to detect any performance difference between cyclists who ate bagels and those who ate energy bars for breakfast before a workout on an exercise bike.

Still, if you're in the habit of heading out to exercise without stopping to eat, an energy bar might be a convenient way to fuel up. If, on the other hand, you're watching your calories, you might be better off grabbing a banana, which supplies 27.6 grams of carbohydrates, 2.8 grams of fiber, and 0.5 gram of fat.

Dr. Habash, hydration also helps you exercise longer and harder, so take extra care to get 8 to 10 cups of water (64 to 80 ounces) a day. Include high-water fruits and vegetables (like tomatoes, peppers, and melons of any kind), fruit juice, milk, yogurt, soy milk, soups, herb teas, and other high-liquid foods and nonalcoholic, decaffeinated beverages.

Curb caffeine. A cup of a caffeinated beverage in the morning or afternoon may make you feel more awake and can even help boost your metabolism. But caffeine is a diuretic, prompting the kidneys to prematurely flush much-needed fluids from your body and divert them away from your muscles and brain. More than a cup or so of coffee (or any caffeine-containing beverage) dehydrates the body, and relying on coffee all day will ulti-

mately tire you out. If you have to have caffeine, follow each serving with one to two extra cups of water, Dr. Habash says.

Snack before you sweat. You wouldn't take a road trip without filling your car's gas tank. The same goes for exercise. Your best snack is made up of carbohydrates because they provide energy during your workout. Also, you digest carbodydrates faster and more easily than dairy or fat, which can cause stomach discomfort during activity. Reach for a banana or other piece of fruit, cereal bar, energy bar, granola, wheat cracker, or whole wheat bread or bagel with fruit spread.

When to eat varies from woman to woman and according to what type of exercise you're doing. Some people digest food faster than others, Dr. Habash says, so they

Don't Bother with Sports Supplements

Working out and eating right take time and attention. Can you lose weight and become fit from taking a pill instead?

"It's human nature to try to get results the easiest and quickest way we can," says Diane Habash, Ph.D., R.D., a bionutritionist and nutrition research manager at the General Clinical Research Center at Ohio State University in Columbus. That's why sports supplements sell so well. But the truth is most people, including athletes, will see better performance from improvements in their training, sleep, and eating habits than from a supplement.

And in some cases, taking the supplement can be dangerous. Here's what to watch out for, based on a review of scientific research conducted by sports nutritionists at the University of Washington and S.P.O.R.T. Clinic in Riverside, California.

ANDROSTENEDIONE. Sometimes called "andro," this steroid, marketers claim, increases muscle and strength, boosts sexual desire, and enhances exercise recovery.

WHY YOU SHOULD AVOID IT: Researchers don't know whether it really does improve performance or whether it's safe. Oral androgens—a related male hormone drug—have been shown to cause liver cancer and heart disease, but researchers don't yet know whether androstenedione has the same effect.

CHROMIUM PICOLINATE. Marketers say this supplement—of an essential mineral needed in trace amounts—increases muscle and helps insulin sensitivity and glucose tolerance while decreasing fat when taken in large doses.

WHY YOU SHOULD AVOID IT: The majority of studies found the supplements to be ineffective. Animal studies even suggest chromium could accumulate in

---

don't feel stomach discomfort when they exercise soon after eating. If you think you digest food faster, it's probably safe to eat a snack or energy bar an hour before exercise. If you think you digest food more slowly, it's best to wait 2 or 3 hours to exercise after eating. It will probably take some trial and error over several workouts to figure out exactly when to have your snack. And if you're going to do activity that jostles your stomach—like running, aerobics, swimming, and water aerobics—allow more time for your food to digest. Same goes for weight-training moves that work your abdominal muscles. But bicycling and walking will be much easier if you've had something to eat beforehand.

Practice recovery nutrition. Your body converts carbohydrates into blood glucose. Also known as blood sugar, glucose is either used immediately, as energy, or stored as glycogen in the liver or muscles for future

cells and cause chromosomal damage. Plus, chromium is found in almost every food, so a varied diet or a multi-vitamin-mineral tablet gives you all the chromium you need.

DHEA (DEHYDROEPIANDROSTERONE). Marketers say this steroid, related to androstenedione, above, increases energy, extends life, increases sex drive, decreases body fat, improves mood, and lowers stress-releasing hormones.

WHY YOU SHOULD AVOID IT: Researchers have found that DHEA is associated masculine effects such as acne and unwanted hair growth, as well as irritability and liver enlargement.

EPHEDRA/MA HUANG. Considered a "natural" version of the dangerous weight-loss drug fen-phen, ephedra is derived from an herb and contains ephedrine and pseudo-ephedrine (amphetamine-like stimulants). Marketers say ephedra (also known by its Chinese name, ma huang) can improve athletic performance, promote weight loss, and increase energy and alertness.

WHY YOU SHOULD AVOID IT: While some research has found that ephedra/ma huang may help with weight loss, the FDA has since 1993 received more than 800 reports of serious side effects that include increased blood pressure, heart rate irregularities, insomnia, nervousness, tremors, seizures, heart attacks, strokes, and death.

HMB (BETA-HYDROXY-BETA-METHYLBUTYRATE). Derived from the amino acid leucine, HMB, marketers claim, increases muscle, accelerates fat loss, and enhances strength and power.

WHY YOU SHOULD AVOID IT: Researchers aren't sure whether it's effective and call for more studies.

use. When you do jogging intervals or pick up the pace on your bicycle, you use stored glucose as fuel during exercise. If you complete 60 minutes of high-intensity exercise today, you can improve tomorrow's performance by beginning to replenish your stored glucose within 15 to 30 minutes of exercise, says Dr. Habash. Help yourself to the same kind of high-carbohydrate snack you enjoyed pre-workout—orange juice, a granola bar, or a banana.

Fill up the tank. Your post-workout snack only begins the process of replenishing your glucose. Within 2 hours after working out, make sure that you have a regular meal. This is your opportunity to replenish your stored glucose and supply your body with other nutrients your body needs, such as protein, vegetables—and, yes, some fat. Enjoy your meal, knowing that you're giving your body the power to create more muscle.

PART 5

THE 40-PLUS RELAX AND RECHARGE PLAN

CHAPTER 16

BREAK AWAY FROM STRESS

Some days, all the yoga in the world can't equal the soothing power of one hot fudge sundae. Or at least that's what we like to tell ourselves.

Ask any woman if a gooey sticky bun will make her feel better when she's stressed, and she'll probably nod vigorously. But truthfully, after the last bit of icing is licked off her fingers, all she'll have to show for it is the same stress—and an extra 500 calories.

Several studies have shown that people under chronic stress tend to gain weight over time. Yet experts say no food on earth can relieve stress—not even chocolate. So why do we keep going back for more?

The biggest culprit is childhood habit. Remember Mom asking, "Would an ice cream make you feel better?" We were trained early on to see sweets and treats as a panacea, so our inner 2-year-old still seeks solace in something from the fridge.

To make matters worse, stress can actually make us hungrier. Researchers at Yale University found that cortisol, one of the main hormones that linger after the stress response, may increase hunger. And women who react more intensely to cortisol eat more calories—particularly high-fat sweets—when they are stressed.

The last third of the stress-eating troika may be the most daunting: a shortage of old-fashioned willpower. Researchers undertook three studies on stress and coping and found that willpower is actually a limited resource. If getting through a stressful day takes all our determination, we have nothing left to resist nighttime noshing, says lead researcher Dianne Tice, Ph.D., professor of psychology at Case Western Reserve University in Cleveland, where the studies took place.

While these theories may offer insight into why we reach for comfort foods, they also offer *solutions*. Some doctors believe if you learn to manage stress constructively, you may automatically lose more weight. That's why relaxing, and recharging your batteries, is the third component of the total Fit Not Fat Plan. As a minimum, shoot for 20 minutes of "me" time a day, and honor this commitment to yourself the way you would a business meeting. When you're setting your Master Plan goals for the week, take special care to note any upcoming events that are likely to foil your best intentions. Do you have a big deadline at work? Are you planning a big party or function? Is it

time to pay your taxes? Write these down on the "big events" lines within your weekly Master Plan (page 76). Calling attention to these hectic days at the beginning of the week will not only help you prepare mentally but also give you time to cushion that stressful event with Fit Not Fat Relax and Recharge strategies.

Once you start to make time for yourself and try some of the following stress relief and prevention hints, you'll begin to understand why taking care of your needs is as essential to losing weight as putting down that sticky bun. Breaking the stress–fat cycle starts with figuring out when you're really hungry versus when you're just stewing and chewing.

Is It Hunger, or Is It Stress?

Repeated diets and binges have left many women with no idea what real hunger feels like, says Elissa Epel, Ph.D., a postdoctoral scholar in psychiatry at the University of California, San Francisco. We're more likely to respond to what's on the clock, the menu, or the agenda to signal us to eat.

One way to define whether you're feeling real hunger or stress hunger is by telling yourself to HALT. That means: Never get too hungry, angry, lonely, or tired—four feelings that can directly provoke stress eating. Ask yourself, "Am I hungry, angry, tired, or lonely?" to help you eat when you need to physiologically, says Dr. Epel.

Don't get too hungry. If you've let yourself feel true hunger pangs, you're actually

FITNESS
MYSTERIES

Why do some women lose their appetite when they're upset, while others turn to food?

Most people initially stop eating during severe stress, due to an appetite-suppressing action upon the release of the first stress hormone, corticoid-releasing factor (CRF), says Elissa Epel, Ph.D., a postdoctoral scholar in psychiatry at the University of California, San Francisco.

If the story ended there, we would all just avoid food during times of stress, yet stress eating is a tremendous problem for many people. Often, people will lose weight in times of severe stress, and then gain weight in the aftermath.

What's more, stress hormones may vary among individuals, which explains why some are stress undereaters and others are stress overeaters, says Pamela M. Peeke, M.D., M.P.H., assistant clinical professor of medicine at the University of Maryland School of Medicine in Baltimore. And according to one theory, women who produce more of the appetite-boosting stress hormone cortisol may tend to eat more *after* stress, possibly because they are producing more appetite-stimulating cortisol relative to their appetite-suppressing CRF.

primed for a stress binge, says Eric Stice, Ph.D., assistant professor of psychology at the University of Texas in Austin. In his research, Dr. Stice finds that those who eat most often—up to six times per day—actually gain the least weight.

If you have trouble finding time for lunch, try Dr. Tice's two-bite rule: "No matter how busy my day is, I force myself to eat two bites of my sandwich—usually that's all the prompting I need to get the rest down." Above all, stay far away from the refined carbs, sugar, and sodas that only make you hungrier, more tired—and more stressed.

Don't get too angry. One study of 23 women found that among several emotions, feelings of tension/fear and anger caused the greatest increase in eating and hunger. Women don't have a lot of practice expressing anger, so a pint of Ben & Jerry's ice cream can make the anger easier to swallow. While food's quick fix provides momentary distraction, you sacrifice long-term benefits—like weight loss—that would help you feel more empowered, says Dr. Tice.

"Eating feels good quickly, but it never lasts," she says. Next time you feel your fuming self reaching for the ice cream scoop, stop and say (out loud), "Food won't help." Pick up a pen and write a note to the person you're mad at, and *really* let him have it—when you're done, tear up the paper. Research suggests your cravings will go away in less than 12 minutes if you focus on something else.

Don't get too lonely. One birthday card features a woman drooling over a banana split, saying, "Some of my best friends are calories." Sound familiar?

Often we try to fill emotional emptiness with dependable, nonjudgmental food—but the solace ends when our hand scrapes the bottom of the cookie box. Food's comforting associations, rather than the food itself, give it power, says Barbara Levine, R.D., Ph.D., director of the Nutrition Information Center of the Weill Medical College of Cornell University in New York City. Before you give in, get on the phone. Call your sister, your best friend—anybody. Social support is one of your most powerful healing forces, but you may give it up when you get busy—exactly the opposite of what's best for you, says Alice Domar, Ph.D., director of the Mind/Body Center for Women's Health at Beth Israel Deaconess Medical Center of Harvard University.

Don't get too tired. When you get depleted, you're usually trying to control too many things at once, says Dr. Tice. Stress-induced fatigue not only physically mimics hunger in the body, it also overtaxes your precious determination. But willpower is like a muscle—it gets stronger with exercise. When stress hits, choose just one weight-loss behavior you can stick with, like drinking more water or crunching on cut veggies instead of chips. "Committing to that one thing will strengthen your will and sense of control," says Dr. Tice.

Shed Stress, Shed Pounds

Lower expectations. Take baby steps. Get support from a friend. Write down your feelings. These strategies will help in *all* stressful situations, but your number one stress hurdle will always be *you*.

"A woman won't be able to take care of herself if she's telling herself, 'I'm not entitled to that,'" says Dr. Domar. "Self-nurture is the basis for all stress relief—without it, we eventually crash and burn." The following key strategies can help you through these I'm-gonna-lose-it moments with your sanity, willpower, and weight-loss goals intact.

THE MORNING RUSH

Forgotten lunch bags, burnt breakfasts, errant keys—weekday mornings can make you feel like the bum steed in an Olympic steeplechase. Preparing your family and yourself to meet the day will never be effortless—but keeping your own needs in mind will make it less stressful.

Greet the day with exercise. Exercise burns up the toxins of the stress response, boosts feel-good endorphins, and lowers cortisol, making it the best stress reliever bar none, says Dr. Epel. Morning exercisers are more likely to stick to a regular routine—before work, the stress of the day can't interfere, and accomplishing a major goal before you hit the showers helps you feel in control all day. Get up 20 minutes earlier to walk the dog at sunrise, or do some yoga on the lawn. (Go on, let the neighbors gawk.)

Make breakfast a breeze. For breakfast on the run, buy a week's worth of single-serving yogurt, cottage cheese, applesauce, baby car-

HOW THEY DID IT

She Learned to Think Before She Ate

Desserts were Grace Penny's best friends, but she often ate them without really thinking. When this retired teacher from Lutz, Florida, learned to stop and ask herself four key questions, she had the tools to help her conquer intense cravings, elevated cholesterol, and high blood sugar.

At 5 feet tall and 205 pounds, I had been carrying extra weight for 35 years and often indulged in sweets thoughtlessly. At work, we had a regular supply of homemade frosted apple cinnamon buns and coffee with milk and sugar. I also loved rich desserts such as cheesecake.

In 1996, I was diagnosed with type 2 diabetes and high cholesterol. I was beginning to feel unwell all the time, and I was aware that my daughter and husband were becoming very concerned about my health. So in May 1998, I signed up for a monthlong stay at Rice Diet Program/Heart Disease Reversal Clinic at Duke University in Durham, North Carolina.

The program introduced me to daily exercise, along with a high-fiber, low-salt, low-fat diet built around fresh fruits, grains, and vegetables. I also learned to think carefully before giving in to a craving by applying the acronym HALT: Am I hungry? Angry? Lonely? Tired? According to the Duke nutritionists, people usually confuse tiredness and hunger more than any other sensations. That was true for me.

Now if a craving hits midday, I take a catnap or a brisk walk. When I find myself yearning for something sweet at night, I call it a day. Rarely do I even remember the craving feeling when I wake up in the morning! I also try to keep my energy high by doing an hour of water aerobics every day.

Within just one week of joining the Duke University program, I was able to go off my cholesterol and diabetes medications and have managed to stay that way since. I lost 50 pounds in 7 months and dropped another 10 pounds over time. Although my ultimate goal is to weigh 115 pounds, I'm worlds better at my present weight of 145.

Four simple questions helped Grace drop 60 pounds.

rots, raisins, and nuts. Prebag portions of high-fiber cereal. Hard-boil a dozen eggs every Sunday and store them in the carton in the fridge. Dump a peeled egg and a pinch of salt in a resealable bag for breakfast on the run.

THE DAILY COMMUTE

Daily traffic jams—second only to teenagers in the category "things I'll never be able to control"—can frustrate even the most intrepid driver. When your commute starts to take its toll, try these mobile attitude adjusters.

Prepare for your entrance. Time your average trip, then leave 5 minutes extra. When you get to work, park in a low-profile spot and spend 5 minutes meditating before you charge inside to your office. Meditating every day may even contribute directly to weight loss. In a preliminary pilot study, Dr. Epel found that after 3 months, men who had meditated lost more belly fat than those who hadn't. Most likely, women benefit in the same way.

Reclaim your time. Make a long commute more enjoyable—fill your car with bird songs, classical music, or mariachi. Listen to books on tape from your local library or start a lending pool with your fellow commuters. Don't subject yourself to the morning shock jock unless you're absolutely addicted.

Listen to yourself. Stress often begins with unconscious beliefs such as "I'm letting everyone down." Start changing that inner nag by making a cassette of five positive affirmations in your own voice. Ann R. Peden, doctor of science in nursing, associate professor in the College of Nursing at the University of Kentucky in Lexington, a psychiatric nurse, and lead researcher on a study of affirmations for the National Institutes of Health (NIH), suggests starting with your negative message and reversing it. For example, "I can't keep up" becomes "I am calm and in control." Say each affirmation three times, and listen to your tape twice a day. Dr. Peden's research shows that affirmations, practiced regularly, strike a major blow to negative thinking.

WORK DEADLINES

Is "mind reader" listed on your business card? Not likely. When massive deadlines loom, the biggest stress is trying to divine what your boss expects from you. The following tricks reduce your reliance on guesswork.

Ask questions. Begin each project with a set of standard questions: When is this due? How long should it be? What information do you want included? Anything you *don't* want to see? Try to get a good mental picture of the finished product before you put your fingers on the keyboard.

Break it down. Working back from the deadline, break down the entire process into minigoals, each with its own target completion date. If you miss any, reevaluate the entire project and shift deadlines appropriately so you don't find yourself caught short at the end. Achieving one goal every day will give you a sense of control, says Dr. Tice.

Own your breaks. Lewis Richmond, a former Buddhist monk and the author of *Work as a Spiritual Practice*, recommends using your bathroom breaks as opportunities to regroup and center yourself. Breathe in for four steps, out for four steps. Try a workplace mantra like "Plenty of time, plenty of energy" or "Plenty of time, plenty of care."

HOUSEHOLD CHORES

Home is where the heart is—and, with it, heartburn. We've all said, "I'll start a weight-loss plan—as soon as I'm caught up." But when in the history of womankind has this ever happened? Our "shoulds" keep us running like rats, slaves to high expectations,

says Dr. Domar. To combat household stress, try the following:

Delegate, delegate, delegate. Before dinner, have everyone sweep through the house—one room at a time—to claim all their stuff and take it back to their room. Train your kids early on to help set, clear, and clean the dinner plates. Praise them for pitching in.

Use chores as mini-meditations. Instead of rushing through the dishes to watch another hour of mind-numbing TV, concentrate on the feeling of your hands in the warm water and appreciate the sparkle of clean glasses in the drying rack.

Do "homework" on Saturday. Don't fritter away your precious weekends on chores that you "should" do but that aren't really necessary. To combat time-wasting perfectionism, set an alarm clock for 3 hours, make a list of priorities, and attack it with gusto. Once the bell rings, walk away and let it go. By giving yourself a deadline, you can focus all your energies without getting distracted by perfectionism.

Commit to a bedtime. No basket of laundry or dirty dish is more important than 8 hours of sleep, says Dr. Domar. Sleep banishes the fatigue that hamstrings your willpower. Face it: The laundry will *never* be 100 percent done. Admitting this can be very freeing. Make peace with lower expectations, and get to bed.

CHILD CARE

One recent study found that mothers of young children have less than 10 minutes a day to themselves. Whether you're Mother Teresa or Mommy Dearest, that dearth of downtime is a surefire formula for burnout. Here are three ways to put the "me" back in "mommy."

Designate a master control center. Instead of mentally scrolling through your to-do list, hang a huge wipe-off board in the kitchen. Write each family member's name across the top and days of the week down the side. Fill in soccer games, drama practices, parent-teacher conferences, and dentist appointments, noting chaperoning or shuttling duties. By managing your own time publicly, you also teach that skill to your kids (and spot where you need help).

Play tag, dominoes, or Frisbee. Or swing on the swings. Feed off your kids' wellspring of energy. Play—that is, any activity that is its own reward—has potent rejuvenating power, says Dr. Domar. Chase your dog around the backyard, count to 100 during hide-and-seek, or jump in the pool for a rousing game of Marco Polo—you'll burn calories, bust stress, *and* instill a love of exercise in your kids.

Carve out sacred "me" time. A daily half-hour spent alone can make the difference between burnout and relative bliss, says Dr. Domar. Deputize your eldest to shield you from incoming calls and sibling spats, and then lock the door and focus on letting the bathwater absorb your troubles.

CAREGIVER OVERLOAD

When you open your home to an aging parent, emotional baggage can take up more space than her ailing body. One national survey found that 25 percent of female caregivers endure emotional stress from their caregiving role. The dual stresses of guilt and resentment can be overwhelming. Try the following tips for some relief.

Establish realistic expectations. When a loved one needs you, you may have a hard time saying no, but if you're not careful, your big heart will overcommit your limited hours. Sit down together and talk about what each of you wants. Focus on the overlaps ("we eat meals together") and negotiate the disparities ("I keep you company all

(continued on page 336)

50 Ways to Raise Your Tranquillity Factor

The best refuge from stress can be the humble, slow accumulation of small moments of respite in otherwise harried days, says Alice Domar, Ph.D., director of the Mind/Body Center for Women's Health at Beth Israel Deaconess Medical Center of Harvard University. Start stockpiling serenity by trying one of these 50 tranquillity tricks every day and adding more as each becomes habit.

1. Start every morning with a touchstone ritual—brewing a steaming pot of your favorite tea or grinding up some fragrant coffee beans.
2. Write something small and achievable on your to-do list and do it—the sense of accomplishment will buoy you.
3. Burn sandalwood incense while you pay your bills.
4. Put a smiley face on notes to yourself.
5. Try a new restaurant once a month.
6. Take a dance class or go to a karaoke bar with your best friend. Be silly. Don't care.
7. Turn the ringer off at 8:00 at night. Screen calls through the answering machine.
8. On busy days, take 5 minutes to walk out the back door of your office building and around to the front.
9. When you start to get down on yourself, whisper softly, "I can do it."
10. In your top drawer, keep a vacation picture guaranteed to make you smile. Take it out when you need it most.
11. Touch a flower, plant, or tree. Take 1 minute to consider its growth from a little baby seed.
12. Give your dog or cat a longer-than-usual belly rub.
13. Keep the TV off for 24 hours. Put Billie Holiday on the CD player.
14. Go to bed before dark.
15. Make a list of 20 things you're grateful for, like "my cat" or "red toenail polish."
16. Drink your morning coffee on the back porch and listen to the birds, even if only for 3 minutes.
17. Say hi to the letter carrier.
18. Make a list of 20 things you'd love to do if you had all the time in the world.
19. Do one of the things on that list, in some form, every week.
20. Have lunch with people who make you laugh.
21. Spend 5 minutes totally alone, totally silent. Listen to the wind in the trees.
22. Buy yourself a $5 bouquet of flowers at the grocery store.

23. Shower by candlelight.
24. Finger paint with your kids—even if they're teenagers.
25. Instead of watching a sitcom, pop in a wedding, baby, or vacation video. Crunch popcorn. Laugh.
26. Make a reservation at a hotel for the night and steal your husband away. Get the king-size bed and the Jacuzzi bath.
27. Visit a farmer's market and buy tomatoes off the back of a pickup truck.
28. Fill a jelly jar with daisies for your desk at work.
29. Hire someone to wash all the windows this spring. Make it a yearly habit.
30. Play tag.
31. Chase the ice cream truck when it heads down your street.
32. Have your husband push you on a swing. Lean back and close your eyes.
33. Go to a baseball game and cheer until you get hoarse.
34. Rent a "chick flick" and commandeer the living room with a girlfriend or two.
35. Call your favorite department store and ask when they're having their next big sale. Then take the day off and shop.
36. Learn how to ice-skate.
37. Bring the Sunday paper to brunch with you. Order a pitcher of coffee and take your time.
38. Jump in a pile of leaves.
39. Make a whirlpool by turning around and around in your neighbor's pool.
40. Body surf.
41. Build a snowman.
42. Say no.
43. Celebrate Memorial Day with a pedicure and a bikini wax and greet the summer in style!
44. Buy cookies when asked to contribute to a bake sale.
45. Start an e-mail chat ring with your best friends from high school.
46. Choose a song you love and set the car audiotape or CD player so it plays as soon as you turn the ignition key every morning.
47. At the salon, ask for extra head scrubbing with your shampoo. Promise a good tip.
48. Run through a sprinkler.
49. Sing in the shower.
50. Put cold tea bags on your eyes and retire to the couch. Put your feet up on the armrest. Think about clouds.

weekend"). After you've fulfilled your agreed-upon expectations, you can always spend more time—but on your own terms.

Look for social proxies. You don't have to shoulder the burden alone. Thousands of services have popped up to help with the growing numbers of elderly who need social outlets, not nursing care. Look into senior day care, community programs, bus tours, library book groups, and Web TV. Ask helpful neighbors to check in on your parent, or swap "sitting time" with a fellow caregiver.

Hire some help. If your parent has moved into your home, you not only have another mouth to feed; you also have more laundry, dishes, etc. That extra work translates to time—two-thirds of caregivers actually lose money in their paid work while scrambling to meet everyone's needs. Rather than get resentful, tell your mom you could spend more time with her if you had less to do—then ask her to pay for cleaning help. She'll probably welcome the chance to make a contribution, and she'll definitely be grateful for a less stressed, more present you.

SPOUSAL SPATS

To have and hold. To honor and cherish. To blame and berate. Okay, so occasionally you both take liberties with your vows. Living with someone for several decades is bound to involve a few tense moments. The key is to remember how much you love each other, despite each other's faults.

Chart your course. Once a year, around the holidays, talk about what you'd like to accomplish together the following year. Being very specific, write down your goals as a couple, as a family, and as individuals. Keep the document in a special place, and celebrate each goal reached with a dinner for two or a family picnic. Your shared mission statement will give you a chance to literally work off the same page and buffer you from periodic conflicts over money and plans, says Ronald Potter-Efron, Ph.D., psychologist and author of *Being Belonging Doing: Balancing Your Three Greatest Needs.*

Divide the labor. Once you know your goals, you can split up the work. Is "keep a clean home" among your goals? If so, what does that mean? How often will you clean, and who will do what? Write down every chore in the house and give each to a specific family member. Knowing who's responsible for what will remove a tremendous amount of stress and resentment.

Show appreciation. Thank him, even if it's on his list of things to do. If he washed the car, tell him it looks great. When he does his share of the laundry, thank him—not because he's "helping you," but to say, "I appreciate you." Chances are, he'll reciprocate—appreciation is a gift that keeps on giving.

CHAPTER 17

ONE-MINUTE MOTIVATORS:
QUICK WAYS TO STAY FOCUSED THROUGH PLATEAUS, BINGES, INJURIES, FATIGUE, AND THE WORKOUT "WALL"

Weight loss, with its inevitable setbacks and frustrations, can feel like the plight of Sisyphus—you nudge that boulder up to the top of the hill with all your high-fiber cereal and broiled chicken breasts, and then—*whoosh!*—a twisted ankle, a fight with the boss, a sleepless night rolls the rock right back over you, crushing your spirit and will.

But contrary to poor Sisyphus, you're actually going to get to the top of that hill, where a thinner you awaits! Plateaus, injuries, and workout boredom may temporarily slow you down, but your most potent ally is your commitment—if you believe you will lose, you will, says Howard Rankin, Ph.D., psychological advisor to the national Take Off Pounds Sensibly (TOPS) organization in Hilton Head, South Carolina, and author of *Inspired to Lose*.

"When your initial motivation fades, you might get down on yourself and think, 'I'm lazy,' but nothing could be further from the

If You're Not Getting Results

Few things are more frustrating than doing all the right things and getting none of the expected results. If you feel like you're not getting anywhere, ask yourself these questions.

ARE YOU WEIGHT TRAINING? If so, you're doing the best thing possible to reverse perimenopausal metabolic decline. Although muscle may be heavier than fat, your plateau is not likely to last. That's because each pound of muscle burns an extra 30 calories a day, even when you're sitting on the couch!

Many women hold off on weight training until they lose some weight because they think cardiovascular workouts are faster at burning calories. But depending on how intensely you work out with weights, your metabolism can stay elevated for as long as 48 hours after you've finished lifting.

ARE YOU ON MEDICATION? Some prescription drugs, like antidepressants, hormone replacements, and steroids, list weight gain as a possible side effect. Check with your doctor to see if your medications may be to blame.

ARE YOU GETTING ENOUGH SLEEP? Sleep not only gives you energy; it also protects your body's muscle-building and fat-burning efficiency. Trade Leno in for an extra hour of sleep and help your body adjust to an earlier bedtime with a soothing shower, a cup of warm milk, and low lights.

ARE YOU EATING BREAKFAST? Your hectic morning schedule could be robbing you of your easiest metabolic rewards. When you skip breakfast, your metabolism slows by 5 percent—definitely enough to keep the last 10 pounds clinging on.

ARE YOU ALREADY AT A GOOD WEIGHT? Excited by the initial results of your weight-loss plan, you may have readjusted your goal downward to a more ambitious weight, a goal that may now be frustrating you. Go back and plug your current weight into a BMI table. If you're at a BMI of 25 or less, ask yourself if you really need to keep losing or if you're just fixated on a number. Sometimes a plateau is actually a good, comfortable weight.

truth," says Dr. Rankin. "Motivation is not a constant—it ebbs and flows like the tide."

Changing a specific behavior takes only 3 or 4 weeks, but it can take up to a year to make that change a firm, entrenched habit. Consider each of the strategies in this chapter another step up the mountain to that magical 1-year mark.

Persevere—Or Break Through—Weight-Loss Plateaus

Although they're heartbreaking, plateaus are a normal, even healthy part of weight loss. Common around the 6-month mark, or after you've lost 10 to 15 percent of your initial weight, a plateau is your body's chance to catch its breath and adjust to metabolic changes.

"Despite how it feels, you're really not running in place," says Madelyn Fernstrom, Ph.D., director of the Weight Management Center at the University of Pittsburgh Medical Center Health System. The best thing to do is grit your teeth and get through it. After a few determined weeks, your plateau *will* dissolve—and, with these tips, possibly even sooner.

Reevaluate your goal weight. If you're within 10 percent of your ultimate goal, you may be at a comfortable weight for your body, says Dr. Fernstrom. But if you still have 30 pounds to go, it's a bona fide plateau. Keep the faith—sticking to your plan for a few weeks will automatically yield results.

Dust off the food diary. After the initial fervor of weighing and measuring, we tend to put food diaries aside. "While we may believe we're eating 1,500 calories a day, in reality we're probably eating 2,000," says Susan Bartlett, Ph.D., assistant professor of medicine at Johns Hopkins School of Medicine in Baltimore. Get a handle on "portion creep" by revisiting your food diary—doing it even 2 days a week will increase awareness of how much you are actually eating and help you trim portions.

Focus on one. "Repeat this to yourself: 'The only pound I have to lose is the next one,'" says Dr. Rankin. It's easy to get overwhelmed with thoughts like "I still have 20 pounds to go!" Rather than focus on where you wanted to be now, look at how far you've come. Losing the next pound is always a question of choices you make today.

Check the schedule. A large percentage of your initial rapid weight loss was, sadly, just water. Actually, most nonwater pounds lost usually add up to $\frac{1}{2}$ to 2 pounds a week, so before you get discouraged, find out your *real* weight-loss rate. Take the weight you were at the 4th week on your program, subtract your current weight, and divide by the number of weeks between week 4 and now—you're probably a lot closer to the ideal than you think.

Add an extra glass. Some women retain more water than others. Flush your body with extra water to release that retained fluid—you just may find those stubborn pounds moving off the scale next week.

Cut down on weighing yourself. When fat is burned up, the empty fat cell quickly fills with water, which is heavier. Until your body releases that water, you will weigh the same—if not more. This frustrating lag plays out on your scale every day, so reduce your numbers anxiety by weighing yourself no more than once a week.

Join a support group—and speak up. Programs like TOPS or Weight Watchers not only give you support; they allow you to support others. You've learned a trick or two that will help someone just starting out, and being seen as a successful person is also tremendously motivating, says Dr. Rankin. One study by researchers from Brown University in Providence, Rhode Island, showed that even online support groups can help you maintain your motivation to lose weight.

Define your weight-loss mission. Let's not kid ourselves—sometimes counting fiber grams gets a little mundane. But your weight loss isn't just about calories. "Ask yourself, 'What's my ultimate purpose? What am I really after?'" suggests Dr. Rankin. He believes that for most women, weight loss is about empowerment. When you can connect to that goal on a daily basis, you're taking control of your life every time you choose a turkey sandwich over a cheeseburger.

Shoot for 10 and hold it there. Research shows that even a 5 to 10 percent weight loss favorably affects cholesterol and triglyceride levels and decreases your chances of developing diabetes. Shoot for 10 percent, and then just maintain for a little while, says Dr.

Fernstrom. Steady maintenance, not losing weight, is *the* key skill in lifelong weight management.

Show it off. If you're truly at a plateau, your body has caught on that you're losing weight and is trying to readjust. Celebrate the fact that you've outwitted nature this far, and get a new pair of pants that silhouettes your figure. Form-fitting clothes are much more flattering, and a great way to alert the people you're close to that you've lost weight.

Chart your progress. On a piece of graph paper, put your weight on the vertical axis and the weeks on a horizontal axis. If you've been following the Fit Not Fat Plan, undoubtedly that line is trending downward. Post it on your bathroom wall and update it at your weekly weigh-in.

Recover from a Binge— Or Head Off the Next One

Everyone binges at one time or another. Thanksgiving is a national binge, points out Dr. Bartlett. The binge doesn't matter nearly as much as how you cope with it afterward. These strategies will minimize the damage during a binge, help you bounce back after one, and head off the next episode before it starts.

DURING THE BINGE

Remove yourself. Get out of the danger zone, says Dr. Rankin. Walk outside. Drive to a friend's house. If you're in line at the drive-thru and suddenly snap to, pull away—fast.

Boot Camps for Women

Grapevines, ponies, and other fixtures of aerobics classes are great for moderate-intensity exercise. But when women get bored or want to reach another fitness level, many join boot camp.

Boot camp classes and programs are miniversions of basic training offered by gyms and spas all over the country to help women improve strength, aerobic conditioning, and endurance. Some are held once a week and others are 1- to 4-week-long programs. Some are for women only, while others are coed.

At the Tower Club Athletic Center in Charlotte, North Carolina, certified fitness trainer Don Evans teaches a 5-day program from 5:45 A.M. to 7:15 A.M. He and his class jog a mile and a half to a football stadium, where they run up and down the stadium stairs, and then do jumping jacks, pushups, situps, and lunges before running back to the athletic center.

Sounds tough—and it is. Some women do only half of the exercises, Evans says. But the point isn't to keep up perfectly. It's to learn how far your body will take you. One of his female students could do only one pushup on Monday but worked up to 15 by Friday. Many women gain so much confidence that they continue to work at a higher intensity on their own, running or doing pushups.

If you think you're up for the challenge, here's what to do.

CHECK YOUR FITNESS LEVEL. Boot camp is intense, so you should consult your doctor before taking the class. If you're not fit, you should work on your fitness before joining such a rigorous program.

RESEARCH THE WEB. To find boot camp programs near you, search the Web for "boot camp and exercise or fitness" or call your local YMCA and other gyms.

MODIFY EXERCISES. If you have trouble doing some of the exercises, modify them. If you can't do regular pushups, do them on your knees. Your instructor should show you how.

KEEP IT UP. If nothing else, boot camp will give you new exercises to add to your personal fitness routine. Many, such as lunges, pullups, and triceps dips, require no equipment.

If you can jar yourself out of the trance of bingeing, you'll have the power to stop.

Minimize the damage. All-or-nothing thinking, like "the damage is already done," can make a binge worse than it has to be.

"It's one thing if you've eaten a bag of chips, but if you then polish off a pint of ice cream, you've added another 800 to 1,000 calories," says Dr. Bartlett. As hypocritical as it may feel, if you've decided you really need a Big Mac, it's always better to order a diet soda with it, then skip the fries, to save an extra 1,000 calories.

Picture your office mate. "Women eat very differently in front of men than alone and usually won't binge in public," says Eric Stice, Ph.D., assistant professor of psychology at the University of Texas in Austin. "Ask yourself, 'Would I eat this in front a male coworker?'" While this may feel uncomfortable, that's the point—to help you realize that food can never be a true comfort or a screen to hide behind.

AFTER THE BINGE

Realize that one binge will never make you fat. "It's what you do next that's most important," says Dr. Rankin. "You could have a 5,000-calorie binge and not gain a pound—as long as it stops there." What you do the other 29 days a month is way more important than that half-hour.

Resume your Fit Not Fat Plan at the very next meal. *Never* punish yourself by skipping your next meal, says Dr. Rankin. That guilt and resulting hunger will only set you on a downward spiral again. Nor should you use it as a free pass for the weekend. "If you slip Friday night, the most common thing is to say, 'Monday morning, I'll start again,'" says Dr. Rankin. "Instead, start with breakfast Saturday morning—or, better yet, a walk on Friday night."

Drink even more water. Your liver is working overtime to digest the excess fat. By drinking several extra glasses of water, you'll help your liver process the fat and help relieve some of that sluggish feeling that weighs you down.

Develop amnesia. First think about why the binge happened (an argument with a friend? stress at work?), and then think about what you learned ("I actually feel worse now than before I ate"). Then *forget it ever happened.* Self-forgiveness is essential to preventing future binges, says Dr. Rankin.

PREVENTING ANOTHER BINGE

Plan out your day. Be very cautious the first few days after a binge, as it's an especially vulnerable time for relapse, says Dr. Bartlett. Put all your guilt energy into planning meals and snacks and doing regular check-ins with your food diary—the planning and recording will keep you accountable and on track.

Eat regularly. Keeping your blood sugar stable helps keep you in control. Skipping breakfast or lunch is a guaranteed recipe for a nighttime binge, says Dr. Stice.

Enlist a buddy. When you head to a party, make a deal with your pal that both of you will avoid fatty dips and chips. Offer to bring cut veggies to ensure your own safe options. Pile up a plate of sweet bell peppers and crunch on them together—you'll feel less deprived if you support each other.

Carry water everywhere. Always check to see if your "hunger" is thirst—humans can survive 40 days without food, but only 4 without water, says Dr. Bartlett.

Have a failsafe. If you feel a binge coming on, reach for a preplanned food, selected beforehand. Something like a bowl of high-fiber cereal and milk takes a few minutes to eat and is very filling—after you've finished, your craving will probably be thwarted.

Talk to a counselor or a doctor. According to the National Institutes of Health, as many as half of all people who struggle with bingeing have been depressed in the past. If this sounds like you, ask your doctor to refer you to a therapist who understands food-related issues. Opening up about your emotions could potentially eliminate all bingeing.

Prevent Compulsive Eating

When a woman eats compulsively—steadily, without thinking—she's usually trying to camouflage feelings of anger and frustration, says Dr. Rankin. Turning her feelings inward, she tries to "stuff" her pain with food. The best remedy is anything that does the opposite, helps her take her internal feelings to the outside world.

Phone a friend. Food may seem to offer comfort and solace, but what we really need is connection. Pick up the phone and call *anyone*. Go to the post office or knock on a neighbor's door just to chat. During every moment you spend with friendly, supportive people, you're loosening your bond with food, says Dr. Rankin.

Resist it just once. Every time you give in to a craving, you reinforce the idea that the food is in control. But every time you resist, you remind yourself that *you* are in control. If overeating at meals is a problem, limit yourself to one single-serving dinner, eat it, and get up and do something else, recommends Dr. Bartlett. "If women do this for even 2 days, they tell me they feel so differently about food," she says.

Bargain down the portions. Rather than go cold turkey on high-fat snacks, start by trimming portions, says Jenna Anding, R.D., Ph.D., assistant professor of nutrition and extension nutrition specialist at Texas Cooperative Extension in College Station. If you normally eat a huge bowl of ice cream, move down to a salad-size dish, then a mug, then a cup, and finally a tiny dessert dish. Every victory over food builds strength for the next time.

Prebag snacks. Compulsive eating often happens when you shove your hand in the bag and lose count of the mouthfuls. Measure out snack foods into preportioned bags or break a large chocolate bar into individual squares, wrap each in tin foil, and store them in the fridge.

Startle yourself. When we eat compulsively, we're in a trance—we're not even tasting what we're eating, says Dr. Rankin. If you sense this is happening, snap a rubber band on your wrist and say "Stop!" out loud. Set an alarm clock to go off at vulnerable times or post a mirror at eye level next to the fridge. Anything that increases your awareness will help you get control.

Tap your feet. The repetitive motion of compulsive eating helps some people focus on work or reading, says Dr. Rankin. Instead, wiggle in your chair, chew some gum, pace around your office—moving that energy into fidgeting could burn up to 500 extra calories a day.

Hit the road. If you're craving ice cream and you really want it, get in the car, drive to Baskin-Robbins, order a scoop, eat it, and go home. "You're using the principles of portion control, so it never gets out of hand," says Dr. Bartlett. You'll also be less likely to indulge if you have to drive a few miles first in order to satisfy a momentary urge.

Shake up your routine. Since compulsive eating is a habit, comfortable and familiar, shaking things up can help you avoid future binges. "The hardest thing to do is break a habit in the same setting," says Dr. Bartlett. Get yourself away from the cupboard, go into another room, and do anything with your hands—fold laundry, play a board game, knit or cross-stitch, or type letters.

Get to the Gym When You're Too Tired to Exercise

Name any other endeavor in which you spend a few hours to gain back years. Bottom line, exercise improves and extends your life. If they were giving out free money at the bank, you'd figure out how to get there, right? Put on those sneakers.

Set it in stone. "Write exercise in on your calendar—in ink—rather than on a to-do list," suggests Harold Taylor, time management expert and owner of Harold Taylor Time Consultants in Toronto. "If it's on the to-do list, it's something to feel guilty about; if it's on the calendar, it's an appointment." Other things will have to "find time" around your most important client—yourself.

Introduce yourself. After you start chatting with other women in the locker room, your morning routine won't be complete without hearing the latest gossip. You're all there for the same purpose—belonging to this community of women will encourage you when your motivation slips, says Dr. Rankin.

Indulge yourself. Before you sign the gym contract, look for a sauna, a steam room, or at least a really satisfying hot shower. Then you can tell yourself you're just going to the gym for a steam—and after you're there, who knows? You may do a 10-minute workout, too.

Make a date. Set up a standing date with a friend whose fitness level matches yours—your mutual motivation lulls will cancel each other out. Research shows that having a dedicated workout partner makes you more likely to stick with an exercise program.

Go off-peak. Take a page from airline travelers and get maximum value during off-hours. Work through lunch, taking advantage of the downtime to be more productive.

FIT |
FLASH

Sniff Your Way to an Easier Workout

Dragging in the gym? Dab a few drops of peppermint oil on your shirt collar.

In a study published in *Journal of Sport and Exercise Psychology*, researchers at Wheeling Jesuit University in West Virginia found that 40 athletes ran faster, did more pushups, and had stronger hand grips when exposed to the scent of peppermint than with other scents or no scent.

"Peppermint boosts mood, so you perform better without feeling like you're working harder," says lead researcher Bryan Raudenbush, Ph.D., assistant professor of psychology at Wheeling Jesuit University.

During the later afternoon hours, you can relish the quiet and have the run of the gym while enjoying your muscles' peak strength hours—from 3 to 6 P.M.

Have a snack. When you run low on fuel, the extra energy demands of exercise lead your body to decide, "She's overdoing it—we need to conserve some fuel by slowing down her metabolism," says Michele Olson, Ph.D., professor of health and human performance at Auburn University in Montgomery, Alabama. That's the last thing you want, so have a protein- and complex-carbohydrate snack, like a hard-boiled egg and a slice of whole wheat toast, 2 hours before you plan to work out.

Put on your shoes. Think baby steps—if you truly don't feel like you can get out the door, just put on your workout clothes. If that feels good, throw on some sneakers. Even if you stay in the house, the clothes will give you an increased range of motion, so you'll probably put more energy into your chores.

Join your company softball team. Regular practice helps condition you for the season, and the inherent motivating forces of teamwork and won games will keep you interested in constantly improving. When you're running around the bases, you'll forget you're exercising.

Go to the source. Plenty of people avoid gyms out of distaste for "workout bunnies." But now that you've made the commitment to regular exercise, guess what. You're one of *them*. Gyms are in the business of making exercise interesting. Take advantage of the classes and the weights and the cardio machines and the nutritional counseling—really milk it.

Be compassionate. When you have more than 30 pounds to lose, it can take about a year for your brain to catch up with your new self-image. You may have thought of yourself as overweight for so long that avoiding the gym is your subconscious way of pacing weight loss. Give yourself time to readjust, listen to compliments, and surround yourself with people who applaud and support "the new you."

Freshen a Stale Workout Routine

Okay, so you're no Jane Fonda. That doesn't mean you're doomed to hate exercise. There are a million ways to move your body, and each one is as valuable and as productive as the other. Try some of these tips to take the "work" out of your workout.

Reclaim your birthright. "Try to link exercise with happiness, social activity, and escape," suggests Peg Jordan, R.N., Ph.D., author of *The Fitness Instinct* in Oakland, California. "Free yourself up to think of movement as your birthright every hour on the hour." Join an African dance class, or try inline skating. Instead of dreading sweat, think of it as calories pleasantly leaking from your body.

Pile on the rewards. Women tend to save rewards for distant, huge goals, like a 20-pound weight loss or three lost dress sizes, says Dr. Rankin. Rather than make goals destination-oriented, make them behavior-oriented. Set a goal to work out three times *this*

Rev Up Your Energy—And Your Workouts

Are your workouts much more work lately? Fatigue during exercise stems from a number of physical and psychological reasons, but usually it's an easy fix. Try these tips to stop the energy drain.

PUMP MORE IRON. As a mineral that helps convert food to energy, iron is essential to keeping energy levels high. But dieting, avoiding meat, and having heavy menstrual periods can put you at risk for low iron. Iron supplements are sometimes risky, so make sure your diet includes 18 milligrams of iron every day—choose lean meats or legumes, leafy greens, and whole grains. Don't forget citrus fruit and other juice with vitamin C, which improves iron absorption from plant foods.

FUEL UP EARLY. Eating the bulk of your calories in the early part of the day will give you the energy you need to make it through daytime workouts. Many women on weight-loss plans find it easier to eat less during the day and more at night—exactly the opposite plan for optimal energy and weight loss.

WET YOUR WHISTLE. Dehydration can seriously drag your energy down. Research shows that even when you drink eight glasses of water a day, 45 minutes of exercise can put you into a dehydrated state. Don't rely on thirst as a measure of need—to prevent exercise fatigue, take a sip of water every 15 to 20 minutes while you work out.

SNACK FIRST. One small study showed that cyclists who had eaten a small meal before their workouts lasted 30 minutes longer than those with empty stomachs. Try yogurt, a banana, or some graham crackers to keep your energy high.

week, and when you achieve it, give yourself a nonfood reward, like a glossy magazine or new nail polish—little indulgences you wouldn't ordinarily give yourself.

Borrow a dog. Or a toddler. "There's nothing like chasing after a 3-year-old to keep you running without even realizing it," says Dr. Bartlett, coauthor of a study of women over 40 that showed lifestyle activity offers weight-loss benefits comparable to structured aerobic exercise.

Sign up for a race. Walkathons and 5-Ks give you goals to work toward, and many women start to see themselves as athletes when they sign up, says Dr. Rankin. When it's for a cause you believe in—like Race for the Cure for breast cancer—raising money, joining with like-minded people, and crossing the finish line can become spiritual events.

Try intervals. Interval-style exercise—Spinning classes, for example—raises your metabolism both during and after the exercise, says Dr. Olson. Steady activity—say, 30 minutes on a treadmill—burns about 6 to 8 calories per minute. A brief, 30- to 60-second burst of intense interval activity burns about 10 calories per minute *and* stimulates your muscles to burn 20 to 30 percent more calories within the same workout.

Make a mix tape. Listening to music eases exercise in three different ways: It distracts you from fatigue, it encourages coordination, and it relaxes your muscles to encourage bloodflow. If music doesn't work, try a book on tape. "Anything pleasurable you can link to exercise will help motivate you," says Dr. Rankin.

Cover all your bases. Do you include each of the triumvirate—cardiovascular, strength, and flexibility—in your workouts each week? A combination of all three keeps your metabolism burning high, your energy level up, and your body injury-free, says Dr. Olson. "It's best to have a variety of plans so you can do something 5 out of 7 days a week," she says.

Bump it to 4. "If you're doing 3 days a week of cardio exercise, that's great for cardio fitness," says Dr. Olson. "But if you're trying to reduce body fat, you really won't target that until you hit 4 or 5 days a week."

Create an exercise menu. Get to know your rhythms, and have an exercise plan in place for each mood. Feeling low? Go for a walk in the park. Keyed up from work? Take a high-energy class. Missing your kids? Bundle them into the car and head for the local soccer field.

Check out a new video. The library's lending period is a great built-in change period. Use one video for 2 weeks, return it, and try a new one. Your muscles will benefit from the variety, and you'll never spend a cent.

What to Do If Your Workout Isn't Working

Just like your brain, your muscles get bored when you do the same workout all the time. Your body will burn fewer total calories after it becomes used to a routine because it quickly adapts to challenges, and works more efficiently on fewer calories. That's great for Olympic athletes, but how do we make our bodies a little *less* efficient?

Change *anything*. Change the intensity, frequency, or duration of your exercise at least once a month—try a harder step class, add one more walk a week, or pause your video and do 5 extra minutes of lunges and jumping jacks. This level of variety challenges your muscles to keep "learning" and meeting new challenges so they can burn more calories and fat, says Dr. Olson.

Up frequency first. By increasing frequency, you'll automatically spend more time burning calories and add another workout time to your schedule, says Dr. Olson. Start with one extra 10-minute walk or weight session per week, and after it becomes a habit, increase the time or the intensity.

Check your expectations. "Within three workouts, the heart already becomes more efficient," says Dr. Olson. Congratulate yourself for running upstairs without losing your breath; celebrate when your thighs no longer rub together. Changes in weight, fat percentage, and muscle development may take a little bit longer, sometimes up to 2 months.

Return to the 1950s. Open the garage door manually, switch the channels *on* the TV, and wash your car (and dishes) by hand. Hang your wash outside instead of throwing it into

FIT | FLASH

Gardening Is a Good Workout

It's 2 o'clock on Saturday afternoon—do you know where your workout is?

If you said it's your garden, you'll burn nearly 30 percent more calories than in the gym, according to a British study.

Researchers studied the caloric expenditure of a 40-year-old woman during two different workouts, one in the step aerobics studio and the other in her backyard. The step class burned an impressive 306 calories, but the yard work—sawing, carrying, and piling debris—blasted away nearly a third more, 392 calories. Better still, she worked in her training heart rate zone, which improves cardio fitness, for twice as much time while gardening—44 versus 24 minutes.

"One day as I headed to the gym, I thought, 'I could just cut the grass,'" says Susan J. Bartlett, Ph.D., assistant professor of medicine at Johns Hopkins School of Medicine in Baltimore. "Now my husband and I regularly vie for who's going to do the lawn!" How many hours on the treadmill leave your house looking more beautiful than when you started?

COOL TOOL

PlateMates

Typically, weights are available in 5-pound increments, whether you're ready for that much additional weight or not. Enter PlateMates, miniweights that magnetically attach to your dumbbells or barbells. They're available in ⅝-, 1¼-, 1⅞-, and 2½-pound sizes.

WHAT THE EXPERT SAYS: "It's a very easy way to add resistance," says Wayne Westcott, Ph.D., fitness research director at the South Shore YMCA in Quincy, Massachusetts. "Most women use solid dumbbells at home or in the gym. PlateMates enable you to attach weight without taking anything apart." (PlateMates don't work with vinyl-, plastic-, or rubber-coated weights, however.)

"It's unreasonable to expect the average woman to jump between 5-pound or 10-pound weight increments," says Dr. Wescott. "At most, you can increase your strength no more than 5 percent between workouts," he says. "In other words, if you're using a 15-pound dumbbell and it's too easy, suddenly lifting a 20-pound dumbbell would require a 30 percent increase in strength. It's too much at once. It's easier to move up in smaller increments."

PURCHASING TIPS: PlateMates are sold in pairs; you'll need one pair per dumbbell in use. Buy two pairs, so you can do exercises that require two dumbbells. Prices start at around $19 plus shipping. For more information or to order, call (800) 877-3322, or visit the company's Web site at www.theplatemate.com. Mention *Prevention* magazine and receive a 10 percent discount.

the dryer. It's estimated that in the past 25 years, laborsaving devices have decreased the number of calories we burn by 800 per day—that's 1.5 pounds per week!

Invest in a trainer. A certified personal trainer can fine-tune your workout for extra results without wasted time and effort. Find a trainer you like, and then schedule follow-up visits four times a year—those dates will give you built-in goals to strive for. One hour of training costs $50 to $70—buddy up with a friend to share the cost.

Hit the weights—right now! Now that she's nearing 40, Dr. Olson dedicates 70 percent of her efforts to resistance training. She says many women over 40 could benefit from starting with weight training even before they start cardio—a stronger woman is less likely to be injured in a step class or while walking. Weight training develops the strength of the all-important core muscles in the trunk, lower back, and hip area, making your body better equipped cardio challenges. To start, substitute strength training for at least one of your regular workouts.

Become a "schlepper." Women may unconsciously avoid extra lifestyle activity if they've already worked out, thinking, "I got my exercise for the day." Take *all* opportunities to challenge your muscles. At the grocery store, grab a basket instead of a cart. Move firewood by hand instead of using a wheelbarrow. Help your college-age nephew move into his dorm.

Bounce Back from Injury

Few things kill motivation more quickly than an unexpected injury. Resting the injured body part is critical—but the rest of you should keep right on going. Tempting though it may be, an injury is no reason to give up and grab the remote. Aquarobics, tai chi, seated table tennis—there's always something you can do.

First, see a doctor. Sometimes injuries like broken toes or shin splints tempt us to avoid the doctor out of the mistaken belief that "nothing can be done." This *isn't* the time for self-healing—get thee to the doctor.

Request a scorecard. While you're at the doctor's office anyway, have her do some blood work—your earlier weight-loss efforts may have resulted in a drop in your cholesterol, triglycerides, and blood sugar levels, says Dr. Anding. Even if your injury tempers your weight-loss rate, you can draw motivation from this hard evidence of how your health has already improved. If your doctor can't squeeze in a quick blood check during your visit, schedule an annual physical exam before you leave the office and you can look forward to having these measurements taken.

Get a referral. Your primary physician may tell you just to rest and "stay off it" for a while; in that case, ask your doctor if a physical therapist can help. She can give you appropriate stretches, show you alternative weight exercises, or introduce you to a new activity, like yoga, that could help your injury heal sooner and may even help prevent a recurrence.

See it as a blessing. Injuries are our body's way of telling us we're doing something wrong—and better to learn your mistakes sooner rather than later, says Dr. Olson. Trying other activities will challenge and shock your body, and you'll get faster results. After you've healed, you'll jump ahead even faster

Reclaim control. Instead of getting stuck in the "poor me" mindset, focus on something you still have total control over: your eating. Now is an excellent time to evaluate your eating habits and look at ways you can minimize this minor roadblock, says Dr. Anding.

PART 6

THE FIT NOT FAT CALORIE COUNTER, SHOPPING GUIDE, AND MENU PLANNER

CHAPTER 18

FIT NOT FAT CALORIE, FAT, AND FIBER COUNTER AND SHOPPING GUIDE

In part 3, Amy Campbell, R.D., a certified diabetes educator and program co-ordinator of the Fit and Healthy weight-loss program of the Joslin Diabetes Center at Harvard University, spelled out exactly what kind of food is fit to eat if women over 40 want to shape up, which foods can make women fat if consumed too often or in large amounts, and others that are fair—not necessarily bad (and possibly even beneficial) when consumed in moderation.

The table that follows offers hundreds of food choices, from breakfast foods to dinners, including some popular restaurant items and examples of brand-name foods found everywhere. They're ranked for their relative value on the Fit Not Fat Food Plan, based on their fat, calorie, and fiber content. Use the table to make smart choices from among the types of foods you *should* eat rather than from the types of foods you *could* eat.

The Fit Not Fat Food Plan calls for roughly 300 calories at breakfast, 400 calories at lunch, 60 calories for an afternoon snack, 555 calories at dinner, and 200 calories for an evening snack. You also get 40 to 45 grams of fat a day, and 30 to 35 grams of fiber a day. Use this chart to help you plan accordingly.

When it comes to fat, the key is to "spend" your fat calories wisely. It makes sense to "save" your fat calories for oils like olive and canola oil (14 grams per tablespoon), pumpkin seeds, or peanuts, which contain beneficial fats, than to blow the same number of fat calories on doughnuts, fried eggs, and deviled ham, all of which contain saturated fat.

As a rule, the more foods you select from the top of each category, the faster you'll reach your fitness goals. (However, keep an eye out for high-fiber foods that may have more calories but pack more of the weight-loss rewards you're looking for.)

Feel free to photocopy these pages and take them along with you to grocery stores, restaurants, the company cafeteria—anyplace that offers opportunities to "eat fit." To find values for the calorie, fat, fiber, and other nutrient content of foods not listed here, go to www.nal.usda.gov/fnic/foodcomp or, in the case of brand-name or restaurant items, Web sites for manufacturers and restaurant chains. Bear in mind that the inclusion of a brand-name food or restaurant item on this list is simply for illustrative purposes and does not endorse or condemn any particular items. No food is forbidden, provided it's part of an overall healthful diet and consumed only occasionally.

CALORIE, FAT, AND FIBER COUNTER

FOOD	CALORIES	FAT (g)	FIBER (g)
Breads, Cereals, and Breakfast Foods			
Rye crispbread, Wasa, 1 slice	30	1	2
Bread stick, plain, 1	41	1	0
Bread, stone-ground wheat, 1 slice	60	1	2
Bread, whole grain, 1 slice	60	1	5
Bread, mixed grain, 1 slice	65	1	2
Bread, pumpernickel, 1 slice	65	1	2
Bread, white, 1 slice	67	1	1
Bread, whole wheat, 1 slice	69	1	2
Bread, oat bran, 1 slice	71	1	1
Bread, raisin, 1 slice	71	1	1
Tortilla, whole wheat, 1	73	0	2
Bread, oatmeal, 1 slice	73	1	1
Pita, whole wheat, 1 (4" diameter)	74	1	2
Pita, white, 1 (4" diameter)	77	0	1
Bread, rye, 1 slice (1.3 oz)	83	1	2
Hamburger roll, reduced-calorie, 1	84	1	3
Hot dog roll, reduced-calorie, 1	84	1	3
Bread, honey bran, 1 slice	90	1	2
Bagel, oat bran, ½ small (3½" diameter)	91	0	1
Tortilla, flour, ¼ c	108	0	1
English muffin, Thomas' Honey-Wheat, 1	110	1	3
Hamburger roll, plain, 1	123	2	0
Hot dog roll, plain, 1	123	2	0
Pita, oat bran, Sahara, 1 (2 oz)	130	1	3

FOOD	CALORIES	FAT (g)	FIBER (g)
English muffin, whole wheat, 1	134	1	4
Cornbread, mix, prepared, 1 slice	152	5	2
Muffin, oat bran, 1 small (2½" diameter)	154	4	3
English muffin, mixed grain, 1	155	1	2
Muffin, blueberry, 1 medium	158	4	1
Croissant, butter, 1 small	171	9	1
Bread, French or Vienna (includes sourdough), 1 medium slice	175	2	2
Biscuit, plain or buttermilk, mix, 1 small	191	7	1
Bagel, plain/onion/poppy seed/ sesame seed, 1 bagel (3½" diameter)	195	1	2
Bread, banana, 1 slice	196	6	1
Bagel, egg, 1 (3½" diameter)	197	2	2
Doughnut, yeast-leavened, glazed, 1 medium	242	14	1
Roll, sandwich, whole wheat, 1	250	4	7
Bagel, blueberry, Lender's, 1 (4" diameter)	264	2	2
Bagel, whole wheat, 1 (4 oz)	291	2	10
Wheatena, cooked, ½ c	68	1	3
Cereal, puffed, Kashi, 1 c	70	1	2
Cereal, All-Bran, Kellogg's, ½ c	82	1	10
Cereal, Cheerios, General Mills, 1 c	83	1	2
Cereal, bran flakes, Post, ⅔ c	85	1	5
Farina, enriched, cooked, ¾ c	89	0	1

CALORIE, FAT, AND FIBER COUNTER

FOOD	CALORIES	FAT (g)	FIBER (g)
Breads, Cereals, and Breakfast Foods (cont.)			
Cereal, Kashi Good Friends, about ¾ c	90	1	8
Cream of wheat, cooked, ¾ c	100	0	1
Cereal, Nutri-Grain, wheat, Kellogg's, ¾ c	100	1	4
Cereal, cornflakes, General Mills, 1 c	114	1	0
Cereal, Fiber One, General Mills, 1 c	123	2	29
Oatmeal, instant, blueberries and cream, Quaker, 1 packet	135	3	2
Oatmeal, old-fashioned, Quaker Oats, cooked, ½ c	148	3	4
Cereal, shredded wheat, Post, 2 biscuits	156	1	6
Cereal, Grape-Nuts, Post, ½ c	190	1	5
Cereal, granola, low-fat, c Kellogg's, ½	217	4	3
Waffle, low-fat, Nutri-Grain, Kellogg's Eggo, 1 (4" diameter)	71	1	1
Waffle, low-fat, home style, Kellogg's Eggo, 1 (4" diameter)	82	1	0
Pancake, whole wheat, dry mix, 1 (4" diameter)	92	3	1
Waffle, oat bran, Kellogg's Eggo, 1	107	4	2
French toast, frozen, ready-to-eat, 1 slice	126	4	1
French toast, Aunt Jemima, 2 slices	240	6	2

FOOD	CALORIES	FAT (g)	FIBER (g)
Crackers and Chips			
Cracker, saltine, 1	13	0	0
Cracker, square, whole wheat, 1	18	1	0
Melba toast, wheat, 1 toast	19	0	0
Melba toast, rye, 1 toast	19	1	0
Cracker, Ry-Krisp, 1 large square	30	0	2
Cracker, graham, plain or honey, 1 (2½") square	30	1	0
Cracker, rye, wafer, 1	37	0	3
Cracker, milk, 1	50	2	0
Crackers, stoned wheat thins, 3	53	2	1
Crackers, saltine, fat-free, Zesta, 5	54	0	0
Crackers, animal, 5	55	2	0
Crackers, stoned wheat, Nabisco Wheatsworth, 5	80	3	1
Crackers, baked, savory, Nabisco Sociables, 7	80	4	0
Cracker, matzo, whole wheat, 1	100	0	3
Crackers, Air Crisps, Nabisco, 32	130	4	0
Crackers, wafers, whole wheat or rye, Nabisco Triscuit, 7	140	5	4
Crackers, vegetable thins, Nabisco, 14	160	9	1
Crackers, classic golden, low-fat, Snackwell's, 6	347	6	2
Tortilla chips, baked, Tostitos, 1 oz	111	1	2
Potato chips, light, 1 oz	134	6	2
Potato sticks, 1 oz	148	10	1

CALORIE, FAT, AND FIBER COUNTER

FOOD	CALORIES	FAT (g)	FIBER (g)
Crackers and Chips (cont.)			
Potato chips, plain, 1 oz	152	10	1
Corn chips, 30 (about 1 oz)	153	9	1
Spreads and Condiments			
Butter spray, imitation, 5 sprays	0	0	0
Margarine, fat-free, Promise, 1 tsp	2	0	0
Fruit butter, apple, 1 Tbsp	31	0	0
Cream cheese, fat-free, Philadelphia brand, 2 Tbsp (1 oz)	39	0	0
Fruit spread, strawberry, Polaner, 1 Tbsp	42	0	0
Cheese spread, pasteurized, processed, Kraft Velveeta, 1 oz	86	6	0
Butter, without salt, 1 Tbsp	100	11	0
Almond butter, plain, no salt, 1 Tbsp	101	9	1
Cream cheese, regular, 2 Tbsp	101	10	0
Tahini (sesame butter), 2 tsp	178	16	1
Peanut butter, reduced-fat, Jif, 2 Tbsp	190	12	2
Peanut butter, commercial, 2 Tbsp	190	16	2
Peanut butter, natural, Smuckers, 2 Tbsp	200	16	2
Mustard, yellow, 1 tsp	3	0	0
Lemon juice, 1 Tbsp	4	0	0
Mustard, Grey Poupon, 1 tsp	5	0	0
Chili sauce, red hot, 1 tsp	7	0	0
Horseradish, 1 tsp	10	1	0

FOOD	CALORIES	FAT (g)	FIBER (g)
Salsa, mild, Hunt's Homestyle, 2 Tbsp	10	1	0
Mayonnaise, fat-free, Kraft, 1 Tbsp	11	0	0
Soy sauce, La Choy, 1 Tbsp	11	0	0
Ketchup, 1 Tbsp	15	0	0
Steak sauce, A.1, 1 Tbsp	15	0	0
Worcestershire sauce, Lea & Perrins, 1 Tbsp	15	0	0
Tartar sauce, fat-free, Kraft, 2 Tbsp	25	0	1
Mayonnaise, light, Kraft, 1 Tbsp	50	5	0
Tartar sauce, Sauceworks, 1 Tbsp	50	5	0
Mayonnaise, regular, Miracle Whip, 1 Tbsp	57	5	0
Syrup, pancake and waffle, light, Aunt Jemima, ¼ c	93	0	1
Syrup, pancake and waffle, original, Aunt Jemima, ¼ c	212	0	0

Milk, Cheese, Yogurt, and Sour Cream

FOOD	CALORIES	FAT (g)	FIBER (g)
Milk, evaporated, low-fat, Carnation, 2 Tbsp	25	1	0
Milk, dry, nonfat, Carnation, ⅓ c	80	0	0
Milk, soy, 1 c	81	5	3
Milk, fat-free, 1 c	90	0	0
Milk, soy, Soy Moo, fat-free, 1 c	110	0	1
Buttermilk, cultured low-fat, 1 c	110	3	0
Milk, low-fat (1%), 1 c	110	3	0
Milk, reduced-fat (2%), 1 c	122	5	0

CALORIE, FAT, AND FIBER COUNTER

FOOD	CALORIES	FAT (g)	FIBER (g)
Milk, Cheese, Yogurt, and Sour Cream (cont.)			
Milk, condensed sweetened, Carnation, 2 Tbsp	130	3	0
Milk, whole, 1 c	150	8	0
Cheese wedge, reduced-fat, The Laughing Cow, 1 piece	50	3	0
Ricotta, reduced-fat, 1½ oz	59	3	0
Veggie Shreds, Cheddar, Galaxy, 1 serving size	60	3	0
Cheese, cottage, low-fat, 1% milkfat, ½ c	80	2	0
Cheese, Parmesan, 1½ Tbsp	88	6	0
Mozzarella, reduced-fat, 1½ oz	108	7	0
Cheese, goat, soft type, 1½ oz	114	9	0
Cheese, feta, 1½ oz	116	9	0
Cottage cheese, creamed, small-curd, ½ c	120	5	0
Cheese, mozzarella, whole milk, 1½ oz	120	9	0
Cheez Whiz, low-fat, Kraft, 2 oz	123	6	0
Cheese, Brie, 1½ oz	142	12	0
Cheese, provolone, 1½ oz	149	11	0
Cheese, Monterey, 1½ oz	159	13	0
Cheese, Swiss, 1½ oz	167	12	0
Cheese, Colby, 1½ oz	168	14	0
Cheese, Cheddar, 1½ oz	171	14	0
American cheese, 2 oz	223	18	0
Yogurt, low-fat, all flavors, Breyers, 8 oz	125	0	0

FOOD	CALORIES	FAT (g)	FIBER (g)
Yogurt, plain, low-fat, 1 c	155	4	0
Yogurt, vanilla, low-fat, 1 c	209	3	0
Yogurt, fruit, low-fat, 1 c	258	3	0
Sour cream, reduced-fat, 1 Tbsp	18	1	0
Sour cream, 1 Tbsp	30	3	0
Sour cream, imitation, 1 Tbsp	30	3	0

Eggs, Egg Substitutes, and Egg Dishes

FOOD	CALORIES	FAT (g)	FIBER (g)
Yolk, fresh, 1 large	59	5	0
Egg, poached, 1 large	75	5	0
Egg, hard-boiled, 1 large	78	5	0
Egg, raw, 1 large	78	5	0
Egg, fried, 1 large	92	7	0
Egg, scrambled, 1 large	101	7	0
Egg substitute: Better 'n Eggs, liquid, Morningstar Farms, ¼ c	25	0	0
Egg substitute: Egg Beaters, liquid, Fleischmann's, ¼ c	30	0	0
Egg substitute: powdered egg, 0.35 oz	44	1	0
Egg substitute: liquid, ¼ c	54	3	0
Omelet, plain, 1 large	93	7	0
Breakfast egg (substitute) with whole wheat pita, homemade, ½ filled pita	223	4	5
Croissant with egg and cheese, fast food, 1 (about 4 oz)	411	28	0
Croissant with egg, cheese, and bacon, fast food, 1 (about 4.5 oz)	454	31	0

CALORIE, FAT, AND FIBER COUNTER

FOOD	CALORIES	FAT (g)	FIBER (g)
Eggs, Egg Substitutes, and Egg Dishes (cont.)			
Biscuit with egg and sausage, fast food, 1 (about 5 oz)	458	30	1
Biscuit with egg and bacon, fast food, 1 (about 5 oz)	458	31	1
Biscuit with egg, cheese, and bacon, fast food, 1 (about 5 oz)	469	31	0
Beans and Bean Dishes			
Soybeans, green, cooked, ½ c	62	6	4
Beans, lima, canned, ½ c	80	0	4
Beans, refried, Old El Paso, fat-free, ½ c	100	0	6
Beans, cannellini, canned, Progresso, ½ c	100	1	5
Beans, pinto, canned, ½ c	103	1	6
Beans, black, cooked, ½ c	114	0	7
Beans, baby lima, cooked, ½ c	115	0	7
Beans, vegetarian, canned, ½ c	118	1	6
Beans, refried, canned, ½ c	119	2	7
Chickpeas, cooked, ½ c	134	2	6
Beans, red kidney, canned, ½ c	151	1	11
Hummus, commercially prepared, 2 Tbsp	46	3	2
Tofu, organic, firm, Nasoya, 3 oz	70	4	1
Three-bean salad, Joan of Arc, ½ c	90	0	3
Veggie Medley patty, Gardenburger, 1	100	0	2
Black beans and rice, Zatarain's, 1 serving (about ½ c)	110	0	2

FOOD	CALORIES	FAT (g)	FIBER (g)
Veggie "burger" patty, Gardenburger, Zesty Black Bean, 1	120	4	5
Beans with pork, Hunt's, ½ c	130	1	4
Pork and beans in tomato sauce, canned, Campbell's, ½ c	130	2	6
Soy "burger" patty, Gardenburger, 1	130	3	5
Tempeh, ½ c	160	9	4
Beans, brown sugar and bacon, Campbell's, ½ c	170	3	7
Chili, with meat, Wendy's, 1 serving (12 oz)	310	10	7
Bean enchilada, 1 (10 oz)	346	9	8
Vegetarian chili, homemade, 12 oz,	450	7	16
Burritos, with beans, fast food, 2	524	21	2

Fish and Seafood

FOOD	CALORIES	FAT (g)	FIBER (g)
Light fish: haddock, flounder, cod (scrod), sole; baked, broiled, or grilled; 3 oz	95	1	0
Perch, Atlantic, baked or broiled, 3 oz	103	2	0
Turbot, European, baked or broiled, 3 oz	104	3	0
Bass, baked or broiled, 3 oz	105	2	0
Snapper, baked or broiled, 3 oz	109	1	0
Tuna, white, canned in water, 3 oz	109	3	0
Salmon, pink, canned, 3 oz	118	5	0
Halibut, Atlantic or Pacific, baked or broiled, 3 oz	119	3	0

CALORIE, FAT, AND FIBER COUNTER

FOOD	CALORIES	FAT (g)	FIBER (g)
Fish and Seafood (cont.)			
Trout, rainbow, baked or broiled, 3 oz	128	5	0
Catfish, farmed, baked or broiled, 3 oz	129	7	0
Fatty fish: tuna, salmon, or swordfish; baked, broiled, or grilled; 3 oz	132–155	4–7	0
Mackerel, jack, canned, 3 oz	133	5	0
Carp fillet, baked or broiled, 3 oz	138	6	0
Fish sticks, crispy, crunchy, Mrs. Paul's, 3 oz	169	6	2
Herring, Atlantic, baked or broiled, 3 oz	173	10	0
Sardines, without skin, canned in water, 3 oz	185	11	0
Fish sandwich with tartar sauce, 1	431	23	0
Lobster, Northern, steamed, 3 oz	83	1	0
Crab, steamed, 3 oz	87	2	0
Crab cake, crustacean, blue, 1	93	5	0
Clams, mollusks, steamed, 3 oz	126	2	0
Oysters, mollusks, Pacific, steamed, 3 oz	139	4	0
Mussels, mollusks, blue, steamed, 3 oz	146	4	0
Scallops, breaded and fried, 6 pieces	386	19	0

FOOD	CALORIES	FAT (g)	FIBER (g)
Beef, Chicken, Turkey, Pork, Ham, Veal, and Lunchmeat			
Beef, top sirloin, lean, cooked, 3 oz	166	6	0
Beef, top round, separable lean only, trimmed of all fat, choice, cooked, steak, 3 oz	169	4	0
Beef, chuck, arm pot roast, separable lean, select, cooked, 3 oz	175	6	0
Beef, steak T-bone, select, trimmed of all fat, broiled, 3 oz	194	12	0
Filet mignon, lean, trimmed of all fat, cooked, 3 oz	208	12	0
Beef, ground, extra-lean, cooked, 3 oz	213	14	0
Beef, flank, lean, cooked, 3 oz	224	14	0
Beef, ground, regular, cooked, 3 oz	244	18	0
Chicken wings, roasted, without skin, 1	43	2	0
Chicken, broiler/fryer, drumsticks, with skin, roasted, 3 oz	112	6	0
Chik Nuggets, meatless, Morningstar Farms, 4	160	4	5
Chicken breast, roasted, broiler or fryer, without skin, ½ breast (3 oz)	142	3	0
Chicken capon, boneless, roasted, 3 oz	195	10	0
Buffalo wings, mild, Pizza Hut, 5	200	12	0
Buffalo wings, hot, Pizza Hut, 4	210	12	0
Chicken, Cornish game hen, roasted, 3 oz	221	15	0

CALORIE, FAT, AND FIBER COUNTER

FOOD	CALORIES	FAT (g)	FIBER (g)
Beef, Chicken, Turkey, Pork, Ham, Veal, and Lunchmeat (cont.)			
Turkey, dark meat, cooked, 3 oz	188	10	0
Turkey, fryer/roaster, leg, without skin, cooked, 1 (3 oz)	356	8	0
Pork, tenderloin, lean, cooked, 3 oz	139	4	0
Pork, fresh, top loin (roast), boneless, separable lean, cooked, 3 oz	165	6	0
Pork, fresh, leg (ham), rump half, lean, cooked, 3 oz	175	7	0
Pork, chops, fresh, loin, boneless, lean, cooked, 3 oz	179	9	0
Pork, sirloin, chops, bone-in, lean, cooked, 3 oz	181	9	0
Pork, shoulder, steak, broiled, 3 oz	193	11	0
Sausage, Italian, cooked, 3 oz	275	22	0
Sausage, Italian, pork, 1 link	353	32	0
Ham, cured, extra-lean, regular, canned, roasted, 3 oz	116	4	0
Ham croquette, homemade, 1	151	9	0
Spam (spiced ham), original, Hormel, 2 oz	172	16	0
Veal, cubed for stew, lean, cooked, 3 oz	160	4	0
Veal, sirloin, lean, cooked, 3 oz	174	6	0
Veal, leg (top round), separable lean, cooked, 3 oz	179	5	0
Veal, breast, whole, boneless, lean, cooked, 3 oz	185	8	0
Bacon, turkey, Louis Rich, 1 slice	34	3	0

FOOD	CALORIES	FAT (g)	FIBER (g)
Turkey breast, smoked, fat-free, prepackaged, Oscar Mayer, 1 serving (about 2 oz)	42	0	0
Ham, smoked, low-fat, sliced, deli, 2 oz	61	2	0
Turkey breast, roasted, sliced, deli, 2 oz	62	1	0
Hot dog, turkey, 1	102	8	0
Pork, cured, bacon, cooked, 3 strips	109	9	0
Hot dog, chicken, 1	116	9	0
Bacon, Canadian style, cured, 3 oz	124	6	0
Hot dog, beef, Oscar Mayer, 1	143	13	0
Salami, regular, sliced, deli, 2 oz	149	11	0
Bologna, regular, sliced, deli, 2 oz	177	16	0
Deviled ham, canned, Armour Star, ¼ c	210	18	0
Olive loaf, chicken, pork, turkey, prepackaged, Oscar Mayer, 3 oz	224	19	0

Vegetables and Vegetable Dishes

FOOD	CALORIES	FAT (g)	FIBER (g)
Lettuce, iceberg, ½ c	3	0	0
Spinach, raw, ½ c	3	0	0
Swiss chard, raw, ½ c	3	0	0
Garlic, raw, 1 clove	4	0	0
Tomato, cherry, red, ripe, raw, 1	4	0	0
Endive, raw, ½ c	4	0	0
Romaine, raw, ½ c	4	0	0
Lettuce, shredded, loose leaf, ½ c	5	0	1
Zucchini, raw, with skin, sliced, ½ c	8	0	1

CALORIE, FAT, AND FIBER COUNTER

FOOD	CALORIES	FAT (g)	FIBER (g)
Vegetables and Vegetable Dishes (cont.)			
Celery, raw, strips, ½ c	10	0	1
Cabbage, raw, ½ c	11	0	1
Broccoli, raw, ½ c	12	0	1
Dandelion greens, raw, ½ c	12	0	1
Tomato, red, ripe, raw, 1 medium	13	0	1
Tomato, plum, red, ripe, raw, 1	13	0	1
Cauliflower, raw, ½ c	13	0	1
Cauliflower, boiled, ½ c	14	0	2
Eggplant, cooked, ½ c	14	0	1
Asparagus, raw, ½ c	15	0	1
Turnip greens, boiled, ½ c	15	0	3
Cucumber, spears, raw, 1 small (about 4.5 oz)	15	0	1
Leeks, cooked, ½ c	16	0	1
Cabbage, cooked, ½ c	17	0	2
Dandelion greens, cooked, ½ c	17	0	2
Kale, raw, ½ c	17	0	1
Snap beans, green and yellow, raw, ½ c	17	0	2
Kale, cooked ½ c	18	0	1
Swiss chard, cooked, ½ c	18	0	2
Sweet peppers:			
Green, red, and yellow, raw, ½ c	19	0	1
Mushroom, pieces, cooked, ½ c	21	0	2
Spinach, cooked, ½ c	21	0	3
Asparagus, cooked, ½ c	22	0	1

FOOD	CALORIES	FAT (g)	FIBER (g)
Broccoli, boiled, ½ c	22	0	2
Collards, boiled, ½ c	25	0	3
Pumpkin, cooked, ½ c	25	0	1
Carrots, raw, strips or slices, ½ c	26	0	2
Okra, boiled, ½ c	26	0	2
Brussels sprouts, cooked, ½ c	30	0	2
Carrots, cooked, ½ c	35	0	3
Tomatoes, canned, stewed, ½ c	36	0	1
Beets, cooked, ½ c	37	0	2
Mushroom, shiitake, cooked, 4 pieces	40	0	2
Squash, butternut, winter, baked, ½ c	41	0	3
Peas, canned, cooked, ½ c	59	0	3
Squash, Hubbard, winter, baked, ½ c	60	1	3
Squash, acorn, winter, baked, ½ c	69	0	5
Corn on the cob, 1 medium ear	77	0	2
Corn, canned, white, sweet, whole kernels, ½ c	82	1	2
Corn, fresh, white, sweet, cooked, ½ c	89	1	2
Rhubarb, cooked with sugar, ½ c	137	0	2
Sweet potato, boiled without skin, 1 medium	159	0	3
Sweet potatoes, candied, home-prepared, 1 piece (4 oz)	155	4	3
Winter vegetable goulash, homemade, 1 serving	222	6	7
Eggplant parmigiana, homemade, 1 serving	319	22	3

CALORIE, FAT, AND FIBER COUNTER

FOOD	CALORIES	FAT (g)	FIBER (g)
Vegetables and Vegetable Dishes (cont.)			
Onion rings, breaded, frozen, prepared, 10	448	29	1
Szechuan vegetable stir-fry with jasmine rice, homemade, 1 serving	478	13	5
Curried stuffed acorn squash casserole, homemade, 1 serving	489	9	14
Vegetable picadillo, tortillas, homemade, 1 serving	536	15	12
Oils, Vinegars, and Salad Dressings			
Oil, vegetable, soybean lecithin, 1 Tbsp	104	14	0
Oil, olive, 1 Tbsp	119	14	0
Oil, canola, 1 Tbsp	120	14	0
Oil, corn, Crisco, 1 Tbsp	120	14	0
Oil, peanut, Planters, 1 Tbsp	120	14	0
Oil, soybean, salad or cooking (hydrogenated), 1 Tbsp	120	14	0
Oil, sunflower, over 60% linoleic acid, 1 Tbsp	120	14	0
Oil, corn, Wesson, 1 Tbsp	122	14	0
Oil, corn, Mazola, 1 Tbsp	125	14	0
Oil, sesame seed, Dynasty, 1 Tbsp	130	14	0
Vinegar, natural rice, Nakano, 1 Tbsp	0	0	0
Vinegar, red wine, Regina, 1 Tbsp	0	0	0
Vinegar, cider, 1 Tbsp	2	0	0
Vinegar, distilled, 1 Tbsp	2	0	0
Vinegar, white, Heinz, 1 Tbsp	2	0	0
Vinegar, balsamic, 1 Tbsp	10	0	0

FOOD	CALORIES	FAT (g)	FIBER (g)
Salad dressing, Italian, reduced-fat, no sugar, Walden Farms, 1 Tbsp	6	0	0
Salad dressing, honey mustard, from mix, fat-free, Good Seasons, 1 Tbsp	10	0	0
Salad dressing, mayonnaise, fat-free, Kraft, 1 Tbsp	11	0	0
Salad dressing, French, fat-free, Kraft Free, 1 Tbsp	20	0	0
Salad dressing, ranch, fat-free, Kraft Free, 1 Tbsp	24	0	0
Salad dressing, blue cheese, fat-free, Kraft Free, 1 Tbsp	25	0	1
Salad dressing, honey Dijon, fat-free, Kraft Free, 1 Tbsp	25	0	1
Salad dressing, ranch, peppercorn, fat-free, Kraft Free, 1 Tbsp	25	0	1
Salad dressing, Italian, reduced-fat, Kraft Light Done Right, 1 Tbsp	26	2	0
Salad dressing, vinaigrette and olive oil, Wishbone, 1 Tbsp	30	3	0
Salad dressing, blue cheese, reduced-fat, Marie's Lite, 1 Tbsp	50	4	0
Salad dressing, Italian, creamy, Wish-Bone, 1 Tbsp	50	5	0
Salad dressing, Thousand Island, 1 Tbsp	59	6	0
Salad dressing, Caesar, Kraft, 1 Tbsp	65	7	0
Salad dressing, French, 1 Tbsp	67	6	0
Salad dressing, vinegar and oil, home recipe, 1 Tbsp	70	8	0

CALORIE, FAT, AND FIBER COUNTER

FOOD	CALORIES	FAT (g)	FIBER (g)
Oils, Vinegars, and Salad Dressings (cont.)			
Salad dressing, Russian, 1 Tbsp	76	8	0
Salad dressing, blue cheese, Marie's, 1 Tbsp	94	10	0
Salad dressing, Thousand Island, Marie's, 1 Tbsp	120	12	0
Soups, Stews, and Chowders			
Broth, chicken, with lemon and herbs, canned, College Inn, 1 c	40	4	0
Soup, chicken gumbo, canned, condensed, made with equal volume of water, 1 c	56	1	2
Soup, chicken noodle, canned, condensed, made with equal volume of water, 1 c	75	2	1
Soup, chicken noodle, canned, ready-to-serve, Progresso Healthy Classics, 1 c	76	2	1
Soup, green pea, instant, Lipton Cup-a-Soup, 1 serving	93	1	4
Soup, tomato garden, canned, ready-to-serve, Progresso Healthy Classics, 1 c	98	1	4
Soup, cream of chicken, canned, condensed, made with equal volume of water, 1 c	117	7	0
Soup, tomato, canned, condensed, made with equal volume of water, Campbell's, 1 c	120	3	2

FOOD	CALORIES	FAT (g)	FIBER (g)
Soup, chicken rice, canned, condensed, made with equal volume of water, 1 c	121	4	1
Soup, minestrone, canned, ready-to-serve, Progresso Healthy Classics, 1 c	123	3	1
Soup, lentil, canned, ready-to-serve, Progresso Healthy Classics, 1 c	126	2	6
Soup, lentil, instant, Lipton Kettle Creations, 1 serving	127	1	5
Soup, cream of mushroom, canned, condensed, 98% fat-free, made with equal volume of water, Campbell's, 1 c	140	6	0
Soup, beef barley, canned, ready-to-serve, Progresso Healthy Classics, 1 c	142	2	3
Soup, vegetarian vegetable, canned, condensed, made with equal volume of water, 1 c	145	2	1
Soup, hearty black bean, canned, ready-to-serve, Progresso, 1 c	170	2	10
Soup, split pea, canned, ready-to-serve, Progresso Healthy Classics, 1 c	180	2	5
Soup, minestrone, canned, condensed, made with equal volume of water, Campbell's, 1 c	180	3	8

CALORIE, FAT, AND FIBER COUNTER

FOOD	CALORIES	FAT (g)	FIBER (g)
Soups, Stews, and Chowders (cont.)			
Soup, cream of celery, canned, condensed, made with equal volume of water, Campbell's, 1 c	180	10	2
Pasta e fagioli, homemade, 1 c	195	5	0
Soup, cream of potato, canned, condensed, made with equal volume of water, Campbell's, 1 c	200	8	2
Soup, cream of mushroom, canned, condensed, made with equal volume of water, Campbell's, 1 c	200	12	2
Soup, creamy potato, homemade, 1½ c (12 oz)	204	9	1
Stew, oyster, homemade, about 1 c (10 oz)	156	9	0
Stew, seafood, homemade, 1 c	177	4	2
Stew, beef and vegetable, homemade, 1 c	194	8	2
Chowder, New England clam, homemade, 1½ c	200	13	1
Chowder, chicken corn, homemade, 1½ c (12 oz)	337	21	3
Potatoes			
Potatoes, canned, Del Monte, 2 medium potatoes	60	0	2
Hash browns, Country Style, Ore-Ida, 1¼ c	75	0	1
Potatoes O'Brien, Ore-Ida, ¾ c	84	0	3

FOOD	CALORIES	FAT (g)	FIBER (g)
Oven fries, home-prepared, baked, 10 pieces	100	4	2
Potatoes, mashed with whole milk and margarine, ½ c	111	4	2
Potato, boiled without skin, 1 medium	116	0	2
French fries, Golden Fries, frozen, Ore-Ida, 11 french fries	120	4	1
Potato, baked with skin, 1 medium	133	0	3
Crinkle-cut potatoes, frozen, Ore-Ida, 11 fries	140	4	2
Potatoes au gratin, homemade, ½ c	162	9	2
Potato salad, made with full-fat mayonnaise or sour cream, ½ c	179	10	2
Potato salad, home style, Joan of Arc, ½ c	179	11	2
Hash browns, toaster, Ore-Ida, 2 patties	192	12	1
Potato pancakes, homemade, 1 medium	207	12	2
Scalloped potatoes, home-prepared with margarine, 1 c	211	9	5
French fries, home style, Burger King, medium order	370	20	3
French fries, Wendy's, medium order	380	19	5

CALORIE, FAT, AND FIBER COUNTER

FOOD	CALORIES	FAT (g)	FIBER (g)
Rice, Rice Dishes, Grains, and Grain Dishes			
Wild rice, cooked, ½ c	83	0	1
Rice, white, enriched long grain, instant, cooked, 1 c	162	0	1
Rice, white, long grain, original, cooked, Uncle Ben's, 1 c	170	0	0
Rice, brown, whole grain, instant, Minute, ⅔ c	170	2	2
Rice, white, boil-in-bag, cooked, Minute, 1 c	190	0	0
Rice, brown, natural whole grain, cooked, Uncle Ben's, 1 c	190	2	2
Rice, brown, long grain, cooked, Minute, 1 c	216	2	4
Rice, brown, medium grain, cooked, 1 c	218	2	4
Rice, white, enriched short grain, cooked, 1 c	242	0	0
Rice, basmati, prepared, ¾ c	275	2	2
Rice cakes, brown rice, unsalted, 2 cakes	70	1	1
Rice pilaf, frozen, Pillsbury, ½ c	110	1	0
Rice and broccoli with cheese sauce, frozen, Rice Originals, ½ c	124	4	0
Rice, peas, and mushrooms with sauce, frozen, Pillsbury, 5.5 oz	130	2	0
Pudding, rice, mix, prepared with 2% milk, ½ c	161	2	0
Rice pilaf, garlic and herb, mix, prepared, Near East, Creative Grains, 1 c	220	5	1

FOOD	CALORIES	FAT (g)	FIBER (g)
Pudding, rice, ready-to-eat, 5 oz	231	10	0
Rice pilaf, creamy Parmesan with rice and pearled wheat, mix, prepared, Near East, Creative Grains, 1 c	280	7	3
Spanish rice pilaf, mix, cooked, Near East, Creative Grains, 1 c	290	6	2
Rice, jasmine, cooked, Rice Select, ½ c	300	0	1
Red beans and rice dish, cooked, 1 c	459	5	9
Cracked wheat, cooked, ¾ c	113	2	4
Bulgur, cooked, 1 c	151	0	8
Tabbouleh, ⅔ c	110	3	5
Couscous, Mediterranean curry, mix, cooked, Near East, 1 c	220	4	3
Couscous, plain, mix, cooked, Near East, 1 c	230	2	2
Couscous, broccoli and cheese, mix, cooked, Near East, 1 c	240	5	3
Risotto with French peas dish, ½ c	314	6	3
Pumpkin squash risotto dish, 1½ c	419	9	3

Pizza and Pizza Sauce

FOOD	CALORIES	FAT (g)	FIBER (g)
Pizza, cheese, thin crust, Little Caesars, 1 slice (from 12" round pizza)	120	6	1
Pizza, pepperoni, thin crust, Little Caesars, 1 slice (from 12" round pizza)	150	8	1
Pizza, cheese, Little Caesars, 1 slice (from 12" round pizza)	160	6	1
Pizza, pepperoni, Little Caesars, 1 slice (from 12" round pizza)	180	8	1

CALORIE, FAT, AND FIBER COUNTER

FOOD	CALORIES	FAT (g)	FIBER (g)
Pizza and Pizza Sauce (cont.)			
Pizza, Thin 'n Crispy Veggie Lover's, Pizza Hut, 1 slice	190	7	2
Pizza, pepperoni, Thin 'n Crispy, Pizza Hut, 1 slice	190	9	2
Pizza, cheese, Thin 'n Crispy, Pizza Hut, 1 slice	200	9	2
Pizza, French bread, vegetable, Healthy Choice, 6 oz pizza	280	4	5
Pizza, cheese, Pan Pizza, Pizza Hut, 1 slice	284	14	2
Pizza, deluxe, Lean Cuisine, 1 pizza	290	6	3
Pizza, sausage, Thin 'n Crispy, Pizza Hut, 1 slice	290	17	2
Pizza, French bread, cheese, Lean Cuisine, 1 pizza	310	6	4
Pizza, French bread, cheese, Healthy Choice, 6 oz pizza	340	5	5
Pizza, cheese, Domino's, 2 slices (from medium pizza)	344	9	2
Pizza sauce, ready-to-serve, Hunt's, ¼ c	22	1	1
Pizza sauce, Hunt's, ½ c	44	0	2
Pizza sauce, chunky, canned, Contadina, ½ c	54	0	2
Pizza sauce, original, canned, Contadina, ½ c	60	0	2
Pizza sauce, with Italian cheeses, Contadina, ½ c	60	1	2
Pizza sauce, with pepperoni, Contadina, ½ c	70	2	1

FOOD	CALORIES	FAT (g)	FIBER (g)
Pasta and Pasta Sauce			
Spaghetti, enriched, cooked, ½ c	99	0	1
Noodles, egg, spinach, cooked, ½ c	106	1	2
Spaghetti, whole wheat, cooked, 1 c	174	1	6
Spaghetti, spinach, cooked, 1 c	182	1	0
Fettuccine, fresh, DiGiorno, 2.5 oz	192	2	2
Linguine, fresh, DiGiorno, 2.5 oz	192	2	2
Macaroni, elbow, enriched, ½ c	197	1	2
Spaghetti sauce, light, Hunt's, ½ c	42	1	2
Spaghetti sauce, mushrooms, home style, Hunt's, ½ c	48	1	3
Pasta sauce, tomato and basil, jar, Classico, ½ c	50	1	2
Pasta sauce, spicy red pepper, jar, Classico, ½ c	60	3	2
Spaghetti sauce, cheese and garlic, Hunt's, ½ c	64	2	3
Sauce, marinara, sweet basil, jar, Classico, ½ c	70	2	2
Spaghetti sauce, three cheese, canned, Contadina, ½ c	70	2	2
Spaghetti sauce, four cheese, canned, Del Monte, ½ c	70	2	3
Pasta sauce, sun-dried tomato, jar, Classico, ½ c	80	4	2
Pasta sauce, Florentine spinach and cheese, jar, Classico, ½ c	80	5	2
Spaghetti sauce, marinara, Prego, ½ c	110	6	3
Spaghetti sauce, no salt, Prego, ½ c	110	6	3

CALORIE, FAT, AND FIBER COUNTER

FOOD	CALORIES	FAT (g)	FIBER (g)
Pasta and Pasta Sauce (cont.)			
Spaghetti sauce, tomato supreme, extra chunky, Prego, ½ c	120	3	3
Pasta sauce, Tomato Alfredo, jar, Classico, ½ c	120	7	2
Pasta sauce, Alfredo, jar, Classico, ½ c	220	20	0
Shells and white cheddar, mix, cooked, Pasta Roni, 1 c	310	13	2
Noodles, chow mein, La Choy, ½ c	349	15	5
Linguine, alla marinara, dinner, Olive Garden, 1 restaurant serving	450	9	0
Fettuccine Alfredo, mix, cooked, Pasta Roni, 1 c	460	25	2
Fruit			
Melons: cantaloupe, honeydew, watermelon, ½ c	20–30	0	1
Berries: blueberries, strawberries, blackberries, raspberries, ½ c	22–41	0	2–4
Apricots, canned with skin, water-packed, ½ c	33	0	2
Cherries, sour, raw, 10	34	0	1
Plum, raw, 1 medium	36	0	1
Oranges, tangerines, raw, 1 medium	37–62	0	2–3
Fruit cocktail, canned, water-packed, ½ c	38	0	1
Pineapple, raw, ½ c	38	0	1

FOOD	CALORIES	FAT (g)	FIBER (g)
Grapefruit, raw, pink and red, ½ medium	41	0	1
Peach, raw, 1 medium	42	0	2
Cherries, sweet, raw, 10	49	1	2
Kiwi, without skin, 1 medium	50	1	2
Applesauce, canned, no sugar, ½ c	52	0	1
Grapes (red or green), seedless, ½ c	52	0	1
Quince, raw, 1 medium	52	0	2
Pineapple, canned, light syrup, chunks, ½ c	66	0	1
Apple, raw, without skin, 1 medium	73	0	2
Mandarin oranges, canned, light syrup, ½ c	77	0	1
Apple, raw, with skin, 1 medium	80	0	5
Dried fruit: raisins, dried apricots, cranberries, prunes, ¼ c	91–124	0	2–3
Pear, raw, 1 medium	100	1	4
Banana, 1 medium	109	1	3
Fruit salad, tropical, canned, heavy syrup, ½ c	111	0	2
Cranberry sauce, canned, sweetened, ½ c	209	0	1
Caramel apple, 1 medium	243	4	4
Figs, dried, 5	269	0	11
Avocado, raw, Florida, 1	340	27	16

CALORIE, FAT, AND FIBER COUNTER

FOOD	CALORIES	FAT (g)	FIBER (g)
Energy and Granola Bars			
Energy bar, Pria, chocolate honey graham, PowerBar, 1	110	3	0
Energy bar, Pria, chocolate peanut crunch, PowerBar, 1	110	4	0
Nutrition bar, chocolate pecan pie, Luna, 1	177	5	2
Nutrition bar, orange bliss, Luna, 1	180	4	2
Nutrition bar, almond brownie, Balance Bar, 1	180	6	2
Nutrition bar, almond crunch, ZonePerfect, 1	190	6	2
Energy bar, cranberry apple cherry, Clif Bar, 1	220	2	5
Energy bar, apricot, Clif Bar, 1	222	2	5
Protein bar, berries and yogurt, GeniSoy soy protein, 1	220	4	1
Energy bar, cookies and cream, Clif Bar, 1	225	4	5
Energy bar, chocolate, PowerBar, 1	230	2	3
Grain bar, banana nut, GeniSoy soy protein, 1	230	3	3
Grain bar, oatmeal raisin, GeniSoy soy protein, 1	230	3	3
Energy bar, chocolate almond fudge, Clif Bar, 1	231	5	5
Energy bar, gingersnap, Clif Bar, 1	233	3	6

FOOD	CALORIES	FAT (g)	FIBER (g)
Granola bar, chewy and soft, peanut butter, 1	101	4	1
Granola bar, chewy, low-fat, Nature Valley, 1 (1 oz)	110	2	1
Granola bar, S'mores, low-fat, Quaker Chewy, 1 (1 oz)	111	2	1
Granola bar, peanut butter, chewy and hard, 1 (1 oz)	114	6	1
Granola bar, oats and honey, Sunbelt, 1 (1 oz)	123	5	1
Granola bar, almond, chewy, Sunbelt, 1 (1 oz)	128	7	1
Granola bar, apple cinnamon, Kellogg's Nutri-Grain, 1 (1.3 oz)	136	3	1

Nuts and Seeds

FOOD	CALORIES	FAT (g)	FIBER (g)
Chestnuts, European, raw, 1 oz (about 2½ nuts)	60	1	2
Chestnuts, European, roasted, 1 oz (about 3½ nuts)	69	1	1
Peanuts, boiled, 1 oz	90	6	2
Corn nuts, plain, barbecue, nacho, 1 oz	124	4	2
Soy nuts, tangy BBQ, Opti, 1 packet (1.07 oz)	150	8	4
Pistachios, dried, 1 oz (about 47 nuts)	156	12	3
Pistachios, 1 oz	158	13	3
Peanuts, dry-roasted, Planters, 1 oz	160	13	3
Pistachios, dry-roasted, 1 oz	161	13	3

CALORIE, FAT, AND FIBER COUNTER

FOOD	CALORIES	FAT (g)	FIBER (g)
Nuts and Seeds (cont.)			
Peanuts, Spanish, raw, 1 oz	162	14	3
Cashews, salted, dry-roasted, 1 oz	163	13	1
Peanuts, Spanish, salted, oil-roasted, 1 oz	164	14	3
Mixed nuts, salted, dry-roasted, 1 oz	168	15	3
Cashews, fancy, Planters, 1 oz	170	14	1
Nuts, mixed, deluxe, Planters, 1 oz	170	16	2
Almonds, unsalted, dry-roasted, Blue Diamond, 1 oz	170	16	0
Almonds, slivered, Blue Diamond, 1 oz	172	14	3
Walnuts, black, dried, 1 oz	172	16	1
Trail mix, ¼ c	173	11	2
Hazelnuts (filberts), unsalted, dry-roasted, 1 oz	183	18	3
Walnuts, halves/pieces, Planters, 1 oz	190	19	1
Pecans, 1 oz	196	20	3
Pecans, salted, dry-roasted, 1 oz	201	21	3
Pecans, salted, oil-roasted, 1 oz	203	21	3
Macadamia nuts, dried, 1 oz	204	21	2
Macadamia nuts, salted, oil-roasted, 1 oz	204	22	3
Pumpkin and squash seeds, salted, roasted, 1 oz	126	6	2
Pumpkin and squash seeds, dried, 1 oz (142 seeds)	153	13	1

FOOD	CALORIES	FAT (g)	FIBER (g)
Sunflower seeds, salted, dry-roasted, 1 oz	165	14	3
Sunflower seeds, salted, oil-roasted, 1 oz	174	16	2

Desserts and Cookies

FOOD	CALORIES	FAT (g)	FIBER (g)
Gelatin, sugar-free, Royal, ½ c (about .09 oz)	10	0	0
Ice pop, 1 (2 fl oz)	41	0	0
Fudgsicle, chocolate, Good Humor, 1 bar	45	1	0
Fruit juice bar, frozen, Dean's, 1	60	0	0
Fruit and juice bar, frozen, 1 (2.5 fl oz)	63	0	0
Ice milk, vanilla, ½ c	68	2	0
Gel Snack Cup, Del Monte, 3.5 oz container	70	0	1
Sherbet, orange, ½ c	102	1	0
Ice milk, vanilla, soft-serve, ½ c	111	2	0
Sorbet, lemon, Häagen-Dazs, ½ c	120	0	1
Cake, angel food, no frosting, 1 piece	129	0	0
Sorbet, whole fruit, raspberry, Edy's, ½ c	130	0	1
Cupcake, chocolate, low-fat, with icing, 1	131	2	2
Tapioca, mix, made with low-fat (2%) milk, ½ c	147	2	0
Pudding, all flavors, cook and serve, Jell-O, ½ c	148	3	0

CALORIE, FAT, AND FIBER COUNTER

FOOD	CALORIES	FAT (g)	FIBER (g)
Desserts and Cookies (cont.)			
Pudding, banana, instant, made with low-fat (2%) milk, ½ c	153	3	0
Danish, apple, Pillsbury's Best, 1	185	9	0
Ice cream, French vanilla, soft-serve, ½ c	185	11	0
Apple strudel, 1 strudel	195	8	2
Cake, sponge, chocolate, no frosting, 1 piece	197	4	0
Doughnut, cake style, 1	198	11	1
Pudding, chocolate, homemade, made with low-fat (2%) milk, ½ c	206	4	1
Custard, baked, homemade, 1 c	209	7	0
Pudding, kiwi-banana, homemade, 1 c	225	6	2
Ice cream bar, chocolate with chocolate coating, Häagen-Dazs, 1	330	24	0
Cookie, gingersnap, 1	29	1	0
Fortune cookie, 1	30	0	0
Ladyfinger, 1	40	1	0
Cookie, sugar, 1	72	3	0
Cookies, oatmeal raisin, fat-free, Entenmann's, 2 (1 oz)	80	0	1
Cookie, oatmeal, 1	81	3	1
Cookies, Fig Newton, Nabisco, 2	120	3	2
Wafers, vanilla, 5	134	6	1
Cookies, chocolate chip, homemade, 2	156	9	1
Cookies, chocolate chip, chewy, Chips Ahoy, 3	170	8	1

FOOD	CALORIES	FAT (g)	FIBER (g)
Beverages			
Seltzer water, sweetened, flavored, Schweppes, 12 fl oz	0	0	0
Soda, cola, canned, Diet Pepsi, 8 fl oz	0	0	0
Tea, diet, lemon/peach, Lipton, 8 fl oz	0	0	0
Tea, green, all-natural/organic, 1 tea bag	0	0	0
Soda, cola, canned, Diet Coke, 8 fl oz	1	0	0
Tea, herbal, brewed, 6 fl oz	2	0	0
Coffee, brewed, 6 fl oz	3	0	0
Soda, canned, Fresca, 8 fl oz	3	0	0
Tea, brewed, black, 6 fl oz	4	0	0
Juice, tomato, reduced-sodium, 5 oz	26	0	1
Fruit punch, All Sport, 8 fl oz	53	0	0
Chocolate milk, sugar-free, powdered, Swiss Miss, 1 envelope	54	1	1
Sports drink, Gatorade, grape, 8 fl oz	60	0	0
Tea, iced, instant, Country Time, 1 tsp powder in 8 fl oz water	62	0	0
Tea, iced, powder, 3 tsp powder in 8 fl oz water	62	0	0
Wine, white (3.5 fl oz)	70	0	0
Juice, carrot, canned, 6 fl oz	71	1	2
Sports drink, Poweraid, lemon-lime, 8 fl oz	72	0	0
Wine, red (3.5 fl oz)	74	0	0
Juice, vegetable, V8, low-sodium, 11 oz	83	0	3

CALORIE, FAT, AND FIBER COUNTER

FOOD	CALORIES	FAT (g)	FIBER (g)
Beverages (cont.)			
Orange breakfast drink, from frozen concentrate, 6 fl oz	85	0	0
Soda, ginger ale, 8 fl oz	86	0	0
Wine spritzer, 8 fl oz	95	0	0
Juice, grapefruit, pink, fresh, 8 fl oz	96	0	0
Rum, 80 proof, 1.5 fl oz jigger	96	0	0
Vodka, 80 proof, ⅕ fl oz jigger	96	0	0
Whiskey, 80 proof, 1.5 fl oz	96	0	0
Beer, light, 12 fl oz	99	0	0
Soda, canned, Seven Up, 8 fl oz	100	0	0
Soda, cola, canned, Pepsi, 8 fl oz	100	0	0
Coffee, instant, Cafe Vienna, General Foods International, 2 Tbsp	100	3.5	0
Lemonade, flavored drink powder, 2 Tbsp in 8 fl oz water	102	0	0
Cocoa mix, powder, 1 oz packet	102	1	0
Soda, cola, canned, Coca-Cola Classic, 8 fl oz	103	0	0
Cranberry juice cocktail, bottled, 6 fl oz	108	0	1
Juice, orange, fresh, 8 fl oz	110	0	1
Tea, raspberry/peach/lemonade, Lipton, 8 fl oz	110	0	0
Soda, canned, Mountain Dew, 8 fl oz	113	0	0
Juice, juicy red, sweetened, Hawaiian Punch, 8 fl oz	120	0	0
Manhattan (whiskey and vermouth), 2 fl oz	128	0	0

FOOD	CALORIES	FAT (g)	FIBER (g)
Cranapple drink, canned, Ocean Spray, 6 fl oz	130	0	0
Cappuccino, iced, Maxwell House Cappio, 8 fl oz	130	3	0
Nectar, apricot, canned, 8 fl oz	141	0	2
Beer, 12 fl oz	146	0	1
Ale, Northstone Amber, 12 fl oz	149	0	0
Martini (gin and vermouth), 2.5 fl oz	157	0	0
Juice, apple-cranberry, canned, Mott's, 8 fl oz	170	0	0
Frappuccino coffee, Starbucks, bottle (9.5 oz)	190	3	0
Ready-to-drink breakfast, Carnation, canned, 10 fl oz	215	3	1
Piña colada (pineapple juice, rum, sugar, and coconut cream), 4.5 fl oz	245	3	0
Meal replacement beverage, Ultra Slim-Fast, French vanilla, 11 fl oz	275	3	7
Nutritional beverage, Ensure, vanilla, 8 fl oz	355	12	0

Miscellaneous

FOOD	CALORIES	FAT (g)	FIBER (g)
Gum, sugarless, Carefree, 1 stick	5	0	0
Pickles, gherkin, sweet, Vlasic, 3	5	0	0
Pickle, spear, kosher, 1	8	0	1
Gravy, brown, instant, ¼ c	10	1	0
Gravy, beef, canned, fat-free, Franco-American, ¼ c	20	0	0
Gum, Bubble Yum, 1 piece	25	0	0
Popcorn, air-popped, 1 c	31	0	1

CALORIE, FAT, AND FIBER COUNTER

FOOD	CALORIES	FAT (g)	FIBER (g)
Miscellaneous (cont.)			
Popcorn cake, 1	38	0	0
Olives, black, 5	42	4	0
Olives, green, 5	50	5	0
Popcorn, with oil, 1 c	55	3	1
Pretzels, fat-free, Newman's Own, 24	90	0	1
Pretzels, fat-free, tiny twists, Rold Gold, 18	100	0	1
Soy protein powder, GeniSoy, 1 serving size	100	0	0
Syrup, chocolate, Hershey's, 2 Tbsp	102	0	1
Pretzels, hard, with salt, 1 oz	108	1	1
Chex snack mix, traditional, bagged, ⅔ c	150	4	2
Soy flour, 1 c	371	6	9

CHAPTER 19

FIT NOT FAT 14-DAY MENU PLANNER

Your new food life begins today! The Fit Not Fat Menu Planner takes all seven steps of the Fit Not Fat Food Plan and translates them into easy-to-prepare, mouthwatering meals and handy, satisfying snacks. Amy Campbell, R.D., a certified diabetes educator and program coordinator of the Fit and Healthy weight-loss program of the Joslin Diabetes Center at Harvard University, designed the menu planner for people with diabetes, for people who have the symptoms of syndrome X, which can put a person at risk for heart disease, and for people who just want to shed pounds and get healthier. (If you have diabetes or high blood sugar, please check with your doctor before starting any new eating plan.)

Based on a daily goal of 1,500 calories, your new plan focuses on convenience and flexibility, allowing you to pick from among the 14 days to select the meal or snack that appeals to you at that moment. Calories and carbohydrates in each of the meal categories are balanced to keep your blood sugar stable and maximize your energy, satisfaction, and appetite control.

In order to keep your metabolism working strongly, you should avoid diets that recommend fewer than 1,500 calories a day. For your most appropriate calorie level, see the chart on page 62. If your weight goal specifies more calories, add an extra afternoon or evening snack—60 to 200 calories—to make up the difference. (For the calorie, fat, and fiber content of hundreds of different foods, see the table in chapter 18.)

Exercise your right to choose, and then mix and match meals for infinite menu combinations. We've included several kinds of yogurts—feel free to select your favorite flavor and eat it every day, or shake up your routine with different flavors that suit your mood. Bon appétit!

Fit Not Fat Menu Planner Approximate Meal Values

We've balanced the calories and carbohydrates in each of the Fit Not Fat Menu Planner's meal and snack categories to make them completely interchangeable, thus maximizing your convenience, choice, and energy. By all means, if you fall in love with the Choco-Banana Smoothie (Day 7), enjoy it several times a week with the blessing of Amy Campbell, R.D., a certified diabetes educator and program coordinator of the Fit and Healthy weight-loss program of the Joslin Diabetes Center at Harvard University and author of the menu plan.

- ▶ **Breakfast:** 300 calories, 45 g carbohydrates
- ▶ **Lunch:** 400 calories, 45 g carbohydrates
- ▶ **Afternoon snack:** 60 calories, 15–20 g carbohydrates
- ▶ **Dinner:** 555 calories, 45 g carbohydrates
- ▶ **Evening snack:** 200 calories, 15–20 g carbohydrates

DAY 1

Breakfast

1 slice multigrain toast

1 teaspoon trans-free margarine (contains no "partially hydrogenated oils")

¼ small cantaloupe

1 cup light-style (artificially sweetened) yogurt

Lunch

Bean Burrito:

  1 6" corn tortilla

  ½ cup cooked pinto beans

  1 ounce part-skim mozzarella cheese (1 string cheese portion)

  ½ cup steamed broccoli

  ½ tomato, chopped

  ½ cup shredded lettuce

  2 teaspoons canola oil (other monounsaturated oils, such as olive oil, canola oil, and peanut oil can be used throughout the menu planner instead)

  ¼ cup salsa

1 medium kiwifruit

Afternoon Snack

8 dried apricot halves

Dinner

⅔ cup brown rice, cooked

1 cup steamed zucchini

Garden salad with 1 teaspoon olive oil and balsamic vinegar

3 ounces broiled salmon

8 ounces 1% milk (low-fat soy milk or rice milk can be substituted for people with milk allergies, but be careful as some flavored soy milks are higher in calories than plain soy milk)

Evening Snack

1 small pear

1 tablespoon peanut butter

NUTRIENT ANALYSIS

1,543 calories, 204 g carbohydrate (53 percent of total calories), 76 g protein (20 percent of total calories), 47 g fat (30 percent of total calories), 11 g saturated fat, 34 g fiber, 1,600 mg sodium, 1,170 mg calcium

DAY 2

Breakfast

½ cup cooked oatmeal

8 ounces 1% milk

2 tablespoons raisins

2 tablespoons chopped walnuts

Lunch

2 slices rye bread

½ cup tuna fish, packed in water

1 tablespoon mayonnaise

Lettuce

Tomato slices

½ cup cucumber spears

½ cup baby carrots

1 fresh peach

Afternoon Snack

2 small plums

Dinner

1 small sweet potato

1 cup green beans, cooked

½ cup yellow pepper strips sautéed with 2 teaspoons olive oil

3 ounces skinless chicken breast, baked

1 teaspoon trans-free margarine

8 ounces 1% milk

Evening Snack

½ large Granny Smith apple

2 tablespoons hummus

NUTRIENT ANALYSIS

1,454 calories, 186 g carbohydrates (51 percent of total calories), 83 g protein (20 percent of total calories), 42 g fat (25 percent of total calories), 8 g saturated fat, 30 g fiber, 1,240 mg sodium, 800 mg calcium

DAY 3

Breakfast

½ small whole grain bagel

1 tablespoon regular cream cheese

1 cup fresh sliced strawberries mixed into 1 cup light-style vanilla yogurt

Lunch

California Veggie Pita Pocket:

1 7" oat bran pita bread

2 ounces roasted turkey breast

½ cup shredded romaine lettuce

½ cup shredded carrots

¼ cup alfalfa sprouts

¼ avocado, cut into chunks

1 tablespoon vinaigrette salad dressing

2 teaspoons Dijon mustard

4 ounces reduced-sodium tomato juice

½ cup fresh cantaloupe chunks

Afternoon Snack

15 frozen green grapes

Dinner

Whole Wheat Pasta Toss:

½ cup cooked whole wheat pasta

2 cups fresh spinach

½ cup canned cannellini beans, rinsed and drained

5 sliced cherry tomatoes

1 clove garlic

2 tablespoons balsamic vinegar

2 teaspoons canola oil

2 tablespoons grated Parmesan cheese

Sauté pasta with spinach, beans, tomatoes, garlic, vinegar, and oil. Top with cheese and serve.

8 ounces 1% milk

Evening Snack

1 cup fresh pineapple cubes

¼ cup low-fat cottage cheese

2 tablespoons chopped almonds

NUTRIENT ANALYSIS

1,523 calories, 203 g carbohydrates (53 percent of total calories), 72 g protein (19 percent of total calories), 47 g fat (28 percent of total calories), 12 g saturated fat, 32 g fiber, 2,800 mg sodium, 1,200 mg calcium

DAY 4

Breakfast

1 slice whole wheat toast

1 teaspoon trans-free margarine

1 teaspoon all-fruit spread

1 boiled egg

½ grapefruit

Lunch

1 cup minestrone soup

3 Ry-Krisp crackers

1 cup celery sticks

1 tablespoon peanut butter

8 ounces reduced-sodium vegetable juice

Afternoon Snack

1 baked apple

1 teaspoon brown sugar

Cinnamon to taste

Dinner

4 ounces broiled shrimp

1 cup "smashed" potatoes (mashed potatoes with the skin)

1 cup red and green pepper strips sautéed with 1 teaspoon olive oil

Garden salad with 1 teaspoon olive oil and balsamic vinegar

8 ounces 1% milk

Evening Snack

2 tablespoons raisins

2 tablespoons chopped almonds

1 ounce part-skim mozzarella cheese (string cheese)

NUTRIENT ANALYSIS

1,507 calories, 184 g carbohydrates (49 percent of total calories), 69 g protein (18 percent of total calories), 55 g fat (33 percent of total calories), 11 g saturated fat, 31 g fiber, 2,000 mg sodium, 700 mg calcium

DAY 5

Breakfast

1 whole grain waffle

½ cup unsweetened applesauce

Cinnamon

2 tablespoons chopped pecans

1 cup light-style vanilla yogurt

Lunch

Baked Stuffed Potato:

1 medium potato, baked

1 cup steamed broccoli florets

2 ounces reduced-fat Monterey Jack cheese

¼ cup salsa

3 tablespoons light sour cream

1 nectarine

Afternoon Snack

10 cherries

Dinner

Vegetable Stir-Fry with Tofu:

    2 tablespoons chopped onion

    ½ cup chopped red pepper

    ½ cup firm tofu, cubed

    ¼ cup chopped green pepper

    ¼ cup snow peas

    ¼ cup cauliflower florets

    2 teaspoons light soy sauce

    2 teaspoons canola oil

    ⅓ cup brown rice

⅓ cup low-fat frozen yogurt

2 small gingersnap cookies

Evening Snack

2 popcorn cakes

1 wedge light Laughing Cow cheese

1 teaspoon all-fruit spread

NUTRIENT ANALYSIS

1,572 calories, 197 g carbohydrates (50 percent of total calories), 79 g protein (20 percent of total calories), 52 g fat (30 percent of total calories), 14 g saturated fat, 27 g fiber, 2,190 mg sodium, 2,100 mg calcium

DAY 6

Breakfast

¾ cup Kashi Good Friends cereal

8 ounces 1% milk

½ banana, sliced

2 tablespoons sunflower seeds

Lunch

Veggie-Tuna Melt:

    1 whole wheat English muffin, split

    ½ cup tuna fish

    1 tablespoon light mayonnaise

    ½ cup fresh zucchini slices

    ½ cup green pepper, diced

    1 ounce part-skim mozzarella cheese

    ½ tomato, sliced

Mix tuna and mayonnaise. Top each English muffin half with half of each ingredient. Place under broiler until cheese is melted.

⅛ honeydew melon

Afternoon Snack

½ cup sliced fresh strawberries and ½ cup fresh blueberries, mixed

Dinner

Tabbouleh:

    ½ cup bulgur, cooked

    ½ cup chickpeas

    ½ tomato, diced

    ¼ teaspoon fresh mint, chopped

    1 teaspoon fresh parsley, chopped

    1 teaspoon olive oil

Mix ingredients together and serve.

Garden salad with 1 hard-boiled egg, chopped, and 1 teaspoon olive oil and balsamic vinegar

1 chocolate Fudgsicle

Evening Snack

½ large Golden Delicious apple, sliced

1 tablespoon almond butter (soy butter can be substituted for people with nut allergies)

NUTRIENT ANALYSIS

1,477 calories, 191 g carbohydrates (52 percent of total calories), 68 g protein (18 percent of total calories), 49 g fat (30 percent of total calories), 12 g saturated fat, 36 g fiber, 1,000 mg sodium, 1,140 mg calcium

DAY 7

Breakfast

Choco-Banana Smoothie:

> 4 ounces 1% milk
>
> 4 ounces plain fat-free yogurt
>
> ½ frozen banana
>
> 2 tablespoons sugar-free powdered chocolate mix
>
> 1 tablespoon peanut butter (or soy butter)

Put ingredients in a blender—blend and enjoy!

Lunch

Chicken Caesar Salad:

> 2 cups romaine lettuce, torn into pieces
>
> 2 ounces broiled or grilled chicken breast, without the skin
>
> ¾ cup croutons

Dressing:

> ½ clove garlic, crushed
>
> 2 tablespoons lemon juice

1 tablespoon balsamic vinegar

1 tablespoon Parmesan cheese

1 teaspoon olive oil

½ teaspoon Dijon mustard

½ teaspoon Worcestershire sauce

¼ teaspoon ground black pepper

5 vanilla wafers

½ cup mandarin orange segments, drained

Afternoon Snack

1 cup honeydew melon chunks

Dinner

⅔ cup couscous, cooked

1 cup brussels sprouts, steamed

1 cup baby carrots, raw

3 ounces pork tenderloin

1 teaspoon trans-free margarine

8 ounces 1% milk

Evening Snack

1 slice raisin toast

¼ cup part-skim ricotta cheese

NUTRIENT ANALYSIS

1,483 calories, 175 g carbohydrates (47 percent of total calories), 90 g protein (25 percent of total calories), 47 g fat (29 percent of total calories), 15 g saturated fat, 17 g fiber, 1,350 mg sodium, 1,200 mg calcium

DAY 8

Breakfast

½ cup bran flakes

1 cup raspberries

8 ounces 1% milk

¼ cup egg substitute, scrambled

Lunch

1 cup lentil soup

1 slice whole wheat bread

1 ounce lean ham

2 cups spinach salad with ½ carrot, shredded

1 tablespoon Italian dressing

1 orange

Afternoon Snack

1 peach

Dinner

Pasta Salad:

1 cup cherry tomatoes, halved

½ cup spinach pasta, cooked

½ cup broccoli, steamed

2 ounces fresh mozzarella, chopped (2 string cheese portions)

2 tablespoons fresh basil, chopped

2 teaspoons olive oil

1 clove garlic, chopped

Mix ingredients together and serve.

8 ounces 1% milk

Evening Snack

Nutty Banana Pop:

½ banana

1 tablespoon light chocolate syrup

2 tablespoons chopped peanuts

Dip banana in syrup, and then roll it in peanuts. Freeze until hardened.

NUTRIENT ANALYSIS

1,447 calories, 177 g carbohydrates (49 percent of total calories), 70 g protein (19 percent of total calories), 51 g fat (32 percent of total calories), 17 g saturated fat, 35 g fiber, 1,700 mg sodium, 1,300 mg calcium

DAY 9

Breakfast

Breakfast Yogurt Parfait:

1 cup plain fat-free yogurt

¼ cup granola

¼ cup fresh strawberries (can use plain frozen strawberries, not packed in syrup)

¼ cup blueberries

Layer ingredients in a parfait glass or a goblet.

Lunch

1 whole wheat sandwich roll

1 soy burger

½ tomato, sliced

Waldorf Salad:

 $\frac{1}{2}$ small apple, chopped

 $\frac{1}{2}$ cup chopped celery

 $\frac{1}{2}$ cup chopped carrots

 1 tablespoon walnuts

 1 tablespoon raisins

 1 tablespoon mayonnaise

Mix ingredients together and serve.

Afternoon Snack

 1 cup frozen papaya chunks

Dinner

 $\frac{1}{2}$ cup corn

 1 cup asparagus, steamed

 Garden salad with 1 teaspoon olive oil and 1 tablespoon red wine vinegar

 3 ounces grilled scrod

 2 Fig Newtons

 8 ounces 1% milk

Evening Snack

 $\frac{3}{4}$ cup pineapple chunks

 $\frac{1}{4}$ cup low-fat cottage cheese

 2 tablespoon sunflower seeds

NUTRIENT ANALYSIS

1,550 calories, 199 g carbohydrates (51 percent of total calories), 85 g protein (22 percent of total calories), 46 g fat (27 percent of total calories), 9 g saturated fat, 29 g fiber, 1,930 mg sodium, 1,100 mg calcium

DAY 10

Breakfast

 $\frac{1}{2}$ cup cooked oatmeal

 $\frac{1}{2}$ small apple, chopped

 1 tablespoon raisins

 Cinnamon, to taste

 2 tablespoons chopped walnuts

 8 ounces 1% milk

Lunch

 1 cup split pea soup

 5 sesame melba toasts

 $\frac{1}{2}$ cucumber, cut in spears

 1 small tomato, halved, drizzled with 1 teaspoon olive oil and sprinkled with 2 tablespoons chopped fresh basil

 1 frozen fruit juice bar

Afternoon Snack

 $\frac{3}{4}$ cup sliced fresh strawberries mixed with 4 ounces orange juice and 1 tablespoon balsamic vinegar

Dinner

 2 small red potatoes, steamed

 1 cup mushrooms, sliced, sautéed with 2 teaspoons olive oil

 1 cup zucchini slices, steamed

 3 ounces broiled swordfish

 8 ounces 1% milk

Evening Snack

10 red grapes

1 oz of your favorite cheese

NUTRIENT ANALYSIS

1,527 calories, 185 g carbohydrates (48 percent of total calories), 77 g protein (20 percent of total calories), 58 g fat (34 percent of total calories), 16 g saturated fat, 25 g fiber, 2,400 mg sodium, 1,100 mg calcium

DAY 11

Breakfast

Strawberry-Banana Soy Smoothie:

4 ounces plain low-fat soy milk

4 ounces plain fat-free yogurt

¼ cup fresh strawberries, chopped (can use frozen if not packed in syrup)

¼ banana, sliced

2 tablespoons wheat germ

Combine ingredients in a blender and blend until smooth.

Lunch

Greek Salad:

1 cup romaine lettuce, torn into pieces

2 ounces light feta cheese

5 black olives

1 small tomato, chopped

2 teaspoons olive oil

1 tablespoon balsamic vinegar

1 7" whole wheat pita

½ cup cantaloupe melon balls

Afternoon Snack

5 dried apple rings

Dinner

Bean Enchilada:

1 flour tortilla

⅓ cup fat-free spicy refried beans

1 ounce shredded light Monterey Jack cheese

1 teaspoon chopped jalapeño pepper

¼ cup salsa

¼ cup shredded lettuce

½ carrot, shredded

4 ounces low-sodium vegetable juice

1 cup light-style yogurt

Evening Snack

1 pear, sliced

1 tablespoon almond butter

NUTRIENT ANALYSIS

1,481 calories, 192 g carbohydrates (52 percent of total calories), 68 g protein (18 percent of total calories), 49 g fat (30 percent of total calories), 14 g saturated fat, 24 g fiber, 3,090 mg sodium, 1,200 mg calcium

DAY 12

Breakfast

½ small whole wheat bagel

1 tablespoon regular cream cheese

1 medium kiwifruit

8 ounces 1% milk

Lunch

Salmon Salad Sandwich:

> 2 slices oatmeal bread
>
> ½ cup canned salmon
>
> 1 tablespoon light mayonnaise
>
> ½ cup diced celery
>
> ¼ cup chopped onion

Mix salmon, mayonnaise, celery, and onion, and spread on bread.

1 medium carrot, cut into spears

1 frozen fruit juice bar

Afternoon Snack

1 medium tangerine

Dinner

½ cup low-fat stuffing

2 tablespoons cranberry sauce

1 cup green beans, steamed

½ cup sliced summer squash, cooked

3 ounces turkey breast, no skin

¼ cup turkey gravy

8 ounces 1% milk

Evening Snack

3 stoned wheat thin crackers

2 teaspoons tahini (sesame butter)

NUTRIENT ANALYSIS

1,529 calories, 187 g carbohydrates (49 percent of total calories), 76 g protein (20 percent of total calories), 53 g fat (31 percent of total calories), 15 g saturated fat, 20 g fiber, 2,300 mg sodium, 1,000 mg calcium

DAY 13

Breakfast

1 cup Puffed Kashi cereal

8 ounces 1% milk

1 cup fresh raspberries

2 tablespoons sunflower seeds

Lunch

English Muffin Pizza:

> 1 whole wheat English muffin, split
>
> 2 ounces part-skim mozzarella cheese
>
> ¼ cup pizza sauce
>
> ¼ cup mushrooms, chopped
>
> ¼ cup green pepper, chopped

Layer half of ingredients on each English muffin half. Broil briefly until cheese is melted.

1 pear

Afternoon Snack

2 small plums

Dinner

½ cup wild rice

½ cup baby lima beans

½ cup stewed tomatoes

1 cup sliced cucumber

3 ounces grilled sirloin steak, trimmed of fat

1 teaspoon trans-free margarine

Evening Snack

2 tablespoons raisins

2 tablespoons peanuts

1 ounce part-skim mozzarella (1 portion string cheese)

NUTRIENT ANALYSIS

1,467 calories, 181 g carbohydrates (49 percent of total calories), 89 g protein (24 percent of total calories), 43 g fat (26 percent of total calories), 14 g saturated fat, 35 g fiber, 1,880 mg sodium, 1,290 mg calcium

DAY 14

Breakfast

Breakfast-on-the-Go:

½ cup All-Bran cereal

1 cup fat-free vanilla yogurt

¾ cup fresh blueberries

2 tablespoons chopped almonds

Mix ingredients together in a small container with a lid for easy travel.

Lunch

1 soy "hot dog"

1 hot dog roll

Garden salad with 1 tablespoon Italian dressing

1 cup papaya chunks

Afternoon Snack

½ grapefruit

Dinner

⅔ cup couscous

1 cup kale, cooked

½ cup beets

3 ounces broiled or grilled chicken breast, without the skin

1 teaspoon trans-free margarine

Evening Snack

½ banana

1 tablespoon peanut butter

NUTRIENT ANALYSIS

1,500 calories, 197 g carbohydrates (53 percent of total calories), 79 g protein (21 percent of total calories), 44 g fat (26 percent of total calories), 9 g saturated fat, 30 g fiber, 1,600 mg sodium, 1,200 mg calcium

INDEX

G

N

O